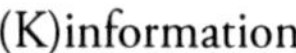
(K)information

Eigene und fremde Welten

The series "Eigene und fremde Welten" is edited by Jörg Baberowski, Vincent Houben, Stefan Beck, Thomas Mergel, and Gabriele Metzler in connection with the Collaborative Research Center no. 640 "Representations of Changing Social Orders: Cross-Cultural and Cross-Temporal Comparisons" based at Humboldt-Universität, Berlin (Germany).

Volume 32

Maren Klotz is a senior lecturer at the Department of European Ethnology of the Humboldt-University, Berlin.

Maren Klotz

(K)information

Gamete Donation and Kinship Knowledge in Germany and Britain

Campus Verlag
Frankfurt/New York

Bibliographic Information published by the Deutsche Nationalbibliothek.
Die Deutsche Nationalbibliothek lists this publication in the Deutsche Nationalbibliografie; detailed bibliographic data are available in the Internet at http://dnb.d-nb.de.
ISBN 978-3-593-50067-6

Cover design: Campus Verlag GmbH, Frankfurt/Main
Printing office and bookbinder: CPI buchbücher.de, Birkach
Printed on acid free paper.
Printed in Germany

This book is also available as an E-Book.

www.campus.de
www.press.uchicago.edu

Dedicated to the memory of my father
Detlef Klotz
(1941–2010)

Content

Acknowledgements

This book is based on my doctoral research, defended 12.10.2012 at the Department for European Ethnology (IfEE) of the Humboldt University Berlin and conducted in Cotutelle Agreement with the EGENIS Centre for Genomics in Society at the University of Exeter. The research was funded through the IfEE and the German Research Council (SFB 640, C4) and—in its early stages—by the University of Exeter and EGENIS.

First and foremost: thank you to the families who participated in this research and were willing to share intimate details of their lives! I would also like to thank the clinics, their staff, and all other research partners. This includes a huge thank you to Petra Thorn, the DC Network, the Infertility Research Trust and various other parties for allowing me to print materials and illustrations.

I am deeply grateful to my supervisors, Christine Hauskeller and Stefan Beck, for their continuous intellectual engagement with my work, for their advice, and for their support. Their fearlessness also made the complex supervision agreement between Britain and Germany possible. Thank you! I am likewise indebted to committee members Jeanette Edwards and Michi Knecht, for their invaluable instruction and warm-hearted criticism. Sven Bergmann, Jörg Niewöhner, Nurhak Polat, Hilke Schellmann, and Moritz Ege have given helpful comments on chapter drafts. I profited from discussions with my colleagues at the IfEE, EGENIS, the SFB 640, and the IfEE STS Lab. I would also like to thank Ruth Dawson, Josephine Go Jefferies, Silke and David Klotz, and Sascha Stingl for their work on the language and layout of this book. Further thanks extend to all those who provided *diffuse and enduring solidarity* during the writing process.

1. Introduction

Much turmoil has surrounded the classical anthropological research topic kinship, most commonly defined as "the relationships arising out of the procreative process" (e.g. Harris 1990, 50). It has led scholars who have spent much of their career writing about kinship as social order or as a simultaneously productive and "bloody" metaphor for connectedness to exasperatedly declare that "there is no such thing as kinship" (Schneider 1984, vii) or that they are "sick to death" of it (Haraway 1997, 265). As a consequence of this creative turmoil, the last 25 years of anthropological research and beyond have given birth to a productive research area often called the new kinship studies. In this research area kinship has been tackled as a generative matrix for relationships of various kinds: a prime site for the negotiation of what a society perceives as the made, and the given, and for the negotiation of what roles are attributed to biological process and physical bodies within practices of human solidarity. In the words of two of the protagonists of the new kinship studies, kinship in the industrial West is to be seen as "a cultural technology not only for naturalizing relationships but also, and at the same time, for the reverse—for transforming naturalized relations into cultural forms" (Franklin and McKinnon 2001, 16). Reproductive technologies, with their capacity for posing ever new biological, social, legal, and ethical questions surrounding *the ties that bind*, have often figured at the center of these research endeavors.

This book focuses on kinship-by-donation in both Germany and Britain, i.e. kinship afforded through clinical donor insemination (DI) or in-vitro fertilization (IVF) with donated eggs.[1] This book analyzes

1 Clinical DI is generally used for family formation in cases of male infertility, or also for lesbian or single women to conceive. It involves an anonymous or non-anonymous man donating his sperm for payment or as a volunteer through masturbating at a

how kinship-by-donation is constituted in different—but entangled—ways in four domains: in the knowledge-practices apparent in affected families; in sperm banks and fertility clinics; within national and transnational regulation; and within intersecting interest group activism. A focal point concerns knowledge-management, studying which aspects of kinship-knowledge are deemed relevant, drawn on in various practices, and made accessible—and which are not. Crucial for the figuration of kinship-by-donation in societies such as Germany and Britain, where some relevance is attributed to genetic relatedness, is what can be known, and how, about the donor. In other words: where gamete (i.e. sperm or egg) donation is clinically administered, as in all the cases researched for this book, the constitution of kinship-by-donation is entangled with the official regulatory regimes of donor anonymity or non-anonymity that are in place.

The *raison d'être* for this research is to make an empirical and theoretical contribution to the analysis of plural late-modern societies and social change. This book does not analyze kinship as "hidden grammar" for society as a whole (as apparent in the older anthropological traditions). It focuses instead on how kinship generates and is generated within diverging intersections of biology, law, care practices and beyond, as called for by recent proponents of the new kinship studies (e.g. Edwards 2009b). This research draws not only on contemporary kinship studies to analyze these diverging intersections, but also on the anthropology of knowledge and on science and technology studies (STS). The research aims to look below broad concepts of *nature* and *culture* and takes reproductive medicine as an anthropological "field experiment" (e.g. Beck 2012; Knecht et al. 2012) for the study of the (re-)formation of relationships in Western societies. This work thereby presents an ethnographic exploration of a recently emerged form of knowing and doing kinship in Europe: by sperm or egg donation, within newly established non-anonymous regulatory set-ups,

sperm bank. The sperm is later injected into the women's vagina or uterus. Egg donation and IVF treatment with donated eggs generally involve far more medically invasive procedures for donors and recipients. The procedure is generally used to help infertile or post-menopausal women to become pregnant. It involves an anonymous or non-anonymous woman donating her eggs for payment, for price reductions in her own fertility treatment, or as a volunteer. The eggs are then fertilized with sperm in a Petri dish, the fertilized eggs are later transferred into the receiving woman's uterus.

and openly talked about in families. The relationships arising out of this very specific procreative process are the object of this study.

The following introductory pages discuss how kinship-by-donation has developed into a regulatory problem (particularly concerning the status of kinship-knowledge) and a publicly visible "experiment" in kinship culture in the last 25 years. It lays out how this research is addressing a specific *desideratum* in kinship studies, through combining a processual and praxeographic approach, using multi-sited ethnography and a comparative perspective. The new kinship studies and their focus on knowledge are then introduced more fully, followed by an overview of the empirical basis and explorative comparative angle of this book. The introduction closes with a recapitulation of the line of argument followed throughout this research.

Kinship-by-Donation in Europe: Regulatory Problem and "Kinship Experiment"

In Europe, kinship-by-donation has long figured squarely among the extended political and social scientific discussions surrounding the social implications and regulatory affordances of the new reproductive technologies (NRTs), or more generally, the so-called new genetics. While egg donation indeed only became possible through the refinement of IVF practices at the beginning of the 1980s, and more widely used towards the end of the 1990s, sperm donation was not particularly new as a practice of achieving a pregnancy. It also was and is not technically challenging, being referred to as "low tech" by many of the German and British clinicians with whom I spoke during my fieldwork. Clinical insemination-by-donor probably had been practiced, most often secretively, for over a hundred years in many European countries (see chapter 6.1 for further historical discussion). And, given that parents usually did not tell their children about being donor-conceived in the past and were in fact often advised not to do so, affected children seldom grew up to tell their story publicly or become political activists on behalf of changed donation practices.

Other questions surrounding NRTs came to figure more strongly within the policy discussions in my countries of research, Germany and Britain. This was partly due to the inherent practice of accommodating so-called missing genetic links and family secrets into everyday life being common in European kinship practices, as many anthropologists and sociologists have shown (e.g. Smart 2011). The policy debates from the 1980s onwards, moreover, did not focus foremost on what children and parents should or would want to know about donors or vice versa. The debates focused mainly on questions surrounding the status of the embryo (e.g. Hauskeller 2004; Jasanoff 2005; Richardt 2003), and, more so in Britain than in Germany, on how legal parenthood is determined by law if donor conception is involved (e.g. Haimes 1990; Katzorke 2008).

For Britain this meant that with the comprehensive regulation of NRTs and the new genetics, which many European countries started to implement at the beginning of the 1990s, a previous *de facto* donor-anonymity became an explicitly *regulated for* donor-anonymity with the Human Fertilisation and Embryology Act (HFE Act) in 1990. In Germany, the Embryo Protection Law issued in the same year outlawed egg donation and did not touch on sperm donation at all. This meant firstly, that many juridical inconsistencies were left in place, for instance those pertaining to potential legal connections between child and sperm donor. And, secondly, that a historically long practiced de facto donor-anonymity remained the dominant practice in German fertility clinics.

However, in the so-called noughties kinship-by-donation, or more precisely the official management of kinship-information within clinically assisted reproduction-by-donor, became a regulatory problem in both countries. It also became a debated example of procreation practice outside the assumed norm of the genetically related heterosexual nuclear family. Thus it emerged as far more publicly visible, in the sense that Stefan Beck has defined a

> "prime Versuchsanordung (an experimental cum experiential system 'in the wild', outside of controlled laboratory settings) [...] producing new subjectivities, new moralities and social obligations, as well as new relations" (Beck 2012, 363).

In Britain, for instance, homosexual and heterosexual parents-by-donation had set up the interest group Donor Conception (DC) Network strongly advocating parental disclosure of the donation and providing families with a tightly-knit network of local groups, annual conventions, and a vast array of advice materials on disclosure to be accessed or ordered through their comprehensive website. Also in Britain, parents and donor-conceived adults took legal action against donor anonymity in 2002 (Rose & Anor vs HFEA 2002). In contrast, in Germany, parents wishing to acknowledge that their children are donor-conceived (a group I will label *disclosing parents*), along with donor-conceived adults, have started to network with each other via specially set-up websites. They have also started to appear in the media, predominantly supporting the non-anonymity of sperm donors. Within a complex matrix of changing family forms, cultural valorizations of transparency and so-called genetic information, patient group formation, new possibilities of DNA testing, and juridical activities, donor-anonymity and the surrounding practices of non-disclosure were challenged. In this process gamete donor-anonymity was officially removed in Britain in 2004/2005 (UK Gov 2004). In Germany donor-anonymity was not as comprehensively discussed within policy and public discourse as in Britain, but nevertheless a new, but less juridically clear regulatory regime of non-anonymity became implemented in 2007 with the so-called Tissue Law (GewebeG 2007). The contemporary ethnographic exploration and analysis of this matrix is one of the central aims of this book.

Research Desiderata

This book sets out to address four *desiderata* in the social-anthropological research on kinship and assisted reproduction. Firstly, existing work in the new kinship studies focusing on how individuals and families do kinship with the help of reproductive technologies has predominantly concentrated on studying snapshot moments of family formation. Such works have thereby convincingly shown how in moments of crisis and medical intervention, actors resort to diverse tactics of naturalization and normalization (e.g. Franklin 1997; Thompson 2001). Only very few studies (see Becker et al. 2005; Edwards 2000) have focused on more everyday life appraisals of reproductive technologies outside of moments of immediate reproductive crises, or on more long-term confrontations that the families concerned might be facing. My work takes a processual approach to address this research gap, both in its research- and its initial sampling-strategy: The families (n=13) who participated were predominantly interviewed several times over a period of a few years. For all of the families the initially successful donor insemination, or embryo transfer in the case of egg donation, already occurred several years before, making the narrative reconstruction of different periods in their becoming families-by-donation possible.

Second, as for instance Jeanette Edwards (2009b, 4) recently criticized, there has been a tendency in contemporary anthropological studies of kinship in Europe and North America to too readily place the observed phenomena in a "biology box" and in a "social box", under-problematizing "what got to be included as biological" and thereby implicitly reifying the nature/culture dichotomy. The approach applied in this book follows Edward's call to "resist the attempt to purify" (2009, 10) kinship and to focus rather on the diverse and flexible practices of its making. For this purpose, the research takes inspiration from relational materialist approaches such as Actor Network Theory (more in chapter 2.3) developed in the interdisciplinary field of STS.

Third and fourth, this study takes a locally and nationally multi-sited approach. Similar previous studies have tended to focus on negotiations of kinship within more singular domains. How kinship is negotiated within regulation, for instance, has been studied from a socio-legal perspective (e.g. Donovan 2006; Sheldon 2005), but not in its intersections with more everyday life practices in families (for a call to change this see Edwards (2006)). My work compares differences and consequent entanglements *between* how kinship-by-donation is constituted in the families, clinics, regulation, and interest groups under study. Moreover, it contributes a qualitative empirical inquiry of reproductive technologies, their regulation, and everyday kinship perceptions *in Germany*, where it has been notably under-researched in comparison to Britain.[2]

2 There are however exceptions to this, mostly coming out of the research cluster (SFB 640) my work was also associated with, for example Beck et al (2007); Klotz and Knecht (2009), Knecht, Klotz, and Beck (2012) or Knecht (2009), but also from elsewhere (e.g. Hauser-Schäublin et al. 2000; Petersen 2000). Timm (e.g 2010; 2011) has not studied reproductive technologies in Germany, but has contributed to an introduction of the so-called new kinship studies and their theoretical concerns into the German anthropological debates and the more historically oriented family studies of German speaking *Volkskunde*.

Studying Kinship and Kinship-Knowledge

One of the constitutive starting points for this book has been my hypothesis that there is a core theme running through the complex entanglements of the above identified matrix of changing family forms, cultural valorizations of transparency and so called genetic information, biotechnological developments and interest group activism. This theme is kinship-knowledge, or rather its social, medical, and regulatory management: what has to be known by whom about sperm and egg donors on the basis of which assumptions about biology? How is this information stored and made accessible? What should children know, and how should they know, about the donation? Or, put more ethnographically, as this research is not an ethical, but a descriptive and analytical endeavor: what is currently known and by whom about the donors? How—and in conversation with which scientific and everyday discourses on biology, heredity, and physiological connections—are these ways-of-knowing validated, represented, and practiced within multiple social relations? Through which familial and institutional practices and infrastructures[3] is this information stored and made accessible? What are children-by-donation told, when and how and by whom? What becomes excluded and silenced? And, ultimately, how is kinship-by-donation constituted within these knowledge-practices—practices of (k)information—in contemporary Western Europe? Answering these questions through an exploratory and multi-sited ethnographic focus on practices of what I have come to call kinship knowledge-management in Germany and Britain is the main aim of this work.

As mentioned above, the study of kinship has a turbulent history within anthropology and has been part of its disciplinary formation reaching back into the 19th century. Two aspects have long been contested: whether kinship, in its anthropologically charted global diversity, is indeed a universal category of human social organization, and how to actually conceptualize the potential link between biological reproduc-

3 As expanded upon in chapter 2.3, by infrastructures I am referring to formal and informal data-management systems crucial for kinship knowledge-management, such as the donor-files in a clinic, but also such everyday life "archives" as photo-albums in families. (For a discussion of the crucial role of infrastructures in the constitution of everyday life e.g. see Star (2002)).

tion, everyday care practices, and socially recognized kinship systems. The recent scholarly works included in the umbrella term, new kinship studies, have incorporated anthropological critiques of ethnocentrism, feminist critiques of anthropology, bioethical discussion on relatedness and privacy, and analyses from STS into a more practice and process oriented perspective of kinship. These works provide the broad theoretical background to this research. They often focus on NRTs' potential for "kinship trouble" (Franklin 2001, 314) or "identity trouble" (Hauskeller 2009, 40) through new relations and new knowledge on those relations coming out of the Life Sciences. New kinship studies contributors have tended to stress the importance of studying how kinship is done—and thereby defined—locally and with attention to rather flexible practices of inclusion and exclusion. Kinship then comes to figure as an "analytical tool" (Bestard 2009, 19; also see Strathern 2005, 7) for studying the formation of relationships and solidarity and the entangled role of "biologies and biologicals" (Franklin 2001).

In this research the analytical tool kinship is employed to describe and analyze how persons in Britain and Germany use gamete donation during a period of transition in which unquestioned anonymity and non-disclosure are replaced by routines of unquestioned non-anonymity and expectations of disclosure. Yet the analytical tool and ethnography's general strength for empirically picking up and reacting to the unexpected have also led me to touch upon the emergence of much wider cultural patterns in this research: namely the rise of transparency and connectedness as moral imperatives, as explored in the concluding chapter. Stripped of universalist or deterministic underpinnings, the study of kinship remains a probe into social life, as relevant a hundred years ago as in this work.

Debates on the role of knowledge or knowledge-practices in establishing kin-relationships also have a long history in cultural and social anthropology (see chapter 2.2). I argue that clinically assisted reproduction-by-donor is different from, say, adoption, IVF or also unassisted reproduction, in the way it brings together the necessity to manage the status of different forms of kinship-knowledge very explicitly: specifically how and which aspects of knowledge about the donor are relevant in official regulation and among parents and children, but also of equal importance, which discourses feed into the clinical "production" of kinship-by-donation (such as, for instance, scientific standards or classifications systems).

Drawing on the works of one of the new kinship studies' founding figures, David Schneider (1968), and using his notion that changing scientific biological knowledge in Western societies is foundational to kinship, Marilyn Strathern (1999) famously claimed that knowledge about biological procreation has the built-in effect of creating relationships through discovery. She therefore called it "constitutive information" and argued that, given the central role knowledge plays on parentage and procreation for people in Western societies, kinship-information cannot be scanned for personal utility by those affected. Rather, it irrevocably contributes to identity formation: "The social effect is immediate" (Strathern 1999, 75). The "constitutivity" of kinship-knowledge is also captured in the title of this research: *k*information.

Both Schneider's original assertion and Strathern's later conceptualization have been taken up and expanded upon within some of the works of the new kinship studies (e.g. Franklin 2001), as discussed in chapter 2. Empirical engagement with Strathern's (1999) concept has been scarce (but see Carsten 2007). It is one of the aims of this research to change this and thereby make an empirical and theoretical contribution to the scholarly debates on kinship-knowledge in anthropology. My research shows that kinship-by-donation is uniquely positioned in forcing the actors engaged in it to address and negotiate explicitly aspects of kinship-knowledge that are often taken for granted or kept private in the making of families. This makes kinship-by-donation a prime site for exploring in close empirical detail what the notion of kinship-knowledge as constitutive knowledge might mean in different societal domains and socio-material contexts. The idiom knowledge-management functions as the term to cover all the complex familial and institutional negotiations of kinship-information that I analyze. The term is borrowed from management theory and organizational studies and has the advantage of stressing the actors' agency and tactical engagement along with regulatory and infrastructural necessities and affordances. I use it stripped of its implicit or explicit rendering of knowledge-as-capital or knowledge-as-substance, which it carries in its originating disciplinary contexts. Rather, taking a pragmatist outlook, I argue that doing kinship and knowing kinship fall together (see chapter 2), yet take different shapes within and across the settings studied. My aim is to show the central role of knowledge-management in the making of families-by-donation in Europe.

Empirical Basis and Comparative Angle

In researching *k*information in four specific domains and in different sites and localities my research shows which aspects of kinship-knowledge are typically foregrounded and hence become constitutive within these domains and within individual families. Thus I encounter multiple axes of comparison, and the structure chosen to account for my findings focuses on three entangled aspects of similarity and difference: comparative axes are the four domains (families, clinics, regulation, interest groups), individual cases, and the two countries, Germany and Britain, as distinct regulatory environments. The narrative position adopted for this comparison is one where familiarity with neither the British nor the German regulatory situation is assumed of the potential reader. The comparative and contrasting aspects of this research then become a methodological tool to capture and analyze local specificities in different field sites and realms of analysis. It is worth clarifying that I do not wish to make claims on generalizable national differences beyond specific national regulations and reactions to these distinct policies. This research presents aspects of a "thick comparison", i.e. a reflexive approach to ethnographic comparing, which "takes seriously that objects of comparison—along with ethnographic fields—are being produced through the research process" (Niewöhner and Scheffer 2010, 4).

One aspect that I chose not to use as a systematic point of comparison, although it is repeatedly touched upon within individual discussions throughout this research[4], is the difference between egg and sperm donation and associated gender-differences in the experience of assisted conception. The individual families I studied were predominantly DI families (partly due to the illegality of egg donation in Germany). To expand the study to cover this specific comparative realm productively and in all its

4 For example in chapter 5.2 pertaining to the clinics and in chapter 8.5 pertaining to virility.

facets would have unduly expanded the pragmatic boundaries set for this work.[5]

The empirical basis of this research is provided through a multi-sited ethnographic exploration, employing in-depth and, as mentioned above, recurring interviews and short ethnographic episodes (such as shared meals or walks) with heterogeneous families-by-donation over a period of several years. The families (D n = 8; GB n = 5) were predominantly found through interview appeals in interest group forums and fertility clinics. The intensity of contact varied, but predominantly consisted of two interviews over a three-year period with e-mail contact in between. Where possible, interaction with families took place more often than the two interviews and in more informal fieldwork situations. The empirical basis of this research is further provided through (in some cases recurring) interviews and informal interactions with clinicians, policymakers, interest group activists, fertility counselors and donor-conceived adults across Britain and Germany. Short periods of ethnographic observation in fertility clinics in both countries were accompanied by the collection and analysis of local and national operating procedures, guidelines and policy documents. Interest group and counseling publications on gamete donation, particularly advice booklets and children's books on disclosure were also analyzed and compared. Further interviews from the "Kinship Cultures" research project (some conducted by myself) with families-by-adoption or -IVF, fertility doctors, and adoption counselors were selectively drawn on as well. Interviews were transcribed verbatim and observations recorded in fieldnotes. All were analyzed in a two-step coding process as suggested by Emerson (1995).

Within the empirically oriented parts of this book, I move back and forth between pointing to practices I identify as typical and pointing to practices I describe in individual detail. The narrative tone adopted in this work is reflexive, and sometimes also experimental or autoethnographic: chapter 2, for instance, experiments with the genre of the ethnographic arrival scene, trying to capture how I arrived at the theoretical and analytical

5 However, in addition to the indeed manifold extant empirical and theoretical discussions of kinship, infertility, and gender within the new kinship studies (Thompson 2005 would be an excellent example), see Klotz (2007) for a limited discussion of UK donor-anonymity and differences between egg and sperm donation. For more systematic comparisons see the works of Almeling (e.g. 2011).

positions constitutive for this research instead of a concrete fieldsite. The (limited) autoethnographic components thread in an additional methodological tool: the author's own "inexperience" with kinship, for example through being raised by parents who foregrounded their personal and political credo that "water" (i.e. chosen ties of solidarity beyond kinship) is "thicker than blood", is used as a tool of defamiliarization whilst probing into taken-for-granted assumptions on kinship. The epistemological position thereby taken throughout this book is one of critical reflexive realism (e.g. Aull Davis 1999), where the researcher's subjectivity is neither eclipsed, nor made visible as an end in itself, but "is a means […] of coming to know, however imperfectly, other aspects of social reality" (Aull Davis 1999, 213). Transparent subjectivity and an associated making-strange of the seemingly familiar are hence used within this research as the anthropologist's well-tried tool for an intersubjectively comprehensible—and thereby accountable—analysis and discussion (e.g. Amann and Hirschauer 1997; Steinke 2000).

Book Structure

I follow my description and analysis of how kinship-by-donation becomes constituted in different ways in the knowledge-practices apparent in families, clinics, regulation, and intersecting interest group activism by firstly tracing my theoretical and conceptual arrival at this research in chapter 2. I use the classical genre of the ethnographic arrival, as touched upon above, to trace three arrival scenes. In scene 1, I trace how I came to identify knowledge-management as one of the key regulatory problems gamete donation poses, because gamete donation disrupts long established recognition practices of parenthood. This section outlines the recent regulatory changes in Britain and Germany. In the second scene, I discuss the term knowledge, its role in the history of kinship studies, and its use in the so-called anthropology of knowledge. I focus on the role of materiality when studying kinship in scene 3.

Chapter 3 gives an account of the research process, the sample, and data analysis. Chapter 4 is the first of five chapters engaging in detail with the fieldwork data. However, the book barely separates into empirical and theoretical chapters: relevant theoretical points and links back to the broader theoretical grounding in chapter 2 are engaged with directly in the relevant empirical sections, and taken up more abstractly again in the concluding chapter.

Chapter 4 is also the first of three chapters (chapters 4, 7, and 8), which put the parents at center-stage, i.e. focus on the domain of the families. While chapters 7 and 8 concentrate on active practices and confrontations in familial knowledge-management, chapter 4 analyzes the broader reflections and opinions of the parents and also reconstructs past-practices. The first section (4.1) follows how the parents defined kinship within their own reflections expressed in the interviews. There it is constituted through three characteristic tensions relating to choice, corporeal continuity, and love. Then I reconstruct what I call the reproductive histories of the parents (4.2). Specifically for the heterosexual couples of my sample, donor insemination appears as a *technology of the last resort*, only to be pursued after the unsuccessful utilization of IVF/ICSI.

Chapter 5 focuses on the fertility clinics and sperm banks I visited in Germany and Britain. The chapter starts (5.1) with details about the regulation of sperm and egg donation in both countries and particularly what role these regulations play—or actually do not play—on the "shop-floor" (Griffiths, 2003) of the different field sites. The section makes visible how kinship-by-donation in both countries was constituted within two differing modes of governance: a tight, yet processual approach in the UK and a "hands off" minimal approach in Germany. The following sections focus on two different pathways of knowledge in the clinical constitution of kinship-by-donation: the medical trajectory[6] (5.2) and the accessible clinical/institutional trajectory (5.3). In 5.2 I analyze in detail the working stages involved in the step-by-step constitution of kinship-by-donation at the clinics. I argue that one of the unique characteristics of kinship-by-donation is how comprehensively it relates to clinical and institutional administration, infrastructures, and scientific standards. This also means that clinical and parental knowledge-management becomes part of the physical constitution of the children born through the procedures, for example through having specific blood groups. Section 5.3 analyzes which aspects

6 I use *trajectory of knowledge* as put forward by Fredrik Barth (2002), which I discuss in chapter 2.2 Barth uses the phrasing to point to the path-dependence of knowledge within entangled practices of validation, storage, and distribution.

of the clinical ways-of-knowing are actually made available to children and parents and thereby underlined as socially relevant. I note that measures for potential access to donor-data were rudimentary in Germany, while the British HFEA at the time of my fieldwork was comprehensively preparing for data access. I also note that the hybridity apparent in the medical trajectory is purified in the Latourian sense (1993) within the accessible trajectory.

Chapter 6 gives an account of the emergent normative canon of knowledge-management within the activities of interest groups and of parents' engagement with this canon. The emergent canon is characterized by an imperative of early disclosure of the donation to the child. I argue that this imperative is mainly framed as a moral question on equal sharing of information, not as a question either of the necessity or of the right to knowledge about genetic relatedness. The first section (6.1) provides a sketch of the historical and still prevalent endorsement of parental non-disclosure by clinicians. It also traces the formation of interest groups in both countries. The section thereby provides an additional historical account of gamete donation, not through focusing on regulation as done in section 2.1, but through focusing on the changing clinical and psychological conceptualizations of disclosure. The subchapter further addresses how recent advice literature and children's books available through the advocacy groups frame kinship-by-donation. In section 6.2 I present my analysis of the parents' experiences with interest group activism and the advice they gleaned from these activities for their own strategies of knowledge-management. The German parents expressed ambivalence regarding their children's later interest in the donation and the donor, a situation I interpret as linked to the uncertain German regulatory status quo.

Chapter 7 focuses on active practices of knowledge-management that families employ within everyday life, and how these practices constitute kinship-by-donation. This chapter (and the subsequent Chapter 8) returns to the first domain of analysis, the families, and makes use of the more long-term process- and practice-oriented data on family life. Both chapters also draw out similarities, differences, and entanglements with the figurations of kinship as identified in the previous chapters. Section 7.1 focuses on the parents' past (during treatment) and present (in subsequent reflections) engagement with clinical information on the donor. I argue that the donor becomes what I call an *administered relation*, where the highly limited and formal knowledge about the unknown donor is used by the parents as a stepping-stone into imagining him or her as a real-life person. I also argue in the subchapter that the notion of an administered relation implies that the parents have to simultaneously re-think themselves within the categories of the clinical information. The second section (7.2) analyzes the parental management of kinship-by-donation through naming practices and terminological decisions: the parents I engaged with all took great care in choosing which kin-words they used and advised others to use, and which ones were systematically excluded. The following section (7.3) traces how the parents disclosed the donation to their children and which tools they used to do this. Chapter 7.4 focuses on subversive practices of knowledge-management. Such wayward practices include in particular the use of the internet and DNA analyses through parents and older donor-conceived individuals to find out about and make (new) relations. I argue that these highly novel socio-material practices show how information on genetic kin-relations cannot be controlled in the present day: kinship, not only but especially by donation, becomes informationally uncontainable.

Chapter 8 is the last of the more empirically oriented chapters. Each of its sections examines everyday confrontations parents faced being a family-by-donation over time, and which tactics of knowledge-management they chose in response. There is a spectrum of confrontations the families encountered, with some being quite common and typical, such as so called resemblance-talk (8.1) and medical history-talk (section 8.2), whereas other confrontations have only been reported by some of the families: discriminatory kinship terminology (8.3); addresses of their non-conformity with the norm of the heterosexual two-parent family (8.4); and everyday life references to fertility as a confirmation of heterosexual love and virility (8.5). In addition, I learned about situations in which the children unexpectedly thematize their donor-conception in everyday interactions and confront the parents with a need for response (8.6). All these confrontations can lead parents to develop *reflexive kinship expertise*: they explicitly interrogate and observe how kinship is constituted in everyday life.

In the concluding sections (chapter 9) I argue that my findings demonstrate a contemporary renegotiation of the values of privacy, information-sharing, and connectedness. I discuss four central results: pertaining to the strong co-implication of kinship-by-donation with regulation (section 9.1); kinship-by-donation's resonance with a cultural pattern I term *transparentization* (section 9.2); kinship-by-donation's foundational link to particularly diverse fields of knowledge-production (section 9.3); and parents' simultaneous multiplication and mitigation of what Strathern (1999) calls the social effects of biological information (section 9.4). In sum, a shift of authority becomes discernible in the way kinship-by-donation is known and managed in Europe; it is a shift, more minute in Germany than in Britain, towards interest groups, parents, and policy-makers, and away from a sometimes high-handed medical profession.

2. Three Conceptual Arrival Scenes: Comparative Vantage Point, Kinship and Knowledge, Kinship Matters

The particular stylistic device of the ethnographic *arrival scene* has been analyzed since the end of the 1980s as one of the typical focal points of the assertion of ethnographic authority and authenticity (Pratt 1986) —ever since "ethnography as the first research strategy within empirical social science had the honor of a literary-theoretical deconstruction" (Hirschauer 2001, 429).[1] Arrival scenes have been analyzed as the classical textual instance for the ethnographer to make him- or herself visible in the text, only to retreat again to narrate her informants' lives in the notorious "ethnographic present" (e.g. Clifford 1986). Of course, authority and authenticity, after what has been called the "reflexive turn" in anthropology (e.g. Faubion and Marcus 2009), have not disappeared, nor have arrival scenes. Only the theoretical grounds on which legitimacy is claimed might have shifted, with arrival scenes or similar literary devices now often signaling situatedness and reflexivity rather than positivist objectivity. Thinking about possible arrival scenes for this book—and what kind of authority they would, inescapably, it seems (e.g. Gay y Blasco and Wardle 2007, 153), assert—I thought about describing how I arrived at my interview partners' houses, and the difficulties I sometimes had getting there. This gives a sense of my aim to meet my interviewees in their homes or other places intimate to them, but also, of course, of the "having been there" identified by Geertz (1988, 1–25) as one of the stylistic devices for signaling ethnographic expertise. I also thought about quoting

1 My translation. Hirschauer is here pointing towards the publication of "Writing Culture" (Clifford & Marcus, 1986) and the ensuing debates. Also see Aull Davis (1999, 216–220); Gay y Blasco & Wardle (2007, 143–153); and Knecht (2009a) for further thoughts on ethnographic arrival scenes.

from some of my more autoethnographic field notes, e.g. how I—not used to spending much time among kin due to a small family and parents who always stressed that "water was thicker than blood"—discovered myself scanning people for physical resemblances at the funeral of my great uncle: thereby invoking a sense of the smaller autoethnographic components of this book and my own entanglements and occasional sense of wonder with regard to my elusive research subject *kinship*. Nevertheless, I decided against anything more than the not particularly elegant rhetorical trick just employed, for another arrival seemed equally important to me: I decided to include three arrival scenes in this book which capture a *theoretical and conceptual arrival*. This was not done to discount the significance of methodology, the relationship with my interview partners, or autoethnography—all of which will have a place for debate in the following chapters. It was done because, as contemplating the final configuration of this book, I was struck by the difficulties of textually representing, through the kind of research steps and associated feedback loops, how one actually arrives at formulating a research question. These steps are, after all, constitutive parts of the analytic process and should not be overlooked within the final representation of the research. In a sense this goes for *all* scientific investigation. It however becomes *particularly salient* for ethnographies, due to the openness of the research set-up to unexpected findings and the central role of the researcher in shaping this open process. In the words of the methodologist David Silverman:

> "We come to look at things in certain ways because we have adopted, either tacitly or explicitly, certain ways of seeing. This means that, in observational research, data-collection, hypothesis-construction and theory-building are not three separate things, but are interwoven with each other." (Silverman 1993, 46)

Hence, I have formulated three arrival scenes, which try to capture how I "came to look at things", and recount my expeditions into literature at the beginning of this book. This section thus tries to fuse background information and literature discussion with a reflexive account of the emergence of my research question. I firstly discuss how the comparison between gamete donation in Germany and in Britain has constituted my research field in specific ways. My own spatial and intellectual movements between the two countries contributed to a particular *comparative reflex* within which the British regulatory situation figures as vantage point. *Knowledge-*

management is identified as a differently shaped regulatory problem in both countries, and as *tertium comparationis* of my research. Secondly, I discuss the crucial role *knowledge* plays for the configuration of kinship. And thirdly, I ask what role *materiality* might play in a research so pointedly centering on knowledge practices—identifying hybrid processes of socio-material articulation and information infrastructures as implicated in kinship knowledge-management.

Scene 1: Knowledge-Management During Gamete Donation as Policy Problem in Britain and Germany

This first scene involves a classical physical arrival, but only marginally. First and foremost it aims at reflexively capturing the research process involved in identifying issues of *knowledge-management* in the realm of kinship-by-donation as specifically shaped regulatory problems in Britain and Germany. This first scene also aims at sketching out these regulatory processes themselves. The physical arrival involved a flight from Berlin to Bristol, the stresses of left-lane traffic during the drive from Bristol to Exeter, and—back to capturing a conceptual arrival—the pursuit of an interdisciplinary science studies degree in Exeter. My studies at the Centre for Genomics in Society alerted me to how genetic knowledge was emerging as a perceived connector of "the molecular body to the phenotypic appearance of a person, and the phenotypic appearance to the person's life history, the bodies (and lives) of her ancestors, and to her current environment" (Hauskeller 2006, 21). Coterminous with entry in 2004 into this specific academic situation, gamete donation in Britain became a much covered and talked about news item; a new law for both male and female gamete donation to become non-anonymous had only just come into force in July 2004, affecting gamete donation from April 2005 onwards (UK Gov 2004). Before that, I had not known anything about sperm or egg donor anonymity or non-anonymity, probably because gamete donation was hardly discussed publicly in Germany. As I later realized, donor-anonymity in Europe is usually a subject of national regulation, whereas in the US, it is essentially decided through market forces. In Europe, there are regimes in place of donor-anonymity (e.g.

Spain, Denmark, and France) and of non-anonymity (e.g. Britain, Austria, and Sweden). There are more EU countries with anonymous regimes than non-anonymous set-ups (for overviews e.g. see European Commission, 2006; Frith, 2001; Jones et al., 2010).

Instigated by the media coverage of the change from donor anonymity to non-anonymity, I did research into what kin-relationships were actually evoked within British policy debates on gamete donation, since the Human Fertilisation and Embryology Act was instated in 1990 to comprehensively regulate reproductive technologies in the UK (Klotz 2006, 2007). I was struck by how much the policy discourse focused on what I later termed *knowledge-management* (i.e. a negotiation of which aspects of kinship-knowledge are validated, drawn on in various practices, and made accessible or inaccessible). Should the donor conception be mentioned on a child's birth certificate? Should donors be anonymous or non-anonymous? Which donor-information should be stored where? How and when could a donor-conceived child find out about this information? How should the health screenings for donors look like? Should they be told about possibly detected "genetic risks"? Should they be held accountable when concealing previously known hereditary diseases running in his or her family? However, my research at the time always lacked a comparative angle. Hence, my arrival at identifying knowledge-management as a regulatory problem started in Britain. This embedded a specific *comparative reflex* in my ethnographic research: because I first came to know kinship-by-donation through looking at the British situation, the German situation figured as *other*. Some of the comparative terms used throughout this book still embody this reflex, i.e. when I speak of the *under-regulatedness* of the German legal situation, instead of calling the British one *overregulated*.

I began to piece together the British regulatory situation and developments: the Warnock Report[2] advising the policymaking processes around the HFE Act of 1990 had actually recommended gamete donor anonymity, because of potential "legal complications and emotional

2 The Warnock Report has been compiled by the Committee of Inquiry into Human Fertilisation and Embryology, chaired by the moral-philosopher Mary Warnock. The committee was instated by UK government in 1982 to put together a report on the social and legal challenges of new reproductive technologies and related biotechnologies.

difficulties" (Warnock and Committee 1985, 15). With the HFE Act that followed, donor anonymity was officially introduced in Britain and all potential legal ties between donor and child cut and the partner of the woman entering fertility treatment named as the legal father (HFE Act 1990 s. 28). With regard to female donation the gestational mother (i.e. a potential mother-by-egg-donation) was named as always being the legal mother of a child (HFE Act 1990 s. 27). In 1990 it was also decided that the Human Fertilisation and Embryology Authority (HFEA), the governmental watchdog organization[3] licensing fertility clinics set up through the HFE Act, was to collect non-identifying information about gamete donors in a national register (HFE Act 1990 s. 31), such as information on the donor's date of birth, his/her ethnic group and physical appearance. This limited data about the donor was to be accessible to children in their late teens. In the original 1990 HFE Act a clause was added which stated the necessity of fertility clinics to take into account the future child's welfare, "including the need of that child for a father" (HFE Act s. 13(5)). Some NHS clinics interpreted this as lesbians and single women being banned from treatment, while others interpreted the section as pointing to the necessity of male role-models or a generally stable family environment (e.g. see Johnson 1999, 66). The resulting access problems for lesbians to donor treatment, led some private clinics to specialize in their treatment, as further explored in chapter 5.

In the late 1990s public voices started to appear during debates around children's rights, arguing against donor-anonymity on the grounds of differing UK adoptee's rights and the importance of information on medical history (e.g. see Turkmendag 2012). In 2001 the UK Department of Health was already internally starting to set up a consultation on the issue of donor anonymity when it was approached by letter from individuals seeking access to identifying and non-identifying donor information, for themselves, or for their donor conceived child, and the establishment of a contact register. Legal action (Rose & Anor vs HFEA 2002) ensued simultaneously with the advancement of the Department of Health consultation. Not wishing to interfere in the ongoing policymaking process, the case was only tried under the question of whether article 8 of the UK

3 The HFEA is officially a non-departmental public body (NDPB) accountable to the UK Department of Health.

Human Rights Act (1998), which guarantees "respect for private and family life, including the right to form a personal identity", could be invoked. The case was decided in favor of the claimants, making it unlikely that donor anonymity would stand under any future legal action (e.g. Liberty 2002). After the High Court ruling in July 2002, the HFEA issued a document in which it praised the efforts of the ongoing Department of Health consultation, and recommended a removal of donor-anonymity (HFEA 2002).

In January 2004, the British government declared that regulations to remove donor anonymity would indeed come into force later in the year (UK Gov 2004). Simultaneously, the then-Minister of Health Melanie Johnson announced a general review of the HFE Act. The new regulations do not automatically apply to donors who have donated under previous regulations and, as in the previous legislation, make no difference between egg and sperm donation. Within the new regulatory framework, children born through fertility treatment using donor gametes have the right to access identifying information about the donor from the central HFEA registry when they reach the age 18, the first possible cases thereby arising in 2023. However, the controversial opportunity of previously anonymous donors registering back as non-anonymous (further discussed in 5.2) makes the 2023 temporal threshold not definite. Under the new regulations the donor can also find out about the number of children he or she helped to conceive, their year of birth, and their gender, by also contacting the HFEA registry. The enforcement of the HFE Act through the HFEA means that how information on the donor is to be collected in the registry, and which forms are to be used to collect and store donor information, is laid out in detail through the meticulous HFEA Code of Practice (HFEA 2009a) and through their centrally formatted donor information sheets (for details see chapter 5).

With the above regulatory framework in mind I took another flight, this time in the other direction, from Bristol to Berlin. I was going back to Berlin to start work as an interviewer in late 2006 on the longitudinal "kinship cultures" research project of the collaborative research cluster SFB 640 on changing representations of social order. I was also already developing my own study on kinship-by-donation then and started to do background research into the German regulation of gamete donation.

What became striking was the extreme level of disagreement, apparent between different expert interviews and within literature searches, on the German regulatory situation. For instance Dr. Dettmaringen, director of the Großstadt-based Sperm Bank Friedhausen, quite vehemently said to me:

"It says in the constitution since 1949 that one has the right to genetic parentage [Recht auf gneetische Abstammung]. And if we had worked entirely correctly within the right to genetic parentage, all sperm bank directors, Germany-wide, would have only collected non-anonymously."

My "birds-eye view" differed significantly: the right to knowledge about one's parentage is not part of the original legal text of the German constitution as it came into force in 1949. Instead, the German *Constitutional Court* ruled in *1989* that they see genetic knowledge as being implicated in the basic right to self-fulfillment (BVerfGE). This case was unrelated to any forms of assisted reproduction—and has only recently been put into legal relation to gamete donation. Interestingly, in the interview passage quoted above, Dr. Dettmaringen did *not* say "the right to knowledge about genetic parentage" (like it is phrased in the case precedent that I assume he is referring to) but simply said "the right to genetic parentage". He conflates *knowing about* kinship with *having* kin, which actually epitomizes Strathern's (1999) point about kinship knowledge being constitutive knowledge (further explored in 2.2).

Similarly, many other actors in the field made references to legal rules, which I did not see as implicated at all, if looked at from a theoretical juridical point of view. However, how did my birds-eye analysis of the German legal situation matter, I came to ask myself, if "rule following on the 'shop floor' of social life" (Griffiths 2003, 1) was entangled with quite different interpretations of regulation? The only straightforward aspect of German gamete donation regulation is that egg donation in Germany is unlawful under the so-called Embryo-Protection-Law of 1990. The original justification for the prohibition within the wording has been the (assumed) psychologically harmful and unprecedented split between genetic and gestational motherhood (ESchG 1990 § 1 + appendage 5). Nevertheless, more recent German bioethical assessments of the ban have tended to focus on the practice of "harvesting" eggs from healthy women who have no medical benefits from the procedure as violating the

Hippocratic oath (e.g. Graumann 2007). Sperm donation in Germany, in contrast, is practiced in a legal grey zone and has never been touched by the regulatory initiatives on new reproductive technologies and biotechnologies, which Europe saw at the beginning of the 1990s—as discussed in the introduction. In fact, knowledge on clinical sperm donation is so limited, even among clinical professionals, that it is not unheard of for clinical personnel to wrongly advise patients that the practice is illegal in Germany, as parents told me during my research. While the British HFE Act and the earlier Warnock Report (1985) comprehensively discuss sperm donation, there is no reference to it at all in the German Embryo Protection Law. As pointed out above, the German law making process firmly centered on abortion and the status of the embryo instead (e.g. Jasanoff 2005; Richardt 2003).

The apparent legal uncertainties with regard to sperm donation in Germany are so extensive, that a precise subsumption even of the uncertainties seems almost impossible (but e.g. see Thorn et al. 2008). What is at stake are both the potential legal connections between donor and child and questions of knowledge-management concerning anonymity and details of data storage: to date, a German donor conceived child could theoretically contest his social father's paternity and instead try to have the sperm donor recognized as a father, thereby instating legal and financial obligations between sperm donor and child (e.g. Rütz 2008; Wendehorst 2008).

During a 2002 reform of the German Civil Code pertaining to paternity disputes—not particularly regulating reproductive technologies—a paragraph was added that a father-by-donation could not later dispute paternity, if he signed a contract that his wife would be undergoing insemination by donor (KindRVerbG 2002: § 1600 (2)). However, this paragraph still left open the possibility—and as mentioned above it is still open—that *the child* could theoretically dispute paternity. Some legal theorists (e.g. Rütz 2008) even suspect a risk for practicing fertility doctors to be sued for financial support or contract breaches by both donor child (to compensate for missed potential child-support payments) and sperm donor (for giving out his information). This situation makes it particularly problematic for lesbian and single women to gain admission to sperm banks. Physicians find it more likely that these women's children-by-donation might later sue the gynecologist. Legal experts of the German

Medical Association are therefore advising against the treatment of anyone other than married heterosexual couples in their professional guidelines (Bundesärztekammer 2006). Practically, some clinics ignore these professional guidelines, although this could produce—but never has—licensing problems on the state level.[4] Legal experts within the gay rights movement are arguing that justifying the exclusion of lesbian couples from clinical gamete donation through references to the ambiguous German legal setting makes no sense juridically (because of changed laws on homosexual parenting and adoption) and suspect an underlying conservative agenda (e.g. LSVD 2007, 34–35).

The legal situation concerning donor (non-)anonymity is similarly unclear: the aforementioned Constitutional Court ruling from 1989 was not applied to sperm donation until the implementation of the EU Tissue Directive (ETD) into German law within the so-called Tissue Law (GewebeG 2007). The ETD is a technical directive geared at, as stated in its full title, "setting standards of quality and safety for the donation, procurement, testing, processing, preservation, storage, and distribution of human tissues and cells" and as such makes no explicit statement on the ethical or legal implications of reproductive technologies. (For one of the rare social scientific discussions of the Directive and its implementation see Klaus Hoeyer 2010). Certainly before the 1989 ruling and for many sperm banks until the implementation of the ETD, a quasi donor-anonymity was the norm within clinical practices. Even though there was no legally instated anonymity, clinical records were mostly destroyed after the official ten year storage period for medical records ended, thereby making it impossible to track down donors.[5] The ETD extended these storage periods of donor records to at least 30 years, making the legal scenario of a grown up child suing for access to donor records more likely. Furthermore, the first ever legal reference to questions of sperm donor (non-)anonymity in Germany is to be found in the German law on organ

4 The German medical profession, just as the legal profession, is mostly regulated through statutory rules of conduct, not state-law. The different German State Chambers of Physicians, who interpret and enforce the guidelines of the German Medical Association, take different approaches to questions of access to DI for unmarried, single, or lesbian women (more in chapter 5.1).

5 This was described to me in personal communication with three German sperm bank directors. The practice is also recounted through Thorn et al. (2008).

donation, which was changed through the implementation of the ETD. There it is stated that "with sperm donation the right of the child to information on its parentage" had to prevail over the principle of anonymity otherwise in place with regard to organ donation (GewebeG 2007 § 14 (3)). Nevertheless, to date it is still juridically unclear how and which information should be made available to children-by-donation, at which point in time, and on what exact grounds. In the absence of a national register it is also unclear how accessing this information might look (e.g. see Bundesärztekammer 2006, A1402). German sperm banks and clinics currently treat access to donor-information by donor-conceived individuals as highly hypothetical in their daily practices, as explored in detail in chapter 5.

There is a small professional association of German sperm bank operators and professionals working in the DI sector, which has published non-binding guidelines (Arbeitsgruppe Richtliniennovellierung 2006) on quality measurements and donor-screenings within this unclear regulatory setting. These guidelines are, however, in addition to their voluntary nature, not as detailed as the binding and, as mentioned above, highly detailed HFEA Code of Practice or the HFEA's internal operating procedures on how to deal with donor-data and access requests (for a detailed discussion see chapter 5). In fact—and note this is my *comparative reflex* at work—the German association does not lay out any protocols in the small section on potential access to donor-data (Arbeitsgruppe Richtliniennovellierung 2006, 18–19) on how to deal practically with such requests.

I returned to Britain for now fully-fledged fieldwork in 2009 and 2010, equipped with the background knowledge on the British and the German regulatory situation sketched above. During my visits to clinics and in interviews with policymakers the central regulation and standardization of donation practices in the UK was underlined. For Germany, it became clear that, despite all the legal uncertainties surrounding it, it was still practically "working". These differing modes of governance will be further discussed in chapter 5. During my return to Britain the HFEA was again reviewing donation policies in detail. This was partly due to a renewal of the HFE Act in 2008. Furthermore, the reviewing endeavors of the HFEA are to be seen as part of the agency's general commitment to evidence based policymaking (more below) as often stressed in its official statements and reports (e.g. see HFEA, 2011a). The changes made to the HFE Act had eliminated the previous mention of "a child's need for a father" and introduced comprehensive regulation of the legal parental status of lesbian partners of women undergoing fertility treatment (HFEA Act 2008, Part I, s. 24; Part II, s. 42–47; for discussion see Gamble and Ghevaert, 2009). The agency was also setting up a voluntary contact register for donor-siblings over 18. The HFEA had also, following parental requests, started to allow parents to access the national register for more comprehensive non-identifying information on the donor, for instance the voluntary personal message left by the donor on the central form to register donors (more in chapter 5) and the number of siblings conceived (e.g. see HFEA 2009b).

For the British regulatory situation it appeared that initial problems on how to manage kinship information (e.g. donor anonymity versus non-anonymity) had given way to new problems of a similar kind: for instance when parents complained to the HFEA officers I interviewed about the agency voluntarily re-registering previously anonymous donors as identifiable, whereas the parents had brought up their children with the narrative that the donor was fully anonymous (see chapter 5.3). Or also when clinicians complained to the HFEA, as I learned both from doctors and from HFEA information managers, that parents were "illegally" networking around clinical donor-codes they had obtained to find half-siblings (see chapter 7.4). Once brought into the limelight of official knowledge-management and not part of long established everyday familial practices of informally negotiating kin-relationships, kinship-by-donation in Britain kept generating new unforeseen problems to be explicitly worked through by evidence based policymaking (EBP). EBP (for social scientific discussion e.g. see David 2002) is a practice firmly rooted in the governmental reforms of the Blair Government in Britain, its founding statement being the Modernising Government White Paper of the new Blair government (UK Gov 1999). Broadly ideologically traceable to the increasing entanglement of policymaking and social science as already discussed in Foucault's governmentality analyses (e.g. Foucault 2000), it is a concept related to the increasing dominance of "audit cultures" (Strathern 2000) in Britain and part of what Miller and Rose (2008) call "governance at a distance" (more in chapter 5). EBP is not yet—despite some calls within German policymaking and political consulting to do so (e.g. see Grabow and Jun 2008)—firmly established within the far less centralized processes of governance in Germany.

Within such comparative fieldwork, gamete donation and the associated practical questions of official knowledge-management emerged as differently shaped regulatory problems and as *tertium comparationis* to be explored throughout this book: in Britain, the "experimental setting" of kinship-by-donation (if one stays with the notion of kinship-by-donation as experiment as presented in the introduction) appeared as controlled and constantly reviewed through regulation. The British medical professionals I interacted with sometimes framed this as "overregulation", while policymakers and also the representatives of interest groups and parents expressed confidence in the approach.

In Germany, gamete donation and associated knowledge-management did not appear as a regulatory problem through complex policy processes making necessary ever new adjustments and deliberations, nor through legal action, as apparent in the UK. Less bound up with regulation, it seemed like a far less controlled "field experiment". Problematizations of kinship knowledge-management were apparent in local opinions and expertise: German clinicians criticized the legal uncertainties surrounding donor-data, anonymity, and the unclear legal connection between donor and child. German parents (as for instance explored in chapter 6) even more vehemently complained about the legal uncertainties surrounding data access—often explicitly making their own comparisons with the British situation. And within the activities of central German political foundations (e.g. Diedrich et al. 2008) and professional associations (e.g. Arbeitsgruppe Richtliniennovellierung 2006; Bundesärztekammer 2006), the legal grey areas surrounding sperm donation and associated questions of knowledge-management were also addressed as needing more central regulation. As recounted above, it had however been the EU Tissue Directive and its implementation, as such not intended for the explicit ethical or social regulation of sperm donation, which had played a decisive part in tipping the scales from *de-facto* donor-anonymity to a fragile and unclear non-anonymity in Germany (also see Klotz and Knecht 2009, 2012).

This arrival scene traced the empirical identification of knowledge-management as *nationally specific* regulatory problems, with gamete donation presenting as tightly controlled in Britain and as minimally controlled in Germany. This section has fused background information on the regulation of gamete donation in both countries with a reflexive discussion of how the research process has shaped the comparative aspects of this book. The "thick comparison" (Scheffer and Niewöhner 2010) presented in the following chapters is characterized by a *comparative reflex* within which Britain figures as vantage point.

Scene 2: Kinship and Knowledge in Anthropology

The second arrival scene does not start with planes or suitcases, but with a text—this arrival, as in fact the third one as well, is only theoretical and conceptual. It takes the shape of an expedition into literature on kinship *and* knowledge. Temporally, its beginnings have to be located after the early stages of the first arrival. Hence, the identification of knowledge-management as regulatory problem for gamete donation is already embedded in this scene. This arrival starts with Strathern's thought-provoking essay "Refusing Information" (1999), which immediately struck me for its relevance to the notion of knowledge-management as policy problem and as being bound up in Britain with the spread of a culture of evidence based policymaking (EBP). Strathern's essay introduces her conceptualization of kinship-knowledge as constitutive knowledge. I would like to recount her argument here, to then lead the expedition into terminological and historical conceptualizations of knowledge and kinship, to end with a discussion of Strathern's points through Janet Carsten (2007) and where the expedition has led myself.

Strathern notes in her essay that since the beginning of the 1990s, kinship knowledge has to be located within a wider landscape of societal debates on knowledge practices: she roughly sketches out the picture of techniques of verifiability of biological kinship information becoming widely available and gamete donor anonymity becoming discussed and centrally regulated in the UK. She also situates these debates within a wider societal drive towards *transparency*, especially within the growing tendency of practices of governance being bound up with large information gathering endeavors (subsequently to become known as EBP).

Strathern argues that this trend is actually informing kinship knowledge-management in Britain. She goes on to discuss that kinship-knowledge can take on a different character depending on the social situation it is implicated in. She differentiates between regulative information and constitutive information. The former refers to kinship-information as being part of governmental practices (e.g. in government administered research) and litigation (e.g. paternity testing); the latter refers to biological kinship-knowledge as an integral part of how Westerners think of themselves as persons: this knowledge is "foundational to personal identity" (Strathern 1999, 68). To make this distinction she draws on John Searle's notion of constitutive and regulative rules. The philosopher of language first introduces the concept in his early work *Speech Acts* when discussing his main hypothesis that language is "rule-governed intentional behavior" (Searle 1969, 16). Searle describes his concept as follows:

"Regulative Rules regulate antecedently or independently existing forms of behavior; for example, many rules of etiquette regulate inter-personal relationships which exist independently of the rules: but constitutive rules do not merely regulate, they create or define new forms of behavior." (1969, 33)

Applied to kinship-knowledge, Strathern wants to make a point about not-knowing—a social status that is, as she notes, currently in the process of being cast as utterly undesirable. She wants to point out that information on kinship in the regulative realm can be screened for relevance in regulatory processes, but knowledge on kinship in everyday life has constitutive effects on one's identity and therefore cannot be refused if found unnecessary:

"Because of the cultural coupling with identity, kinship knowledge is a particular kind of knowledge: the information (and verification) on which it draws is constitutive in its consequences. (…) Kin persons who find out about ancestry acquire identity by that very discovery." (Strathern 1999, 68)

Personal kinship-knowledge situates Westerners in a web of relationships, which are entangled with one's subjectivity. The change, which this web undergoes if personal kinship-knowledge changes, is of major significance to Westerners' sense of self. Strathern's point is not to therefore argue *against* notions of transparency in the realm of gamete donation or similar domains it is rather, in her own words, "a plea for attending to contemporary complexity" (1999, 64) by questioning transparency as a value in its own right or simply taking it for granted as another step in an enlightenment project.

Strathern, in my "arrival text", speaks of knowledge as being in effect subject-bound ("a sensory or mental construct referring to an individual's perceptive state"), while information is object-bound in the sense that "someone must be informed so that information implies communication" (1999, 311). Of course, both terms are highly complex in their various disciplinary employments, contestations, and divergent definitions. In much of the information and organizational studies literature, hierarchical definitions between information and knowledge are used, with knowledge ranking higher in validity, applicability, and complexity (e.g. Liew 2007). What has come to be known as the anthropology of knowledge has not reveled in the separation of the two terms or on hierarchies, but also reflects a notion that knowledge is more complex than information. And, similar to Strathern, that knowledge in contrast to information is about a person's practices of sense-making. Kirsten Hastrup, for instance argues that from an anthropological perspective knowledge is "organized information about ways of living in the world and modes of attending to the world" (Hastrup 2004, 456), including not only explicit knowledge, but also embodied implicit knowledge in the sense of Michael Polanyi (1973). And Fredrik Barth—tentatively—defines knowledge as "what a person employs to interpret and act on the world" (2002, 1).[6] I follow Hastrup's and Barth's definition of knowledge, which would make kinship-knowledge, tentatively defined *what a person employs to interpret relations arising out of reproduction and modes of attending to these relations.*[7] I explicitly use

6 In the reply to his article's comments (Barth 2002, 16), the author argues that he "intended less than to 'define' knowledge positively ('what a person employs to interpret and act on the world... etc.'). It is enough for us to recognize that it is where persons engage in such tasks that we should look for empirical manifestations of knowledge".

7 I am aware that Hastrup is rather critical of Barth. However, I do not share her criticism that he "tends to overlook the issue of what can be known under particular historical circumstances", and simply views knowledge as an out there to be discovered substance, nor that he implicitly presupposes "a rather anachronistic concept of culture as an essence that is installed in individuals in equal measure by birth and belonging" (Hastrup 2004, 457). In fact, I understand Barth as explicitly writing *against* the concept of culture, for he views it as essentializing and tries to build up the anthropology of knowledge in contrast to this tendency: "The image of culture as knowledge

the terms knowledge and knowledge-practices in the chapters to come as synonyms to connote an action-oriented notion of knowledge, as indicated in Hastrup's and Barth's approaches, and also in pragmatist concepts of knowledge. Dewey and Bentley have pointedly argued that "knowing and identifying, as ways of acting, are as much ways of doing, of making [...], as are chopping wood, singing songs, seeing sights, or making hay" (1945, 231). Relational materialist approaches within STS have similarly underlined, often in explicit engagement with the legacy of American pragmatism, that knowing is a practice (e.g. Mol and Law 2004). The anthropological perspective I have taken on board during my expedition further implies using the term knowledge in a *descriptive*, rather than in a *normative* philosophical sense.[8] However, this still implicates that knowledge is characterized by social practices of validation, or, in other words, by what people "accept as real" (McCarthy 1996, 2). In the case of Western kinship-knowledge, it is science providing these means of validation, as further discussed below.

When viewing knowledge not as an out there to be discovered substance, but as a relational practice, bound up with human actions and historically derived "modes of knowing" (e.g. Hastrup 2004, 456), the separation of information and knowledge becomes rather elusive. Being interested in how knowledge-practices, through infrastructural and interactional affordances, take on specific trajectories, separating the two terms might actually undermine my own attempts of analyzing such affordances and relations. I therefore employ the term kinship-knowledge *both* to refer to how persons find out about, think and act upon relations arising out of reproduction *and* to refer to what about these relations is stored, made accessible or non-accessible and communicated. I occasionally use the term (kinship-) information synonymously.

Nevertheless, there are representational restraints. Capturing the relationality and action-orientation of knowledge is not always precisely possible. When writing, there often needs to be "a temporary objectification

---

abstracts it less and points to people's engagement with the world, through action. It acknowledges the fact of globally continuous variation, not separable into homogenized and mutually alien cultures. It alerts us to interchange and to flux. 'Knowledge' is not characterizable as difference..." (Barth 1995, 66).

8 For an excellent empirical example of this approach in the anthropology of knowledge see Ward Goodenough (1986).

of relational knowledge" (Hastrup 2004, 458). Furthermore, knowledge is always, but in differing, socio-materially determined ways, reductive and selective (e.g. Hastrup 2004, 456). These ways of reduction and selection, in my four domains of study (family life, clinical practices, regulation, interest group activism), are the object of my study—to make use of the previously discussed temporary figure of objectification for the sake of clarity.

Which methodological and conceptual tools did the expedition acquire upon arriving at the anthropology of knowledge? Firstly, one has to stress that the latter is a rather loose body of scholarly works. Dominic Boyer argues that it "would be difficult to locate anthropological research that did not, at some level, speak to and about human knowledge" (2005, 141). In contrast to the sociology of knowledge, with its clear lineage of influential individuals (first and foremost Karl Mannheim) and theoretical move over time from a distinct focus on social determination *of* knowledge to social construction *through* knowledge (e.g. McCarthy 1996), what is referred to as the anthropology of knowledge does not have a similarly clear genealogy. These scholarly works focus on the status and comparability of knowledge both within anthropology's objects of investigation and anthropology's own scholarly output—often combining questions regarding the two in reflexive musings on ontology and epistemology (as pointed examples see Boyer 2005; Hastrup 2004).

Such works commonly conceptualize their specific focus on knowledge as being driven by an interest in comparison and social processes. Culture and knowledge are *almost* used synonymously here. Rather than focusing on notions of diffuse sharing, such as encapsulated in most concepts of culture, one should rather be able to focus on logics of distribution, power, and difference through focusing on knowledge instead (e.g. Barth 1995, 65; 2002, 1; Boyer 2005, 141, 148; Crick 1982, 303). The anthropology of knowledge is thereby still following a project at the heart of anthropology, with a genealogy going back to scholars such as Émile Durkheim, Marcel Mauss, and Evans Pritchard: "After all, some would wish to define our basic concept of culture as a process of acquiring and displaying knowledge—of rules, values, and beliefs", as Malcolm Crick puts it (1982, 287).

Within this loose field of research, only Barth proposes a concrete empirical research program. He compares different traditions of knowledge across societies in a relativist, descriptive fashion—essentially exploring the vastly different trajectories or pathways of knowledge. When asking questions about the shape, path-dependence, validation criteria, and the convertibility of knowledge, he proposes to observe the interplay of three mutually constitutive aspects of knowing: firstly, a knowledge tradition's "corpus of substantive assertions about the world" (Barth 2002, 3). Secondly, he proposes to analyze its communicative media. In his own examples this could for instance mean that a certain corpus of knowledge is only communicated through verbal poetic images. I propose to extend this focus on communicative media from a perspective only capturing questions of representation to also capture more socio-material affordances of material storage and infrastructure (more in scene 3 below). Thirdly, Barth proposes to take into account patterns of distribution of knowledge within social relations. He underlines that his analytical program does not advocate to study these three points separately, but to rather observe how "these three faces of knowledge appear together precisely in the particulars of action in every event of the application of knowledge, in every transaction in knowledge, in every performance" (Barth 2002, 3). Through the detailed discussion of these three aspects of knowlege, Barth manages not only to describe local modes of knowing convincingly and vividly, but also to offer some potential explanations for forms of change and other forms of path-dependence. My own references to "paths" or "trajectories" of knowledge are made with the Barthian notion in mind, as pointed out in the introduction.

The expedition has taken me to a place where kinship-knowledge is studied in how it is validated, stored and communicated, and distributed relationally as a practice. Yet, my interest in kinship-knowledge is by no means a new phenomenon within anthropological scholarship, just because knowledge-management for kinship-by-donation is quite a contemporary phenomenon. I therefore want to guide the expedition into a brief exploration of anthropological kinship studies—before returning to a discussion of Strathern's concerns as taken up by Carsten (2007). As pointed out in the introduction, the study of kinship (historically predominantly for so-called Non-Western groups) has co-evolved with the professionalization and institutionalization of socio-cultural anthropology in Britain, the USA and Germany (e.g. Knecht 2003). Such studies of kinship have always been fuelled by differently configured interests in social order and modes of solidarity. Virtually every influential anthropologist in the past has worked on kinship, whether historical figures such as Henry Lewis Morgan and Johann Jacob Bachhofen, working before the institutionalization of socio-cultural anthropology are concerned, or influential modern anthropologists such as Franz Boas or Bronislaw Malinowski. Yet, underlying theoretical assumptions for anthropological studies of kinship all over the world have varied and changed widely. Roger Keesing has already argued in the 1970s with some disillusionment about anthropology's key concept:

> "Despite a century of effort, no anthropologist has succeeded in producing a satisfactory general theory of the systematic relationship between kinship classifications and social organization." (Keesing 1975, 102)

He further argues that despite the vast anthropological records on "formal blue-prints of kinship structure—lists of clans, rules of marriage and residence, kinship terminologies", little is actually known about how kinship is or was done in everyday lives for these groups (Keesing 1975, 121). Particularly how to conceptualize the contingent interrelation between biological reproduction and social perceptions of relatedness has occupied anthropologists since the beginning of kinship studies with the early ethnologists 200 years ago, as again discussed in scene 3 below.

Today, with reproductive technologies posing ever new social and legal questions about kinship "at home", kinship studies have seen a new rise in popularity, particularly in English language anthropologies. They now push far beyond the classical and controversial claim that kinship is the key concept to analyze the social organization of so called primitive societies. One of the many aspects uniting the works of these so-called new kinship studies (e.g. see Carsten 2003; Edwards 2000; Edwards et al. 1999; Franklin 1997; Franklin and McKinnon 2001; Strathern 1992a, 1992b) is that kinship is analyzed as something which is done rather than just given. It is not referred to as a "hidden grammar" in a Straussian structuralist fashion. A further characteristic of the new kinship studies is their feminist interest in denaturalizing assumptions on gender and kinship. The empirical interest in studying reproductive technologies is motivated through their assumed potential for innovating how kinship is "done" and making explicit otherwise typically implicit questions on the nature of or in kinship (more below).

This practice-turn in kinship has its historical roots in the scathing critique through 1930s and 1940s British social anthropology of particularly German speaking anthropology, as lost in evolutionism and without empirical foundation (e.g. Harris 1990, 11). Its early forms were particularly driven forward through Raymond Firth's (e.g. 1954) attempts at a more processual perspective on kinship, and then later Pierre Bourdieu's (1976) comprehensive formulation of his theory of practice. Recent works in the new kinship studies mostly draw on the younger theoretical perspectives of feminist anthropology and its critique also of the functionalism of British social anthropology (e.g. see Fishburne Collier and Yanagisako 1987) and on perspectives developed within interdisciplinary science and technology studies (e.g. Franklin and McKinnon 2001; or Goodman et al. 2003).

German language studies on reproductive technologies fully or partially rooting themselves within this scholarly tradition are rare (but e.g. see Beck et al. 2007a; Hauser-Schäublin et al. 2000). The historical family studies of German *Volkskunde* provide yet another distinct scholarly tradition of focusing on kinship "at home", but have started to incorporate elements of the aforementioned practice-turn (e.g. Lipp 2005). While particularly the British new kinship studies have their roots also within social history (Peletz 1995), the German attempts at establishing a new kinship studies perspective in their research have been criticized for lacking historical perspective, and lacking conversation with historical family studies (Timm 2011). Nevertheless, recent empirical and theoretical discussions of kinship and family out of the German language folklore studies context (which has also provided a partial disciplinary home for this study) reflect a stronger coming together of French, German, and English language scholarly traditions (e.g. see Heimerdinger 2011; Timm 2010, 2012).

From the perspective of the new kinship studies, as many excellent overviews (e.g. Carsten 2003) and detailed discussions (e.g. Franklin 1997; McKinnon 2001) of the chronicle of kinship studies have been put forward and it would be tautological to recount this history in detail.[9] I

9 For an excellent collection of historical key texts see Jack Goody (1971). Michael Peletz (1995) provides an impressively concise general overview of kinship studies in anthro-

shall instead turn to discussing approaches to the specificities of kinship *and knowledge* below. Whether differing (seen from a Western perspective) kinship systems could be explained by the natives' lack of knowledge of the "true facts" of relatedness has been one of the most controversially discussed topics in kinship studies. This is already apparent in the very early works of Morgan, who assumed a relationship between biological relatedness and "knowledge of the existence of some or all of these relations between persons" (Schneider 1984, 53). Morgan hoped this could give some explanations for the vast differences in kinship systems he encountered. Durkheim, as the founding father of kinship studies for the French-speaking academic world, argued in contrast that there was no intrinsic relationship between the forms kinship took and knowledge on biological relatedness. Instead, beliefs about a common origin or other forms of beliefs, which would instate moral and jural obligations in a group, were to be seen as key (as for instance analysed through Schneider 1984, 100; or, more general, Segalen 2001).

A more recent significant engagement with questions of knowledge and kinship has been anthropology's very own virgin birth debate: a controversy which revolved around Malinowski's assertion that the Trobriand islanders had "no glimpse" (Malinowski 1948, 230) of physical paternity and that this, very roughly summarizing, could explain the absence of a genitor in their kinship system (for insightful discussions and recapitulations of the debate see Franklin 1997; McKinnon 2001; Pulman 2004/5). Delaney, in a late comment on the debate itself, pointed out that the earlier

pology. David Sabean and Simon Teuscher (2007) provide an outstanding historical analysis of kinship in Europe. In a tour-de-force through six centuries they describe how changing property-systems, state-formation, and the emergence of new social classes were *co-constituted* with historically changing kinship practices. They e.g. argue that in the 19th century horizontal kinship structures gained immense importance within strict endogamic marriage practices. Patrilineal inheritance was meanwhile losing importance, making way for more dynamic patterns of capital circulation. They see these capital flows within the closely-knit horizontal kinship structures as intimately related with the formation of new social classes. Their analysis provides a counter-narrative both to the *grand narrative* of the sociology of the family (i.e. that the industrial revolution and modernization was accompanied by a de-emphasis of kinship and a stress on the nuclear family) and of evolutionist and/or *othering* tendencies within some branches of anthropology (namely that closely-knit and strongly endogamic kinship structures are either archaic or what "the others do").

preoccupation with physical paternity in the Western sense and the concentration on whether there was a *lack* of knowledge or not, obstructed Malinowski's and other earlier male anthropologists' view from realizing that the Trobriands have or have had a highly *divergent* cosmology within which Western ideas of begetting carried no cultural significance:

"I began with the question whether certain 'primitive' peoples did or did not know physiological paternity. That question has not been answered, but I think I have shown that the question was misconceived. I have argued that paternity is embedded in an entire matrix of beliefs about the world and the way it is constructed. […] From the most intimate to ultimate contexts, from physical to metaphysical realities, an entire world is constructed and systematically interrelated. The same, I believe, is true for the Trobrianders, but it's a different system." (Delaney 1986, 510)

Phrased for my own research: kinship and knowledge are highly intertwined. Kinship is not something one has or does not have, but it is bound up with specific knowledge practices. However, *which* forms of knowledge (i.e. practices of validation, representation/storage, and distribution in the Barthian sense) come to bear on kinship—giving it a particular figuration —is a question of particular situations and associations.

Within studies of kinship, Western social scientists—especially in the last 20 years—have turned to describing the significance of *specific knowledge practices* for kinship "at home". Family secrets, for instance, have only recently been treated as currently playing—and maybe even more so in the past—a vital part in the figuration of Western kinship (e.g. Davidoff et al. 1999; Smart 2011). Moreover, it is *scientific* knowledge, Western scientific knowledge on genetic relatedness to be precise, which plays a significant role within Western concepts of kinship, as first formulated through Schneider (1968). Schneider is an important early figure for the new kinship studies and has turned kinship from a universally assumed organizing principle within anthropology to a phenomenon in need of empirical analysis in differing constellations (e.g. see Schneider 1984, 198). He put forward an early anthropological study of kinship perceptions in the industrial West with his monograph "American Kinship" (1968). There he was pioneering in arguing—taking a strictly symbolic approach—for a study of "nature" for its symbolic role within Western culture:

"So much of kinship and family in American culture is defined as being nature itself, required by nature, or directly determined by nature that it is quite difficult, often impossible, in fact, for Americans to see this as a set of cultural constructs and not the biological facts themselves." (Schneider 1968, 116)

As discussed by proponents of the new kinship studies (e.g. Franklin 2001), Schneider never clarified within which relationship he saw the symbolic dimensions of biology with what he calls "the biological facts". He did however famously argue, as pointed out in the introduction, that scientific knowledge was foundational to kinship-knowledge:

"If science discovers new facts about biogenetic relationships, then that is what kinship is and was all along, although it may not have been known at the time." (Schneider 1968, 23)

Taking up Schneider, Sarah Franklin has discussed how biology produces new knowledge about kinship and underlines the curious constitutiveness, siding with Strathern, of this information: "Knowledge itself can make kinship appear" (2001, 306). Franklin then stays with the idea that kinship-knowledge comes from the natural sciences to mockingly enquire, invoking Donna Haraway's examples of genetic manipulation: "But what if 'science discovers new facts about biogenetic relationships' that enable a fish to be crossed with a tomato?" (2001, 314) This is of course the crucial point of the new kinship studies, as for instance comprehensively discussed by Strathern (1992a): that while anthropology has a history of reveling about the relationship of kinship and nature, the question of nature in kinship is now "accompanied by a denaturalization of biology itself from within" (Franklin 2001, 303).

Bound up with the life sciences, Western kinship-knowledge is not only about stories of ancestry, practices of documenting family life and local—sometimes inherently "ungenetic"—practices and narratives around what-makes-a-family. It is also knowledge about DNA sequences, digitally or paper filed, contested and verified, used by families, patients, other medical and regulatory actors, and subject to technological interventions. Those scientific and regulatory practices involving and re-making kinship-knowledge are of course intensely resonant with wider societal and political questions. These wider questions not only come to figure within molecular biology (as briefly explored further below and also see Hauskeller 2006) or medicine (as apparent in risk profiling based on genetic testing and/or medical history, differently discussed by e.g. Featherstone 2006; Finkler 2001; Konrad 2005), but also with policing (for instance through DNA profiles and familial searching in forensics, e.g. see Haimes 2006; Sturdy 2009) and the politics surrounding colonialism, migration, and race/ethnicity (e.g. see Duster 2003; Kittles and Royal 2003; TallBear 2003). Strathern discusses how these complex entanglements often play out as a balancing act between potentially differing concerns:

> "The problem is evident: how to balance the fact of sharing information that may lead to better medical outcomes with the privacy that an individual expects. The balance is particularly acute when it comes to relations with other family members. Information that one family member has may be important for others, and the 'web of moral responsibilities' that characterizes such relations becomes an example of a more general issue of balancing 'social and individual interests'." (Strathern 2005, 36)

In other words, the individual and relational aspects of these ways-of-knowing (together with its high status) make kinship-knowledge simultaneously intensely private, intensely political and intensely collective.

The rise of molecular framings of kinship-knowledge as a powerful cellular language provide the Strathernian notion of the constitutiveness of this knowledge with a twist. Lilly Kay (2000), but also see Evelyn Fox Keller (1995), has provided an excellent historical account of how genetic sequences came to be seen as containing "information". Kay meticulously recounts how DNA sequences successively came to be known as "language" and the genome as an "information system" in molecular biology from the 1950s onwards. However, there never was a clear experimental applicability of this notion, which is apparent for instance in the fact that the so-called DNA code was not cracked cryptoanalytically, but experimentally by biochemists. Still, what Kay calls "the information discourse" (i.e. the powerful scientific legacy of the mathematical theory of communication informing cybernetics and information theory), materially, discursively, and socially committed biologists to specific research paths. The idea of DNA being itself information puts the idea of kinship-knowledge as constitutive knowledge in a slightly different light: the notion of kinship-knowledge "writing" and thereby literally assembling the body would imply that it is constitutive in an additional sense than that referred to by Strathern—not only constitutive of kin-relationships and identity, but materially constitutive. Yet, as established earlier in this expedition, which modes of knowing become part of kinship-knowledge is a question of particular situations and associations. Whether the informational framing of DNA sequences as discussed by Kay plays a role in the figuration of kinship in my domains of study—or whether it is different scientific discourses possibly becoming foundational to kinship in the Schneiderian sense—becomes an empirical question.

As pointed out in the introduction, there actually has been little empirical engagement with the concept of kinship-knowledge as constitutive information (Strathern 1999), with Carsten (2007) as one notable exception.[10] She discusses how the concept could be extrapolated when empirically engaging different scenarios of what people do with acquired kinship-knowledge. She also explicitly links her thoughts on kinship-knowledge to questions of globalization and new politics of information:

> "One much commented upon feature of globalization is an increased access to information. If new kinds of information, and a new speed of access to it, characterize the so-called 'global society,' then how do new kinds of kinship information and kinship knowledge affect Western practices of kinship, or a Western 'sense of self'?" (Carsten 2007, 403)

Carsten takes this question as a starting point to discuss anthropological research on adoption, pre-natal testing, family secrets, and egg donation. This leads her to build on Strathern's work by pointing out three features of how the constitutive character of kinship-knowledge might play out and become managed in everyday life. She firstly cautions against Strathern's tendency mainly to discuss the constitutive force of kinship information as a contemporary phenomenon, bound up with new reproductive technologies, DNA testing and new practices of governance. Carsten points out that secrecy and the uncovering of secrets has been a dominant theme within Western kinship for a long time—and that the idea of kinship information coming with built-in constitutive effects when implicated in certain social situations can also be applied to other past and contemporary

10 Konrad's (2005a) ethnography of anonymous exchange relations between ova donors in Britain is another example of extensive empirical research on kinship-knowledge and the relations it engenders, however without making explicit connection to Strathern's concept.

kinship practices. She secondly points out that, in addition to questions of relationships and identity/personhood, acquiring kinship-knowledge can sometimes be seen as an act of "reasserting agency over past events […], because there is a sense that being 'deprived' of knowledge also connotes lack of agency" (Carsten 2007, 416). Thirdly, she points out that persons can also actively manage (while going along with Strathern that they cannot outright refuse it) kinship-knowledge, by "creating spaces to accommodate or limit the 'constitutive force' of new information" (Carsten 2007, 419), for instance by not following up all available information, but only certain aspects, or by leaving long periods of time between different stages of the search.

It is exactly such tactics of active management, which is this book's focus. I have chosen to speak of *knowledge-management* in this context, just to add a last remark on use of terminologies to this second arrival-scene, to be able to refer to these active processes in families, clinics, regulation, and interest group activism with one consistent conceptual umbrella term. In conversation with an interest group activist and concerned mother, she pointed out that knowledge-management potentially sounded "too technical" to refer to practices in families. I agree that it is a technical term, which brings with it a specific and in parts problematic legacy. The expression *knowledge-management* is widely used within management and organizational theory, where it refers to "the generation, representation, storage, transfer, transformation, application, embedding and protecting of organizational knowledge" (Schultze and Stabell 2004, 551). Just as knowledge has developed into a social science "buzzword", the concept of *knowledge economy* (e.g. Reinecke et al. 2010; Stehr 1994) has fostered the development of a field of applied theories on how to practically manage knowledge-as-capital on the company shop floor (e.g. Nonaka and Takeuchi 1995). This view of knowledge as an objective economic resource —although resonant in some of the clinical and governmental knowledge practices described in this book—evidently does not overlap with the anthropological approach introduced above. I suggest speaking of knowledge-management stripped of its implicit or explicit rendering of knowledge-as-capital or knowledge-as-substance, which it carries in its originating disciplinary contexts. By using the same term for all domains under study instead of using different concepts (say, information-management in the clinics and knowledge tactics in the families and patient groups) I hope to bring into focus the potential entanglements *between* domains. Furthermore, the term also connotes active practices, and—probably most importantly—it connotes that material and immaterial information infrastructures might be involved (more on materiality in 2.3 below). Hence, despite the concerned mother's valid criticism, I arrived and stayed with the highly etic expression *kinship knowledge-management* throughout this research.

I would like to close this second arrival-scene, which took the shape of a theoretical and conceptual arrival, by recapitulating that I became alerted to Strathern's (1999) concept of constitutive knowledge with the conceptualization of knowledge-management as concrete policy problem for kinship-by-donation already in hand. I took with me the notion of a constitutive character of kinship information for personal identity and relationships in the West. I also took with me the notion that kinship-information is increasingly becoming regulatory-information, bound up with litigation and evidence based policymaking. I then turned the course of the expedition to concepts of knowledge in anthropology and to the debates on kinship-knowledge in the history of the discipline. The expedition advanced to a conceptualization of knowledge as practice and not substance, despite representational restraints of making this notion clearly visible. The expedition further progressed to a conceptualization of knowledge as empirically approachable in how it forms trajectories characterized through entangled practices of validation, representation and storage, and distribution through social relations. The expedition arrived at the notion that even if kinship-information cannot be refused by those personally affected, it can be actively managed. Analyzing *how* this active management might constitute kinship-by-donation in families, clinics, regulation, and interest group activism, is the approach followed in this book.

Scene 3: What's the Matter with Kinship?

This final scene is again a conceptual and theoretical arrival. The scene's starting point is not a particular text, as in the last arrival, but a question: what's the "matter" with kinship? Through the literature explored in this final scene *knowledge* is not taken as departure point for an expedition, as done above, but *materiality*. This is done to capture analytical considerations, which were for some time only running parallel to my research into kinship and knowledge, but eventually converged in the final configuration of this book. The arrival-question has many layers: Christopher Harris has taken it to arrive at a witty definition of kin-relationships in Western societies, when he argues that "persons related by kinship 'matter' to each other" (Harris 1990, 75). He thereby captures not only the emotional aspects of kinship, but also two further decisive aspects of European folk models of kinship. Europeans are assumed to believe that they share *matter*—blood or genes—with their consanguine kin. And both affinal and consanguine kinship (and the law codifying these practices) organizes the flow of yet another form of *matter*, namely money and possessions.

My expedition into the question, however, starts with a simpler take on it as it occurred to me during my undergraduate studies and my first encounter with anthropological kinship-studies: what's the matter with kinship? As in: why is it so complicatedly discussed in anthropology? Is it not obvious that kinship must be the most important organizing principle everywhere, because, after all, sexual procreation is universal and babies die if not looked after? Schneider soon provided a first answer on the arrival question for me through his own query: what is it "about reproduction that makes it so salient that it is given a central place among the privileged institutions? Why not, for example, the customs surrounding eating, or a dozen other things universal to human beings and equally vital?" (Schneider 1984, 193). Schneider has strongly criticized traditional anthropological kinship studies as imposing their "own folk culture" (1984, 193) on the non-Western groups they studied through privileging kinship and associated ideas on duo-genetic relatedness. He has demonstrated empirically (in his study of the Yap of Micronesia) and through his theoretical discussion that kinship as a privileged social order cannot be universally assumed. His critique also does not stop at influential (and not straightforwardly evolutionist or biologistic) figures such as Bronisław Malinowski (who argued that kinship only functions as a fulfiller of primary needs, but is not in itself biological)—or Durkheim (who argued that kinship was to be seen as only social). About the former Schneider scathingly wrote:

"it is not clear just what the relationship between form and function is, […] most particularly in its failure to specify just precisely what functions impose just precisely what constraints on which cultural forms, or just precisely what functions do determine just precisely which cultural forms, or even just where and why certain functions are independent of which cultural forms." (Schneider 1984, 161)

And the latter, Durkheim, he criticizes for postulating that kinship is social, without then explicating how it could be recognized or differentiated from other forms of solidarity if not by an imposed implicit reference to biological reproduction:

"When Durkheim said that 'kinship is social or nothing' he did not mean that it lost its roots in biology or human reproduction; only that it was now to be treated as a social fact, not a biological fact." (Schneider 1984, 191; also see 101)

Schneider has thereby touched upon a second dimension of my arrival question: what's the matter with kinship? As in: what role does biology play in it? This dimension of the question not only accompanied me through the beginnings of my interest in kinship studies, but of course also when thinking more concretely about how to study kinship-by-donation. As discussed above, in his own symbolic-anthropological study *American Kinship* Schneider has not reveled in the relationship between biology as "cultural construct" and what he calls "the biological facts themselves" (e.g. Schneider 1968, 116). Further, socio-cultural anthropology as a discipline seems predominantly to have given up its quest for a universal answer to the query, as apparent in the disillusioned quotes by Keesing (1975) in chapter 2.1. The new kinship studies have instead underlined how kinship should be seen as a generative matrix for relationships of various kinds. Kinship is conceptualized as a prime site for the negotiation of what a society perceives as the made and the given, and for the negotiation of what role biology and physical bodies are attributed within (or contribute to) practices of human solidarity. Locally studying these negotiations—as also done within this book—should then provide local empirical answers to this layer of the arrival-question.

In her insightful text *The Matter in Kinship* Edwards (2009b) criticized that within these empirical queries exactly what *matters* in European kinship has been left unscrutinized and taken for granted without closer situational study. She argues that too often "'the biological' was bracketed off and deemed outside or beyond the concern of anthropology of a social or cultural bent" (2009b, 3) and, further, that the "limits to constructivist accounts became apparent as what got to be included as biological remained notably under-problematized" (2009b, 4). This, according to Edwards, has led to a scholarly tendency to actually keep the so-called nature-culture divide, which the new kinship studies so explicitly set out to challenge (e.g. Goodman et al. 2003), implicitly intact in many of its writings. Edwards argues that ethnographers should meticulously unpack how kinship "matters" empirically. The task would not be to purify it as either social or biological—for kinship "belongs in neither one nor the other" (2009b, 9). Instead, anthropologists should set out to analyze in what socio-material practices kinship is locally enacted and how notions of the made and the given are (re-)produced through these practices. Edwards further cautions that ethnographers' concept of "nature" or "biology" might actually be more fixed and geneticized than the notions found in informants' accounts and practices, or in laboratories and scientific texts.

Singular in demonstrating how an empirical answer to the arrival-question that takes seriously the concerns discussed above could look like are the works of Charis Thompson on an US-American fertility clinic (Cussins (Thompson) 1998; Thompson 2001, 2005, 2009). Thompson's studies compellingly *combine* anthropological kinship studies with STS. Her works have been praisingly mentioned by prominent STS scholars for demonstrating how a relational-materialist approach could be operationalized for a comprehensive empirical study (Latour 2005, 207; Mol 2002, 43). To try and conceptually capture the fundamental hybridity of kinship, Thompson introduces the term "ontological choreography", which she defines as the:

"dynamic coordination of the technical, scientific, kinship, gender, emotional, legal, political, and financial aspects of ART clinics. What might appear to be an undifferentiated hybrid mess is actually a deftly balanced coming together of things that are generally considered parts of different ontological orders (part of nature, part of the self, part of society). These elements have to be coordinated in highly staged ways so as to get on with the task at hand: producing parents, children, and everything that is needed for their recognition as such." (Thompson 2005, 8)

In an unlikely but gripping combination of theoretical influences (from Butler's gender performativity concept to Actor Network Theory), Thompson analyzes how many matters (hormones, gametes, ultrasound, drugs) in an infertility clinic in the USA are in interplay with hegemonic gender and kinship constructions, personhood, and specific modes of production: she shows how at the end of the choreography—despite the many questions raised through the different reproductive technologies used—legitimate parents emerge. She makes an argument for both an underdetermined "social" and "nature":

"All kinds are specified and differentiated by strategic naturalization and socialization, depending on which part is underdetermined at a given time and place." (Thompson 2005, 12)

What I find ambiguously handled in Thompson's excellent ethnography is what ontological status she attributes to the matters she describes as part of the choreography. Do the matters "kick back"—as Barad (e.g. 1998) phrases the common (although divergently formulated) anti-constructionist approach within relational-materialist quarters of STS? Or are matters rather to be seen as underdetermined parts of a choreography of legitimization driven forward *not* through a hybrid interplay as for instance entailed in Mol's (2002) work, but ultimately through the powers of discourse, as for instance clarified by Butler about ontology and epistemology in her research?[11] Thompson's studies, in my view, leave the answer to this question open. They remain the most extensive empirical engagement with my arrival-question within anthropology and STS.

Although unique in their strong empiricism, Thompson's works have not been the only engagements of the new kinship studies with parts of STS. As touched upon above, the new kinship studies have developed in parts out of the intersections between feminist anthropology and feminist studies of science, as particularly driven forward through Franklin (e.g. see 1995, 2001) and also Strathern's (e.g. 1992a) quite unique legacy. Nevertheless, as part of Edward's previously cited call to not too readily place the produce of ethnographic work on kinship "in a 'biology box'" and "in a 'social box'" (2009b, 4) a new alliance with a specific relational materi-

11 For example see Butler (GEZEIT 1994) in an interview on epistemology and ontology and on the reception of her book "Gender Trouble" (1990), as cited through Regina Becker-Schmidt and Gudrun-Axeli Knapp (2000, 92).

alism in STS has been proposed through Joan Bestard (2009) with Actor Network Theory (ANT). The latter proposes to stay out of "boxes", with its emphasis on hybridity and resistance to "purification" in the sense of a clearly discernible separation between human and material world (e.g. Latour 1993). Bestard, invoking ANT approaches, but not attempting a comprehensive empirical ANT analysis, puts forward to study kinship as a network: "for instance a network linking a gamete, a woman who is an egg donor, a legal mother, a name, a town and an identity" (Bestard 2009, 21). A point where Strathern, Latour, and Bestard align is that the relation in a network implies "relata"—or "mediators" in Latour's sense—and not autonomous entities or individuals simply connected (e.g. Latour 2005, 39, 106; Strathern 2005, 40). This leads Bestard to argue, in yet another convincing take on my arrival-question, that kinship is a network through which constant interactive mediations between matters are taking place. These mediations could "colonize different areas of social life" without these processes being subsumable under purified concepts, such as *geneticization*, or *culturalization* (Bestard 2009, 27). [12]

To date, however, no comprehensive kinship study has been attempted within the ironically raised "rules for ANT membership" (Latour 2005, 10–11). Those rules, according to the controversial gospel of Latour, are comprised of the explicit inclusion of non-human actors; making no reference to broad explanatory concepts, such as *the social* or *context*; and staying abstinent from established forms of political critique.[13] Instead one should make intersubjectively comprehensible the mediating nature of the relata in a network (e.g. 2005, 61), but only by analytically "walking on foot" (i.e. only following actors and not broad concepts or assumptions when tracing a network) (2005, 178) and, lastly, leaving untouched what Latour calls "mute" phenomena (i.e. established figurations, which can-

12 *Geneticization* is a concept coined through epidemiologist and science studies researcher Abby Lippman in the early 1990s, for instance see Lippman (1992). As taken up for more comprehensive discussion in chapters 7 and 9 and touched upon throughout this book, *geneticization* refers to a growing currency of genetics as explanatory model within different social arenas. The concept assumes this influence to be dangerously determinist and colonizing of other, more politically just, emancipatory, or actively chosen social relationships and explanatory models.

13 Latour argues one should not confuse ANT with a "postmodern emphasis on the critique of the 'Great narratives' and 'Eurocentric' or 'hegemonic' standpoint" (2005, 11).

not be penetrated through the ANT empiricism that is methodologically geared at open processes of assemblage) (2005, 31).

Devising a kinship-study within this framework, at least outside of the fertility clinic and focusing on everyday family life, would be a challenge and of questionable analytical gain to both ANT and the new kinship studies. In everyday life kinship would oftentimes be "out of the social world—in the ANT sense" (Latour 2005, 31). The recent and not so recent mediations, which would have given kinship its figuration during a particular everyday event (say through religious beliefs, property regimes, or scientific discoveries) would stay silent and would hence not be addressable by staying "on foot" (i.e. visibly empirically connected) anymore. The emotional and intersubjective elements characteristic of doing kinship in everyday life, in contrast, could only be analyzed through comprehensively enhanced ANT methodology and vocabulary (e.g. Latour 2005, 212–213). The expedition thus seems to stall when trying to follow the ANT. Or, in other words: The set-up up of my study, which was devised to address the somewhat neglected *interrelatedness* of the constitution of kinship in different domains (as explored in the introduction) and which follows several family-cases, figures squarely with an orthodox ANT approach as proposed above.

However, there is an expansion of the arrival question suggesting itself: what's the matter with kinship-*knowledge*? As in: what matters, quite literally, in knowing kinship? Proponents of ANT and similar relational-materialisms have demonstrated incredible empirical and theoretical strength in analyzing the interplay of *matters* in making scientific knowledge. They have focused on how scientific legacies, particular scientists, instruments, laboratory practices, and the physiologies and things under study "enact" (Mol 2002) or "articulate" (Latour 2004) science within material-semiotic mediations.Such an understanding of knowledge, the expedition found, could be of help to my ethnographic exploration. In other words: a relational-materialist approach to the ways in which we come to know relatedness would help do justice to the above cited valid concerns to resist a purification of kinship. It adds to the previously explored Barthian notion of knowledge through not losing sight of physiologies and things as mediators. Such considerations thus mark the point at which the second and the third conceptual expedition join forces. (This I already hinted at in my earlier proposition to extend Barth's focus on media of representation to modes of storage and infrastructural affordances). Medically administered and nationally regulated, kinship-by-donation is partly known through large institutional information infrastructures. Susan Leigh Star, both relational-materialist ally and scathing critic of ANT (e.g. see 1991), has worked intensively on what she calls "boring aspects of infrastructure" (2002, 110) in a more interactionist and politically oriented perspective of STS. With infrastructures she refers to the taken for granted material structures and materially incorporated classification systems on which everyday life "runs". She argues:

"Study a city and neglect its sewers and power supplies (as many have), and you miss essential aspects of distributional justice and planning power [...]. Study an information system and neglect its standards, wires, and settings, and you miss equally essential aspects of aesthetics, justice, and change. Your ethnography will be incomplete." (Star 2002, 17)

Star and her collaborator Geoffrey Bowker have analyzed how through socio-material feedback loops, information system infrastructures and communities of practice[14] mutually constitute each other. They call this process *convergence* (e.g. Bowker and Star 1999; Star et al. 2003). This leads to the disingenuous everyday life perception that infrastructures (and the associated classification and ordering systems) simply mirror the world, whilst they actually contribute to its making. Thus, where Barth is not concerned with how knowledge "matters", Star argues that knowledge actually takes on specific pathways or trajectories in the Barthian sense exactly through the material (and immaterial) constraints of information infrastructures: "knowledge is constrained, built, and preserved" (Star 2002, 110) within these infrastructures in particular ways (also see Levinson 2010, 163–188). In contrast to Latour, Star (2002) underlines the importance of empirically attending to what is "not said" and "cannot be said" through specific infrastructures and the associated communities of practice, thereby analyzing through reflexive ethnographic observations

14 The term "community of practice" has its origins in the anthropology of learning of Jean Lave and Etienne Wegner (1991). It refers to a community, for instance a particular profession, which shares certain conventions, and formal and tacit knowledge on certain tasks.

how social practices are framed through exclusions partly embedded within taken for granted infrastructures.

To conclude, this last expedition has aroused a curiosity about the mediating nature of physiologies, things, and infrastructures within [k]information. I arrived at the literature on kinship and STS with a question: what's the *matter* with kinship? Different dimensions of the question took me on a short expedition through kinship and its relationship to materiality. The expedition explored the assumed European folk model of kinship, which combines a stress on biological and economical *matters*. The expedition further concluded that biological *matters* do not causally produce kinship as a privileged form of social order. That the hybridity of *matters* should be more closely considered when studying figurations of kinship was concurred with en-route. And—as the last path explored—information-infrastructures were suspected to *matter* in constituting kinship-by-donation in particular ways.

3. Fieldwork and Data Analysis

This book presents an ethnographic exploration into how kinship-by-donation is constituted within practices of knowledge-management in contemporary Western Europe. It focuses on families-by-donation, clinical practices, regulation, and interest group activism in Germany and Britain. Recounted as a conceptual arrival in the previous chapter, the exploration combines research approaches from the new kinship studies, the anthropology of knowledge and STS. The book thus focuses on knowledge-practices, their validation, material storage/representation, and distribution within social relationships. I investigate which aspects of kinship-knowledge are validated, drawn on in various practices, made accessible or inaccessible, foregrounded or silenced.

My analysis in this book is based on multi-sited ethnographic fieldwork, which I subsume under the methodological label *ethnographic exploration*.[1] The label refers to the realization of qualitative interviews, short

1 Given that my periods of observation were rather short (i.e. shared meals or walks with families and only few weeks of "hanging out" in the clinics), I have deliberately chosen not to employ the label *ethnography*. Although many excellent methodologists argue *against* restricting the label of ethnography to works based on extended participant observation (e.g. Faubion and Marcus 2009, 5; Gay y Blasco and Wardle 2007, 10) and for instead including *all* empirical research in theoretical conversation with the discipline of anthropology, I contend there is value in underlining that an ethnography is strongly based on observations, given the different data this yields (e.g. Hirschauer 2001). The label of *ethnographic exploration* thus captures better, in my view, the mixed-methods approach most appropriate to my specific research interests for this work. One methodological side-note: in addition to the numerous English language debates on what ethnography is (e.g. see Ingold 2008), fieldwork traditions and methodological discussions get even more complex when also taking into account the German-language debates within European Ethnology. Discussing the role of ethnography within *Europäische Ethnologie* in detail would be beyond the scope of this work,

periods of ethnographic observation, and the collection of various written and visual materials. A mixed-methods approach was chosen because the practices of interest in this research are "so spread out that they are hard to study [solely] ethnographically for a limited number of researchers", in Annemarie Mol's and John Law's (2004, 59) words, who take a similar approach in their research. Therefore, as I was interested in following the *entanglements* between practices of kinship knowledge-management in families, clinics, regulation and interest groups, I opted for a multi-sited and mixed-methods approach.

In this chapter I describe what this ethnographic exploration looked like and thereby provide an overview of my fieldwork process, the collected materials, and how I analyzed them. This is done in a brief and straightforward manner, because more detailed discussions of individual cases, the (sometimes conflicting) nature of individual data, or my role in the field are given in detail when relevant in the empirically oriented chapters themselves. In this chapter I first give an overview of the process of data-collection and resulting fieldwork materials. I then describe how I analyzed the materials and how I chose to represent this analysis. In this last section I also make general remarks on language-use throughout the book.

Overview of Data-Collection and Resulting Fieldwork Materials

My ethnographic exploration has led me into the homes (or in some cases other preferred places, such as favorite cafes) of the 13 British and German families-by-donation who participated in this research (for an overview of the family sample see figure 3.1). The families were found through interview appeals in fertility clinics, interest group internet fora, and snowballing among my social circle. Some interviewees were recruited as part of the longitudinal study of the previously mentioned "kinship cultures" project at the Humboldt University (Project C4, SFB 640). This meant

but see Utz Jeggle (1984) for an account of fieldwork traditions in German folklore studies on their way to become European Ethnology. For more recent methodological contributions to European Ethnology for instance see Dietzsch et al. (2009) or Göttsch and Lehmann (2007). Gisela Welz (e.g. 1998) has strongly contributed to a translation of the international methodological debates on multi-sited fieldwork into German-speaking European Ethnology.

that in a minority of cases other interviewers were involved as well.[2] When quotes from their work are used in the individual chapters, this is indicated.

Figure 3.1: Overview of families engaged with

Family (Pseudonym)	Method of Conception	Why assisted conception?	Approx. age of couple	# of children (approx. age)
		Germany		
Arnulfs	DI (known donor) for 2 children; 3 children from previous heterosexual marriage	lesbian couple	late 30s	♀/♂: 5 (2–16y)
Dünkes	Surrogacy in USA (with egg donor)	gay couple	early 30s	♀: 1 (3y)
Feldmans	DI	male infertility	mid 40s	♀/♂: 2 (3–6y)
Liebs	DI (in USA)	single-mother-by-choice	early 50s	♀: 1 (12y)
Müllers	DI for 2nd born son; natural conception of 1st born	late onset male infertility	mid 40s	♀/♂: 2 (5–12y)
Schneiders	DI (via Danish sperm bank)	male infertility	mid 40s	♂: 1 (6y)
Stegers	DI	carriers of genetic disorder	late 30s	♀/♂: 3 (2–5y); 1 deceased firstborn
Tönschs	DI	male infertility	early 40s	♀/♂: 2 (1–5y)
		Britain		
Greenwoods	DI	male infertility	late 30s (f), late 40s (m)	♀: 1 (5y)
Kings	DI	male infertility	mid 50s	♀/♂: 2 (>20y)
Hamptons	DI	male infertility	late 30s	♀/♂: 2 (3–6y)
Nakamuras	Egg donation	Post-menopausal single-mother-by-choice	early 60s	♂: 1 (6y)
Taylors	1st born: Egg donation; 2nd born: natural conception	female infertility	mid 40s	♀/♂: 2 (teenagers)

Sampling criteria for the families, in addition to being families-by-donation, were their willingness to participate in my study and their willingness to stay in touch over longer periods of time. Given that many parents-by-donation still decide not to disclose the donation to their social circle at all (see section 6.1 for a detailed discussion), openness to a researcher is of course not self-evident, and finding interviewees proved

2 Mainly Michi Knecht, but also Sabine Hess. I also profited from having insight into the data collected by an independent study group of students, lead by Frederike Heinitz and supervised by Michi Knecht. The outcome of their study is to be found under Knecht et al. (2010).

challenging, necessitating repeated attempts. I also aimed for compiling a sample of *heterogeneous* families-by-donation in terms of family forms and reasons for using gamete donation. This enabled me both to explore typical experiences between families and to tease out specificities of individual cases and methods of conception.[3] I make no claim here or in the empirically oriented chapters about the representativeness of my family sample in the statistical sense of the word.[4] Instead, my diverse sample gives interpretive insight into individual and sometimes shared experiences of particular families-by-donation and their knowledge-practices.

Most families replied to the appeals posted on the interest group sites. Because of that, my family-sample is not restricted to a specific region of Germany: I simply travelled (by train) to the families willing to speak to me. In Britain it was restricted to England out of pragmatic travel considerations, but not to one specific town. My self-selected interviewees' socio-economic status ranged from lower to higher middle-class. The majority of participants had university-entrance diplomas and many, but not all, academic degrees. Not all interviewees who here figure as *German* or *British* necessarily had been born with this nationality. The label instead refers to their country of residence. Where specificities of the families (such as nationality, physical appearance, or education) are made relevant in my interpretation of individual situations analyzed or interview passages quoted, this is indicated in the empirically oriented chapters itself.

The intensity of contact with the families varied, but predominantly consisted of two 2–3 hour long interviews over a three-year period with e-mail contact in between. Where possible, families were interacted with more often and in more informal fieldwork situations. First fieldwork contacts started in 2007, most in 2009, last contacts took place in 2013. Most children at the first interview were around three, but some considerably

3 Through this comparative framework, concentrating on typicalities and specificities of cases, but not on prolonged individual case-discussions, some of the highly unique cases (such as the Dünke family: two gay men who had used an egg donor and a surrogate mother in the USA) are only marginally drawn on within the discussions provided in the chapters. The absence of such a detailed case-discussion however does not mean that the interviews did not feed into the analysis of my fieldwork materials as laid out below.

4 However, the findings on typical experiences in many chapters of this book could of course be operationalized in hypotheses to be tested within larger quantitative studies.

older. The rationale for recurring contact was to enable a more processual analysis of the family's experiences over a longer period of time, as laid out as one of the research *desiderata* in contemporary studies of kinship (see chapter 1). Most interviews were conducted as conjoint interviews with couples, because this was preferred by most interviewees and because it enabled more informal and interactive contact. Children were seldom present during formal interview situations (but instead sleeping or playing), but interacted with extensively outside of the immediate interview situation.

For the first family interview I always used an interview manual, consisting of specific themes. I firstly discussed in detail with the families what had led up to their use of gamete-donation. The extended reconstructive accounts of infertility, decision-making processes, and experiences with doctors then mostly turned into animated discussions of family-life. Where possible, I let my interviewees then lead the interview process, myself ticking off if we had already discussed topics included in the manual. Themes covered in addition to the family's reason for using gamete donation and their detailed experiences before, during, and after donation treatment, were the disclosure decision; experiences with and opinions on the regulation of gamete donation; experiences with being a family-by-donation in everyday life; reactions of their social circle; a discussion of parents' general views on kinship; and what role contact to the extended family played in their everyday life. By minimizing my role in conducting the conversation through letting my interviewees lead the conversation, I avoided prompting my research partners into specific conceptualizations, an effect that is generally desired within qualitative interviewing (e.g. Helfferich 2005; Rubin and Rubin 1995). Themes that had not been covered "naturally" at the end of the session were then asked about through prepared interview questions. I note in the passages quoted in the empirically oriented chapter below, whether certain themes were prompted or not and how.

I taped all interviews. They were later transcribed verbatim by myself or a research assistant. I also wrote field notes on each interview contact, specifically trying to capture those aspects of the fieldwork-situation not discernible in the later interview-transcript: notes on the environment we met in; which objects seemed to play a significant role for the interview situation (such as photographs); how I felt in the interview situation and what I viewed as important interactive and affective dynamics (for excellent discussion and practical advice on the work with ethnographic field notes e.g. see Emerson (1995)). Where possible, I also collected additional materials from the families, such as copies of their treatment contracts, children's books or self-help materials they were referring to.

Families were often interested if I had children myself or any personal experience with gamete donation or adoption. As customary for anthropological fieldwork, which proceeds to research relationships through entering into relationships (for theoretical discussion e.g. see Strathern 2005), I openly engaged with all questions about my personal life or personal opinions ("no children, but so-far voluntarily, no personal or family history with assisted reproduction"). My self-selected interviewees typically perceived my fieldwork as a chance to reduce taboos surrounding their family form or as a welcomed chance to talk to "an outsider" about their experiences. The roles they attributed to me in our interactions varied. Where relevant to the meaning of a passage quoted, I discuss such processes in the empirical chapters directly.

In the course of the interview or during our follow-up meetings contact usually became more informal with the families: we shared meals, stayed up late and finished a bottle of wine, ordered pizza or went to the playground. Some of my interviewees offered that I could stay overnight when I came to visit. I sometimes experimented with methods to employ in subsequent family-contact, such as passing out paper and pens and letting families depict themselves. All contact was reflected on in further field notes. Although finding families willing to participate had not proven easy, when rapport had been established no conflicts occurred.

The clinical parts of my exploration took place in three fertility clinics and further associated sperm banks. Two clinics were located in Germany (Sperm Bank Friedhausen and Fertility Centre Luisenburg) and one was a larger clinic with several units in Britain (Largecity Fertility Hospital). The clinics and associated sperm banks are introduced in detail in chapter 5. Fieldwork in the German Friedhausen clinic and in the British Largecity clinic consisted of short periods of ethnographic observation, amounting to roughly one week's "pure" observation time in each clinic. I observed practices in the laboratories, at the walk-in clinic reception desks where donors were greeted, the donor recruitment, and the clinical administration. I was never allowed to be present during private consultations between patients and physicians or donors and physicians. In Luisenburg I was given tours of the clinic and spent some time in the sperm bank, but was not allowed to just "hang out". In addition to the observation periods, all three clinics were visited recurrently (before and after the ethnographic episodes) to conduct more formal interviews with personnel ranging from administration and laboratory assistants, counselors, embryologists and biologists, to the clinic's owners and managers. All formal interviews were recorded and transcribed verbatim; more informal interactions and periods of observation were recorded in field notes. From the clinics I collected large amounts of internal written materials pertaining to my interest in knowledge-management and associated clinical infrastructures; these included examples of donor and patient files, screenshots of administrative software, user manuals and operating procedures. I also collected publicly accessible information on the clinic, such as brochures and screen-shots of website-contents.

My sampling criteria for the clinics were that they specialized in gamete donation programs and were willing to participate in my fieldwork. Obtaining access and continuous contact proved to be challenging. The clinics pushed hard for formal interviews instead of granting comprehensive access to observe practices. This often led to situations where a senior member of staff agreed to periods of observation, and the junior member of staff in charge of "booking me in" with personnel being confused about what I actually wanted to do and trying to reduce fieldwork time to interviews again. Communication was generally challenging regarding the setting of appointments or reaching agreements on visiting times. My solution to break-downs in communication was writing formal letters via mail for such negotiations, because they were more likely to be answered. Phone messages or e-mails were often left unanswered. However, one additionally approached British clinic never returned phone-calls, e-mails, or formal written letters.

In interview situations or during the agreed periods of observations, contact with clinicians was always friendly and informative. In personal communication clinical personnel mostly expressed interest in my research and apologized for being so hard to reach. In such situations it became clear that the fertility clinic as a work place and as an institution under strict privacy regulations led to the problems in communication: workflows could not be interrupted for longer periods of time, records needed to be kept confidential, and most of the personnel did not have continuous access to communication devices, because they were busy in consultations or with laboratory tasks.

To further understand the practices of clinical and governmental handling of data on donors and patients I also interviewed and stayed in e-mail contact with two officers at the British Human Fertilisation and Embryology Authority (HFEA) and a representative of the charity and awareness organization National Gamete Donation Trust, financed by the British Department of Health. The HFEA officers were in charge of overseeing the central registry for gamete donors, accessing requests to this registry, and working on the HFEA policy-making approach concerning gamete donation. Access for more observational periods of fieldwork was sought here as well, but not granted due to data protection measures. I was, however, allowed to look at internal operating procedures and staff manuals.

Data on interest group activism, but also much useful background information on clinical practices and parental knowledge-management, I drew from my long interviews and extensive further e-mail contact with two prominent German and British gamete donation experts influentially involved with family activism: Olivia Montuschi of the British interest group Donor Conception Network and Petra Thorn, prominent German fertility counselor and workshop convener (see chapter 6). They are the only research partners in this book who have, with their consent, *not* been anonymized, given their highly unique expert status. I conducted internet searches on interest group activism and monitored (publicly visible) networking endeavors on the internet. I stayed in e-mail contact with some interest group activists moderating individual websites. Because most of my parental interview partners also participated in interest group activism, they could provide additional insights. Since interest group activism often led to the publication of large amounts of written materials—guidebooks, children's books, brochures, etc.—these materials were also ordered and analyzed, as well as scientific publications from the counseling sector.

Moreover, I draw on two interviews with adult donor-conceived individuals in Britain who replied to my call for interview partners, although

I had stated I was looking for families. These long interviews proved to be so interesting in the additional viewpoints they raised that they are recurrently drawn upon within the empirical chapters. To further complement those perspectives, I also researched the viewpoints of German donor-conceived individuals, but mainly via their internet and media activities and through the research contact a colleague had established with one German donor-conceived person.

Lastly, as a member of the "kinship cultures" project of the Humboldt University (SFB 640 C4), I could draw on further interviews my colleagues and I conducted with families-by-adoption, with families-by-IVF, with German clinicians in other clinics than my field sites, and with various experts on reproductive technologies and adoption in Germany. These interviews were part of the larger longitudinal study conducted in the project (e.g. see Knecht et al. 2011), and in that sense sometimes, but not always, separate from my own research project. We, for instance, jointly invited a notary to give a talk on documentation practices surrounding DI in Germany, or my colleague Michi Knecht attended several workshops for "rainbow" families (i.e. families involving homosexual individuals and couples) run by a gay rights organization and provided me with her field notes. My colleague Sulamith Hamra and I repeatedly conducted conjoint interviews with families-by-adoption (e.g. see Hamra 2007; Klotz 2009). These last materials did not all find entrance in the detailed coding process of my data as described below, but all contributed to the general interpretative framework of this research.

I additionally kept a diary to record more personal thoughts on kinship or autoethnographic ideas and episodes, noting my feelings on kinship during family unions and two funerals that took place in my own family during my research. This was done to reflect on my own "inexperience" with kinship: being raised by *sixty-eighter generation* parents who took great care to "embed" their children among their friends, sometimes also codifying this through godfather or godmother status, but hardly keeping any contact to consanguine kin. In fact, the quotes in chapter 1 on "water being thicker than blood" were quotes I was consistently raised with. Some of these autoethnographic reflections are used within the empirical chapters. These personal notes moreover served as "tools" to aid the continuous analytical loops between making-strange and making-familiar crucial to ethnographic fieldwork processes "at home" (for discussion e.g. see Amann and Hirschauer 1997; Steinke 2000).

All in all, collected materials amounted to approximately 40 interviews for my core-sample of families, clinicians, policy-makers, and interest group activists; and my field notes totaled roughly 200 pages. An additional approximately 30 interviews and further diverse field notes resulted from the collective project activities although these latter materials were not subject to a detailed coding process.

Data-Analysis and Writing

The data my fieldwork generated contained aspects of knowledge-management discernible in interactive practices and reflections *within* the interview situation itself. It contained notes on observed practices, as well as recordings of and notes on *accounts of* practices and events that took place at other times in other situations. Additionally, textual and visual materials provided further understanding and contextualization of these data. Accounts of practices were *not* approached from a strictly constructivist perspective, where interviewees are not seen to generate data giving insights beyond the shared interview situation. They were instead approached from what I would describe as a cautiously realist perspective. Such a methodology has for instance been suggested by Mol (e.g. 2002, 20) as particularly appropriate for research such as mine: dealing with sometimes extremely private, sometimes institutionally guarded, or also rare and occurring by chance practices impossible to capture comprehensively through participant observation. In other words, this perspective is to be seen as methodological compromise between my practice-oriented research interests and the impossibility of being able to observe all these practices myself. The approach also fits into the general ethnographic tradition of taking actors seriously as experts about their everyday lives (for a discussion of the history and presence of the participant/researcher relationship e.g. see Färber 2009).

Preliminary data analysis took place in close interchange with my colleagues from the "kinship cultures" project, starting from first fieldwork encounters in 2007 and onwards. Collected materials and transcripts were imported into a shared data-pool with the Atlas.ti software for qualitative data analysis. The materials were loosely indexed according to recurring themes and patterns on how kinship was "done". We continuously held meetings and within these meetings further developed the collectively used index-system, which resulted in a combination of inductive and deductive codes.[5] Sampling of my research partners took place simultaneous with this process of preliminary data analysis. It was guided as such by my emerging research interests, a process described as "theoretical sampling" in Grounded Theory (e.g. Strauss 1987, 16).

After having arrived at my final research interests, as recounted in chapter 2, and after having conducted approximately two thirds of the data-collection process, I changed to a more detailed process of data-analysis. For this I imported all of my research materials, along with the collected photographs, regulatory documents, scanned brochures and children's books, into a new "hermeneutic unit", as Atlas.ti archives are called. Materials were now analyzed in an inductive two-step coding process, as suggested by Emerson et al. (1995), who try to combine the minute Grounded Theory methodology with more reflexive approaches to data analysis, as advocated in anthropology. This process ensured an immersion in the data, along with a simultaneous analytical distancing and disruption of premature interpretation through the coding process —whilst, however, not presuming that an exhaustive break between the researcher's subjectivity and the produced data was possible (or in fact desirable).

In practice, this meant I proceeded from an open coding phase to a focused coding phase lasting about five months, before I started to actually "write up" the research in roughly twelve months. Open coding was conducted on a subsection of interview-transcripts and some of my clinical field notes. I proceeded with the most general questions. What can I find out from the materials collected, about (k)information? Are there particular connections forged? Materialities coming into play? Regulations being drawn on? Do I notice the exclusion of particular themes? Reading through my fieldwork materials time and time again, in printed form or within the Atlas.ti interface, I slowly started to note down first thoughts on

5 Taking part in these meetings were, in differing constellations, not only Michi Knecht and Sabine Hess, but also Sulamith Hamra, Nevim Cil, Nurhak Polat, and Stefan Beck.

these questions within emerging codes and memos that I attached to the specific fieldwork passages. From this process resulted a first framework of open codes.

Subsequently, I took time to reflect on the newly written memos and codes, and on how I had started to organize my fieldwork materials through this process. From this I began to develop the structure of this book. This is captured in the organization of the individual chapters and the materials presented in them. To illustrate, I, for example, grouped all open codes pertaining to aspects of what I discuss as "outside confrontations to families" in chapter 8 in a code-group "confrontations". Each code in this group was named according to individual confrontations, such as for instance "resemblance-talk". These re-named and grouped codes I re-integrated into Atlas.ti, thereby developing a final coding framework. Subsequently, the large majority of all existing fieldwork materials, not only a subset such as during open coding, became coded and "memoed" within the new focused framework. After completing this second coding phase I decided on the final layout of the book, using the memos—by then quite comprehensive—on different emerging lines of analysis for orientation.

Representation

Empirical accounts given in the book are held in the past-tense, to avoid the *a*temporality of the by now notorious "ethnographic present" (e.g. Clifford 1993). Clinical practices were for instance changing perpetually through company mergers, the move of one of the clinics to a different building, and newly introduced technologies. The clinical routines I am discussing at length thus provide an analysis only of practices observed during a specific time, as preserved in my fieldwork accounts in the past-tense. In other words, things might be different "now". And families, including the growing children, were of course also dynamic and not expected to just remain "frozen" in opinions voiced at specific times or in specific situations.

All research partners named are anonymized, not only by changing their names, but also by changing other potentially identifying markers, such as, for example, where they live. In this I followed university regulations, but also my own interest in not unduly exposing families, children or clinical staff by their personal opinions. Only interest group experts Olivia Montuschi and Petra Thorn were, as mentioned above, not anonymized, because their highly specific position in the field would have made anonymization impossible. My quotes of their words were authorized by them. The British HFEA as an institution was, of course, not anonymized, but the officers who spoke to me were.

Kinship terminologies used, within this research or elsewhere, imply certain relationships and positionings concerning the nature in—or of—kinship. This is apparent in the different emotive and legal connotations in terms such as social father, biological father, genitor, and donor. My research partners adopt various terminologies; how their work with words relates to their kinship knowledge-management is analyzed throughout this book, but particularly in chapter 7.2. For myself, I speak of mothers, fathers, and siblings for those individuals taking on classical kin positions in families-by-donation and speak of donors and donor-siblings when referring to those persons related to the families via the practices of clinically administered gamete donation. Where such positions overlap or are less clearly separable, namely in "rainbow families" (i.e. families involving homosexual individuals and couples) and in one single-mother family, I use both terms. In rare sections of this work, where it is crucial to make clear in one idiom which donation technique has been used, I use expressions such as *mother-by-sperm-donation*, but most generally try to abstain from such terminology, for it implicitly suggests that the person's role as parent (or child) is determined through the method of conception. I thus consciously do not employ expressions such as *social father* in the research.

I am not employing the term *Euro-American* (as common within the new kinship studies, see Edwards (2006) for discussion of its different meanings) in this book. Instead—if not specifically referring to Germany and Britain—I employ the terms *European* and *Western*. *European* roughly refers to the geographic region and its inhabitants. *Western*, again an even fuzzier and even more contested term, refers to Europe and North America, but also more generally to a scientifically permeated, enlightenment-driven, (post-)colonial hegemonic culture with European origins. I am avoiding the label Euro-American, mainly because I find its synonymy with the currency *Euro* misleading.[6] Finally, I wish to add a note on language-use in this book: occasionally I use purposefully unusual English language in this work. For example, when I try to make an action-oriented approach to knowledge visible in language-use this is denoted by phrasings such as "ways-of-knowing" instead of knowledge; or when I employ terms such as "resonance", "co-implication", "co-construction", etc. it is in order to convey complexity and non-causality.

The epistemological position taken throughout this research is one of critical reflexive realism, as for instance advocated through social-anthropological methodologist Charlotte Aull Davis (1999). Such a position implies rejecting the radical postmodern claim that ethnographic research is only a textual activity without relationship to a world "out there", outside of the text. My take on reflexive critical realism thus appreciates the idea that there is a physical reality, but one mediated through actors' perceptions and socio-material interventions (as also largely advocated through the relational materialist quarters of STS, e.g. see Barad (1999); Latour (2005); Mol (2002); Pickering (1995)). A position of critical reflexive realism however welcomes the postmodern stress on paying attention to how research is textually represented. After Aull Davis (1999, 213–214) my research and its representation follows a threefold mediation of reality: firstly, with and between actors and materialities in the field; secondly, in analysis and writing: in interpreting others' perspectives and practices, one's own perspective and practices, and finding ways to represent these perspectives and practices textually; and thirdly as textual end-product, where mediation between author and reader takes place. Objectivity, in the sense of stopping these mediations, is not possible. What is possible is to critically interrogate such mediations; reflexively make them part of the fieldwork process and ultimately intersubjectively comprehensible within the textual representation of the research. This is my approach in the following chapters.

6 In fact, among German language readers of earlier drafts of this work, the label *Euro-American* (roughly used as proxy for *Western*) recurrently caused confusion whether I was referring to the *Euro-Zone*, which was especially contested at the time of writing, and what *America* then had to do with this.

4. Knowing Kinship-by-Donation as Parents: Reflections and Histories

This chapter focuses on how the parents in my family sample defined kinship during our interviews and on how they became families-by-donation. It is the first chapter to engage closely with my fieldwork data. While the subsequent chapters 7 and 8 both focus on detailed familial practices of knowledge-management, this chapter analyzes broader parental reflections and reconstructs what I came to call the reproductive histories of the families I engaged with during fieldwork.

The first section (4.1) follows how parents constituted kinship within their reflections in the interviews. I have chosen to allocate these parental definitions such a prominent place within the arrangement of the book chapters *not* because I am suggesting that parents are here voicing axiomatic kinship values informative of *all* the later practices discussed. I have chosen rather to give prominence to my informants' own opinions on the elusive subject of *kinship* in the ethnographic tradition of treating informants as experts of their own lives and cosmologies.[1] I analyze what my research partners typically came to describe: kinship as a relationship characterized by three tensions surrounding the theme of *choice*, the theme of (corporeal) *continuity*, and the theme of *love*.

In the following section (4.2) I focus on typical reproductive histories of my familial research partners. The data I am analyzing for this reconstruction are the parental accounts of this process, their more detailed descriptions and performative re-enactments of past situations, but also other remnants of the treatment process, such as the contracts the parents set up with the clinics and other clinical information materials handed over to me by the parents. When analyzing these data more constrictions

1 For a recent discussion of the informant/researcher relationship in the history and presence of anthropology and European ethnology see Färber (2009).

than in the previously analyzed reflections of how kinship-by-donation can be known, and hence done, become apparent. I shall argue that for all heterosexual families in my sample, donor insemination (DI) only became achievable as the last step within a hierarchy of reproductive interventions. Within the reconstructions of their reproductive histories, DI figured as what I call a *technology of the last resort*, in comparison to the "hope technology IVF" (Franklin 1997b).[2]

The frictions produced between the parental definitions of kinship as being quite flexible and only marginally grounded in biology and, in contrast, their reproductive histories evoking prolonged periods of repro-technological interventions for a genetically related child are not interpreted as a simple learning process or adjustment of values through the parents. I rather show how the socio-material arrangement of DI through the clinics contributed just as much to make donor insemination a *technology of the last resort*, as did the parents' later abandoned wish for a shared corporeal continuity. This overall chapter thus provides a broad contextualization of the concrete practices of parental knowledge-management to be analyzed in subsequent chapters. It does so by analyzing the meaning parents attribute to kinship when asked to give their own definitions years after having become a family-by-donation and by reconstructing practices leading up to this decision.

2 Franklin's analysis is not meant affirmatively. She for instance argues: "Although IVF is ubiquitously celebrated as offering 'hope', it is this very hope which can cause the desperation it is said to alleviate. The search for a resolution through IVF, then, can be seen to create precisely the irresolution it was meant to eliminate" (Franklin 1997b, 183). Her point is rather that IVF unfolds a specific socio-material logic, within which "hope" is a central idiom: hope in scientific progress, in the success of the treatment, in a child. This actually produces various dilemmata for the women undergoing treatment, for instance long liminal stages of treatment where other life plans are put on hold and IVF "just takes over" (e.g. 131–168). It also raises questions regarding agency and choice for the social status of being involuntarily childless, because—in theory—IVF can be pursued over and over again.

4.1 What is Kinship? Characteristic Tensions of Choice, (Corporeal) Continuity, and Love

Towards the end of most of the first interview sessions conducted with parents, when I felt we had established a sense of joint reflection rather than following a strict questionnaire structure, I asked my research partners to share their views on kinship with me: how they personally defined it and what role they thought it played in society. This section analyzes these conversations. The meal that many families had kindly served me was finished by then, oftentimes a bottle of wine as well—or the cup of coffee if I came to visit during the afternoon. When I asked for parents' personal definitions and appraisals of kinship, I always added that I was interested in them getting "a bit philosophical", that there was "no right or wrong" and I did not expect any "text-book definitions", but rather liked them to just reflect and think out loud. I posed my question on personal definitions of kinship in such a way, because I had noticed during previous exploratory family-interviews[3] that interview partners tended to only enjoy reflecting on kinship when they were absolutely sure that I did not expect them to come up with readily quotable definitions. Interview partners mostly also investigated how they saw biology as implicated or not implicated in kinship within these reflections, without myself specifically prompting them to comment on notions of heredity.

Following my overall approach to analyzing how kinship becomes known situationally within diverging practices and socio-material configurations, my argument in this subchapter is not that the reflections analyzed below show axiomatic kinship values necessarily informing all of my research partners' practices. Rather, I am analyzing the definitions and reflections given to me as specifically situated knowledge-practices in themselves. They are set at a point in time years after conceiving through gamete donation and put forward not in an everyday situation, but in an effort to answer the ethnographer's question in an interview situation, which by that point had often turned into an animated joint discussion. I shall however touch upon resonances—and sometimes frictions—which the definitions of kinship "distilled" from these situated knowledge-

3 With families-by-adoption or -by-IVF, conducted for the collaborative research cluster SFB 640/Project C4.

practices produce within other domains and practices analyzed in this book.

When I first asked the parents to reflect more generally on kinship, all of my interview partners invoked a sense that kinship was something that probably had played a "bigger role for people in the past" and was "nowadays" often being replaced by friendships, which—for the majority of interviewees—were "just as important" or "definitely more important". The following quote by German father Philip Steger is typical for this notion:

> Philip Steger: "You do not have these extended families anymore. Society has got more flexible, more mobile above all. Not only throughout Germany, but worldwide. One just has to see that one creates one's family wherever one lives, artificially, in a sense, with friends. And that obviously works… […] Although I think for older people, that is still a bit harder."

My German and British informants all seemed to agree with the *grand narrative* of the sociology of the family that kinship was a social institution slowly being replaced by other forms of solidarity and today concentrated predominantly on the nuclear family.[4]

When first analyzing the interview passages and field notes I had marked with the code "kinship definitions/ reflections" I noted a theme was that they were characterized by seemingly contradictory statements. Thus I concentrated on the ambivalences expressed through these contradictions, when, literally, trying to fit the printed out fieldwork materials together like a puzzle. I foundthat they were typically centering on the ambivalent roles that choice, continuity, and love played within kinship in general, and within kinship-by-donation in particular. Below I shall explore each of these characteristic tensions in more detail.

Firstly, when trying to put forward how they would define kinship, a common theme was that my German and British research partners reflected ambivalently on the notion of choice within kinship. Typically, interviewees addressed kinship as a paradoxical relationship both inflexibly given and simultaneously, actively chosen. An example of the expression of this ambivalence is the passage below from my first interview with the

4 For a historical counter argument to this narrative of the sociology of the family see Sabean & Teuscher (2007), as also mentioned in chapter 2.2.

German-Brazilian Tönsch family, who had used sperm donation to conceive a year earlier:

Maren Klotz: "I would like to ask you a question and to possibly get a bit philosophical, to just reflect your views for me a little bit. What is… or makes kinship, in your opinion?"
Dörte Tönsch: "Well, one cannot choose it… I have a relatively small family. […] And I have never really been a family person. […] I guess in situations of crisis one remembers that one does have relatives, who would actually…. Well, who would stand by you and not suddenly decide that they want nothing to do with you. It is nice, that there is something like that, and important. But other than that, my family, that is my son and my partner. And any kin beyond that, hmmm, I actually pretty much choose…"

Kinship becomes known as a relationship one cannot choose, but still does. The notion that it was a relationship one could fall back on in crisis and that it was a "diffuse and enduring solidarity"—to evoke Schneider's (1968) definition of kinship—was commonly touched upon in interview situations. However, whether this was a notion one personally agreed with and what it might mean in terms of reciprocity and choice within one's own lives was critically interrogated. The passage below quoted from the end of my first interview with the German family-by-sperm-donation, Müller, is also a typical example of this situational negotiation. The passage is also typical for the common tendency that couples into the interview sessions often tended to discuss my questions at length with each other (also see chapter 3), starting to lead the interview process through their interactions:

Marcel Müller: "Family is important to me, but only as far as that's something mutual. […] If nothing comes from my family—nothing comes from me. I've become tough like that. […] Some people say blood is thicker than water and if family needs me I am there, no matter what. But that is where I have said, this rests on mutuality!"His wife Silke Müller, addressing me: "So he says whether something comes back makes all the difference. That's not how it is for me, actually, because family is family, yes. No matter how nasty they might behave or if people argue: […] blood is thicker than water and those are relatives, one cannot choose them. They are simply there. And that is actually important to me".In the interview situation from which the quotes above were taken, Silke and Marcel Müller expressed diverging views on the fixity or flexibility of kin connections. They thereby interactively performed the characteristic tension surrounding the role of choice for kin relationships within the interview situation itself.

Secondly, beyond these typical expressions of kinship being ambivalently positioned between chosen and given, a further characteristic theme in the definitorial reflections offered to me in the interviews was that of continuity: my interviewees described kinship as providing continuity, and thereby making a connection between persons and between bodies, often implicating different times and particular geographical regions. The notion of kinship being a (corporeal) continuity or connection was, however, characteristically only addressed as an ambivalent sense of coherence or connection, not as a causal or substantial connection definitorially interrogated in detail. In the first interview with the Feldman DI-family in Southern Germany, father Uli Linde-Feldman for example started his definitorial reflections on kinship with an assertion that he is from the Southern German region Swabia, and therefore kin relationships were quite important to him. He winked at me and switched into the Swabian accent to say "kinship rates high for the Swab". Another German mother, Melanie Steger, made a similar statement, but invoked Northern Germany, instead of Southern Germany as placing a particular stress on kin connections in everyday life, and as being typical in "having a lot of family celebrations". Marcel Müller, in yet another example of this tendency, which was typical particularly among my German interviewees, also invoked his sense of connectedness to a particular region in Poland. Masuria had been his father's family home before being driven out of Poland in the upheavals at the end of World War II and Nazism. Even though Marcel Müller had for a long time only heard about Masuria through his father's childhood memories, he still said that, "if you have such a long family history with a region, and you hear about it all the time, something just sticks with you, my family is connected to Masuria". Instead of offering me any more general kinship definitions, Marcel Müller vividly evoked what he knew about his family's history. When reassured that I did not find he was going off-topic by telling me these stories, but that I instead welcomed more detailed explorations, he also showed me historical materials he had collected on his family, such as a long family tree (see section

7.2). I then asked Müller where he thought his already declared interest in family history stemmed from and he mused:

Marcel Müller: "I just think it is great, it is exciting, a childhood dream, somehow: where do I come from, where am I going, this is what has been… My grandfather, for example was part of one of the crusades-"
His wife Silke jokingly intercepts that, surely, this could not have been his grandfather. He laughs and adds: "Well one of the grandfathers, with a sword…" All three of us burst out laughing at their kitchen table.

Müller described kinship as connecting persons to places sometimes through different layers of time, adding to a sense of coherency in his life.

Müller also added that he did not find this sense of connectedness had "anything to do with biology, zero". When asked for personal definitions of kinship, most of my interview partners generally downplayed that heredity played a significant role. Typical was for instance the assertion of British interview partner Holly Greenwood: "Of course, the genetic aspect of kinship is not particularly important to me, otherwise we would have not decided to use donor sperm". In fact, Lena Konrad, mother and co-mother in the Konrad rainbow-family, was the only interview-partner among all the members of the 13 families I spoke to who clearly characterized kinship and family as biological when she answered my question on personal definitions of kinship with the contention: "family, that's first and foremost 'blood' for me", going on to qualify that her definition followed a fairly classical model of kinship with affinal and consanguine ties.

Yet, ambivalent notions of experienced, or also missed, continuities between *physical bodies* were typically explored within the definitorial reflections of most of my German and British interview partners. Dörte Tönsch, for instance, reflected on how she found it fascinating to watch how children, genetically related or not, were often taking on mannerisms from their parents. This remark prompted the dialogue below between her husband and her:

Miguel Tönsch: "I guess that's what you learn from these situations, it [kinship] is not about genetics, it is about how you treat a child. How you raise a child, what it learns from you, that is the most important thing. That's where resemblance comes from, the real, true human resemblance. Being built in a certain way, that's just nonsense…"
Dörte Tönsch: "Or language… When I first heard your [to Miguel] father talk,

I knew where your language was coming from, your passionate, argumentative language…"

The Tönschs, in the passage above and also in subsequent conversations I had with them, quite poetically evoked a joyful sense of continuity between bodies and persons without invoking classical notions of heredity. All families I interviewed did at some point put forward observations on physical resemblances between them and their children. They also told me a lot about others confronting them with talk on perceived physical resemblance (see section 8.1 on *resemblance-talk*).

British interview partner Tim Hampton, father of two DI conceived children, was very eloquent in conveying during his definitorial reflections the typical ambivalences surrounding kinship as (corporeal) continuity. He firstly pointed out to me that friendship was just as important to him as family, but added that he also really "valued" his "genetic connections". However, he added, this in turn did not mean that he would somehow experience an impairment in connecting to his children, whom he could actually not "imagine feeling any less close to". In the passages below Hampton reflects for me what he thinks about genetic connections:

Maren Klotz: "Could you explain some more what you meant with valuing your genetic connections?"
Tim Hampton: "The men on my father's side of the family are all athletes. You know, we can all hit a ball, we can all run around, we've all enjoyed sport. And… I don't pass that onto my son. I pass on the fact that I enjoy sport. I don't pass on any hand-eye coordination to him and I'm, I'm sorry about that."
His wife Sarah joins in that she has very good hand-eye coordination as well and smiles. They joke around about him being thankful for that. She then teases him that he just wants his children "to be like him".
Tim Hampton: "No, it's actually quite a simple thing: my dad can hold a tune, I can hold a tune, but I am not passing that on. Not that anyone necessarily would… A few raw materials that might have given them some pleasure. It's really not wanting him to be like me! The sport thing, I know how much pleasure I've got out of it and I would just have wanted to give them at least some raw material, so that they might choose".
Sarah and Tim go on talking about in which ways they would actually like their children to be like them and agree that they would want them to be like them in how they know "right from wrong, and treat people".

Hence in the situation partially captured through the quotes above, Tim Hampton reflects about the breaking-off of one form of continuity particularly brought about through heredity. This he imagines to provide, particularly for his older son, "the raw materials" for potentially similar joyful physical experiences. But within the interview situation, kinship becomes known through other forms of (corporeal) continuities as well: enjoying sports, how his partner Sarah might still be able to "pass on" those "raw materials" that are important to him, and through shared values.

The third theme brought up by my parental interviewees, when asked how they would personally define kinship, has been love. All of the parents I spoke to stressed that it was first and foremost love, or an emotional connection, that was crucial for kinship when reflecting on how to define it. Uli Linde-Feldman, for instance, reflected quite typically: "I guess that's an important aspect when talking about kinship. I mean, the daily relationship with the children and this intense love one feels for them." However, the fathers especially of children conceived through DI in my sample, took these reflections as a prompter to tell me about some ambivalences regarding this theme. They actually laughed in hindsight about their past fears that an emotional bond to their children actually might not develop. Most said that they occasionally still wondered if they would feel differently for a child not conceived through DI, and concluded these reflections with the assertion that they simply never would be in the position to compare.

The two fathers in my sample who did have both the experience of conceiving with DI and without any medical interventions talked quite extensively about making such comparisons themselves and also about how other fathers-by-donation were very interested in their ability to compare. Philip Steger, who had gone through the horrendous experience of losing his first daughter to a double-recessive hereditary disease when she was not quite one year old, and only after this tragedy had children through a sperm donor tested for the disorder, for example recalled an afternoon during an interest group meeting: one of the attending fathers said that he loved his child, but, from a logical point of view, would never know whether he would love "a child that is my own more". Philip Steger was attending the meeting at a point in time when his wife and him had yet to make the final decision for or against using a sperm donor. He told me how he recalled noting down the other man's question in his head during the meeting. He then added:

Philip Steger: "You see, today I can answer it and I can only say: there simply is no difference at all. It was exactly the same feeling from the beginning onwards, as if she was *really* my child, in quotation marks—actually, it's difficult to put this right..."

In the passage above Philip Steger is confirming how the bond to his first DI conceived daughter feels just as strong as that to his deceased daughter. Moreover, he is also struggling with language during the comparison. I would argue that he makes reference to an implicit norm of genetic relatedness and the absence of this in his family through invoking "as if" and "really", but then performatively underlines that he does not want to perpetuate that implicit norm by adding the "quotation marks" and breaking off the sentence (also see section 7.2 for an analysis of kin terminologies as part of constituting kinship-by-donation). A similar situation of both negotiating the right language to use and discussing the ability to compare different kinship connections arose when talking to Marcel and Silke Müller. The Müllers conceived only their second son with donor sperm, because Marcel Müller's medically unexplained azoospermia had only appeared late in life. Below they are quoted talking about other infertile men's interest in Marcel's ability to compare his feelings for his two sons:

Marcel Müller: "In the group meetings I experienced something... I would not call it jealousy, it's not jealousy. But the men are looking at us with something like an interest and admiration. When chatting to the guys, they were like: 'Wow, you have something we don't have, but now you're one of us. But you still have your own, you have your own, but still...'"
Silke Müller (cuts in): "But there's no difference between the two [children], because..."
Marcel Müller (amused protest): "-no, no, no, I didn't mean to say that".
Silke Müller (laughingly): "Yeah, yeah, I only meant to clarify, thank you!"
Maren Klotz: "So you think that, probably, they, the other men, are interested in having the comparison?"
Marcel Müller: "Yes, the men, from what I have picked up, you see".
Silke Müller: "Yes, that's no issue for the women".
Marcel Müller: "For the men it's really really important".

In the passage above, the Müllers convey their impression that interrogating whether biological relatedness makes an emotional difference for kin ties was common among the men they met in an interest group for families-by-donation. Silke Müller put forward that this was, however, only of importance to the infertile men, not to their partners. She also underlines that her husband does not feel differently for their two children. At the same time she keeps him from adding qualifying remarks on his feelings, through her interruption. The interruption comes at a similar point in conversation as where Philip Steger, as earlier quoted, breaks off his description of comparing kinship bonds. Marcel Müller at the beginning of the quote above is also struggling with how to phrase the comparison between a child conceived with and without DI ("...but you still have your own, you have your own, but still..."), seemingly situationally marking the tension entailed in such a comparison. All parents not in a situation to compare noted how they could not imagine that they would feel "more" for a child without the assistance of a donor, but also addressed an ambivalence in that they would "just never know" if there was a difference.

In summary, within the specific knowledge-practice of reflecting on what kinship "is" in the ethnographic interview situation, parents suggest that it was a specific relationship. This relationship, if one summarizes their often seemingly contradictory reflections, was typified through three characteristic ambivalences to do with choice, (corporeal) continuity, and love. Kinship was evoked as making connections and thereby establishing continuities between persons, bodies, places, and through times. However, these connections are simultaneously marked by choice, and its absence, by unquestioned love and its interrogation.

Edwards (e.g. 1999; 2000; also see 2006), in her rare and gripping everyday life ethnography of a small contemporary town in the North of England and its people's practices of relating to the past, each other, and technological change, has argued that it is actually characteristic of European kinship to create relationships within quite flexible negotiations of what is perceived as flexible or given. She, for instance, argues about her fieldwork materials:

"While kin relationships are on the one hand thought to be enduring—you can always choose your friends but not your family—they are on the other hand also thought to be fragile, easily disrupted and require great patience and tenacity to sustain in an appropriate manner." (Edwards 1999, 55)

Her observations are resonant with the tensions negotiated within my interviewees' reflections of what kinship "is". Nash (2005), when discussing Edwards' and her own work on kinship has summarized that it is exactly this ambivalence by which kinship takes its powerful capacity to make and sustain relations. This ambivalence means kinship is neither monolithically fixed, nor straight forwardly mapped by biological procreation. Kinship rather takes its endurance from making connections, "evoking the fixity and certainty of the natural and making use of the flexibility of the social" (Nash 2005, 452). Hence, it is exactly its flexibility and ambivalences—in my fieldwork materials these are characteristically to do with choice, (corporeal) continuity, and love for kinship-by-donation—which makes kinship an elusive subject for definition by abstract enquiry during an interview situation.

4.2 Reproductive Histories and DI as a Technology of the Last Resort

I now want to change genres regarding the analysis of my fieldwork materials to produce, and think about some frictions. In the above section kinship has emerged in an encompassing connective ambiguity. This is due to the particularities of being asked very open questions in an interview-situation, but also because of the realities of the caring families-by-donation that have let me into their lives for short periods of fieldwork time: families that had long overcome the often extremely difficult periods *before* the birth of their children. In this section I juxtapose the previous reflections on kinship with an evocation of how kinship-by-donation, in this case particularly clinical sperm donation, becomes known when analyzing what I have come to call the reproductive histories of the parents I spoke to. These reproductive histories, i.e. the experiences and socio-material practices which have led up to becoming families-by-donation, I reconstructed through analyzing what my interviewees told me when asked "how they became the family they are today" and then narratively walked me through this process. I further reconstructed these histories through analyzing more performative evocations of past experiences and practices during the interviews and informal interactions, when couples often reenacted detailed past exchanges they had had with each other or clinicians. And lastly, I also analyzed some of my interviewees' treatment contracts or advice materials handed over to me, and additional information I sometimes had on the clinics they used.

Those parents who used sperm donation as a single mother (Maria Lieb) or as a lesbian couple (the Konrads), or those who used surrogacy as a gay couple (the Dünkes) and ova donation as a post-menopausal single woman (Shoko Nakamura) and as a young couple with female-side fertility problems (the Taylors) all had highly individual reproductive histories. I shall touch upon particularities of their cases in the following chapters. In this section I will, however, concentrate on the reproductive histories of my heterosexual interview-partners who have used DI to conceive (the Feldmans, the Müllers, the Tönschs, the Schneiders, the Hamptons, the Kings, and the Greenwoods, all because of male infertility; and the Stegers because of the genetic disease in their family). I shall do so, because I found that there were striking similarities. When analyzing these, kinship-by-donation emerges as a way of doing kinship firmly positioned as the last possible step in a succession of intensive repro-technological interventions.[5] Thus, if IVF is often enacted as a technology of "hope" producing long liminal treatment phases (Franklin 1997), kinship-by-donation here becomes known as a *technology of the last resort*—without this, however, being attributable to one-dimensional forms of geneticization. Below I shall discuss how I came to this interpretation.

When reconstructing and analyzing the reproductive histories of the German and British DI families, I learned that the DI treatment always came last—*after* ICSI.[6] In hindsight, ICSI and the related biopsies of the

5 For a comprehensive discussion of "logics of intervention" during unwanted childlessness—analysing a broader sample of kinship-by-IVF, kinship-by-adoption, and kinship-by-donation—see Knecht et al. (2011). We discuss two typical treatment trajectories: the *escalating* and the *direct-maximal* treatment-trajectory, which were part of different normalization strategies of assisted conception among users *and* doctors.

6 ICSI—Intracytoplasmic Sperm Injection—is an advanced variant of IVF where the nucleus of a single sperm is inserted into the retrieved egg cell with a special pipette. ICSI enables successful fertilisation with the sperm of virtually infertile men—due to

men's testicles to try and recover sperm cells were typically discussed as a physically, emotionally, and socially invasive procedure, e.g. as "hellish and recommendable to no one" (German father Marc Schneider). German mother Nadine Schneider, for instance, told me that she quit her job due to the periods of depression she experienced during hormonal stimulation for the IVF/ICSI procedure. Another German father felt like he was "at the butchers" during his testicle operation. And British interviewee Tim Hampton recalled, still visibly uneasy about this painful time, the phone call after his failed[7] biopsy "which puts you in pretty serious psychological discomfort, after the operation left you in pretty serious physical discomfort. It was a pretty unpleasant time, a pretty unpleasant time". And his wife Sarah added that they spent about three months mourning that they would never be able to have children "together" after that phone call, withdrawing from their circle of friends and drinking quite a lot of alcohol.

In vitro fertilization's seemingly socio-materially in-built and gripping imperative of "having to try" (e.g. Franklin 1997, 170), no matter what the emotional, physical, and economic costs might be, also emerges in the recollections of my interview partners. German-Brazilian father Miguel Tönsch, for instance, who so poetically reflected on kinship being about corporeal continuities through shared experiences and not about "being built a certain way" (see 4.1 above) and who resisted a so-called physical matching to his DI-child (discussed in 7.1) nevertheless argued:

> Miguel Tönsch: "I think the chances for the operation were not so well and I don't like operations. But still: 'Ok, if we do not try this, maybe we will regret it later? We might say 'Oh, why did we not try?' So yeah, we did it, it did not lead to anything, not even the cause [of my infertility] was established, now it's over."

All of my German and British interview partners opted for such a period of trying before making the decision to use DI. Donor insemination was typically addressed as a technology, which could only follow after these attempts. The German mother Berit Linde-Feldman reflexively commented

low sperm counts or immobile sperm, for instance. It also implies that fertile women have to undergo the invasive IVF/ICSI procedure so they can conceive with the sperm of their "infertile" partner. The sperm for ICSI is either retrieved through masturbation or in cases of severe male infertility through an operation to recover potential sperm cells directly from the testes.

7 Meaning that no sperm cells could be retrieved through the operation.

that she did not believe DI could be anything else than what I have started to call a *technology of the last resort*, even though her before quoted husband Uli had said to me that—in hindsight—he was not sure whether they should not have skipped the biopsy and attempts at ICSI altogether, since it had been such an unpleasant experience.

Berit Feldman: "I think that probably… -one has to grow into it [DI]. One has to exhaust every possibility before and when nothing works anymore—you can make that step. That's probably why people still in the IVF/ICSI process might say that DI is not an option for them. Because this is evidently that way, as long you still have the option of a genetically related child."

All parents expressed how they had mourned that they could not have children "together" and how this had been a motivation for trying IVF/ICSI earlier. Typically, this was not addressed in reference to any hereditary considerations or wishes, but in terms of what I would describe as the desire for a shared emotional and physical connection and continuity between lovers through a genetically related child.[8] During the interviews, most parents also did not reflect long on this theme, which seemed only commonsensical given the wish had not been fulfilled and they had made the decision to become families-by-donation after all. Only German-Brazilian couple Tönsch reflected longer on this in our second interview. Dörte Tönsch then put the desire for having a child together into the following words:

Dörte Tönsch: "Well, we did say then, okay, we will try whether we really cannot find any sperm cells. I had already heard that there is the possibility, with a biopsy and ICSI, to still make it work. Because—obviously—it is always the biggest wish that you would have a child… -a child that's from both and who looks like both."
Miguel Tönsch (laughingly): "The mixture, right?"
Dörte Tönsch: "Yes, exactly, this mix is what interests you. How does it turn out?"

The possibility of having "at least" the—in a sense still shared—physical experience of a pregnancy through DI was then typically acknowledged to me as a relief and as setting DI apart from adoption. DI still provided the "full experience" for his partner, in Tim Hampton's words.

The reproductive histories of my research partners however showed that the wish for a corporeal continuity between lovers had only been one

8 Edwards in her before cited ethnographic research (1999, 2000) also makes note of how a child is viewed to "embody the relationship between the two parents" (2006, 134).

factor in turning DI into the last step of an irreversible succession of reproductive interventions: the clinics, in how they advertised their services, set up their contracts, interacted with patients and booked them into treatment pathways, all very much contributed to the enactment of DI as a *technology of the last resort*. The Tönsch's treatment contract (see clipping 4.1), for instance, starts with a passage that the couple is opting for DI after it has been informed by the doctor that "the possibility of an own child has been medically exhausted". Hence, the clinic was not even acknowledging the option of couples opting for DI *before* ICSI in their contract. As analyzed in more detail in section 5.2, German and British clinics were often actually presenting "failed IVF/ICSI" as the "indication" for a DI treatment for heterosexual couples in their information materials and on their websites.

Clipping 4.1: Section of the Tönsch's treatment contract with a German sperm bank (Source: Tönsch family)

1. Das Ehepaar hat sich entschlossen, die Erfüllung des beiderseitigen Wunsches nach einem gemeinsamen Kinde mit Hilfe der instrumentellen donogenen Insemination, d.h. der Übertragung von Spendersamen, zu verwirklichen und beantragt hiermit deren Durchführung in der Praxisklinik für Fertilität.
2. Das Ehepaar blieb bisher kinderlos und wurde ärztlicherseits darüber unterrichtet, daß die Aussicht auf ein eigenes Kind nach Ausschöpfung aller Möglichkeiten nicht verbessert werden kann. Die Eheleute sind nach eingehender Prüfung zu der Überzeugung gekommen, daß die donogene instrumentelle Samenübertragung als Behandlung der Kinderlosigkeit ihrer Ehe medizinisch angezeigt ist, weil sie nicht auf Kinder verzichten oder ein Kind adoptieren wollen.

In hindsight, several parents described feelings of despair and loss of control during their IVF/ICSI treatment phase, after which the DI treatment then felt "like a walk in the park" (Nadine Schneider). Parents typically referred to themselves as "naïve" during the ICSI phase and as having found themselves in a wake of clinical practices within which they felt like they had lost agency and, temporarily, the ability to make informed decisions. These conceptualizations of my interviewees were highly resonant with Franklin's (1997) ethnographic accounts of how IVF "just takes over". German mother Nadine Schneider, as a typical example, recalled how they "stumbled into the process of the ICSI treatment somewhat, naïvely at first, or uninformed". Or Silke Müller said with slight disbelief in her voice about their treatment decisions:

Silke Müller: "In the clinic, we relatively quickly entered into a form of machinery. You did not have time to think: 'Do I really want this?' It had already been done, then. You already have the appointment for the biopsy. And that's when you realize the consequences: why do a biopsy? Do I actually want an IVF treatment? Is that a way for us? We had not actually familiarized ourselves with this…"

The "machinery" came to a halt by itself, because no cells were recovered during the biopsy of Marcel Müller's testicles, just as had been the case for Tim Hampton. For the Hamptons, the clinical push towards IVF/ICSI even continued into the DI treatment: now it was IVF with donor sperm that was being suggested. Sarah Hampton, for example, described how she did not get pregnant during the first two inseminations she had had. Then—although determined healthy by her local gynecologist—the clinical personnel kept pressuring her to use IVF/ICSI with donated sperm. Already having to come to terms with Tim's medically unexplained azoospermia, the Hamptons had taken pride in the fact that at least "there was nothing wrong with Sarah". The passage below is only one of many examples of the couple's re-enactment of situations encapsulating the push towards IVF/ICSI treatment they experienced. This push even included a phone-call from one clinician to Tim Hampton so he would encourage his wife into IVF, which the Hamptons later officially filed a complaint about.

Tim Hampton to his wife: "…and you got repeatedly frustrated, didn't you, that (Pause), that, it wasn't regularly acknowledged that you were alright!"
Sarah Hampton: "But all they are worried about, it seems, is their statistics, getting you pregnant…"
Tim Hampton: "Yeah."
Sarah Hampton: "…the quickest and the most successful—as far as they are concerned that's IVF, so…"
Maren Klotz: "So that's why-?"
Sarah Hampton: "-they get you on that road, because then they are able to use those stats and show a pregnancy, and that's how you definitely feel that you are being treated there (…)"
Tim Hampton: "Sarah very calmly gave her story: there is nothing wrong with me, we want to stick with DI and the doctor said 'oh, the expense of more' [conventional DI treatments] and we said, we'll bear the expense. The money is not a

problem. We want to carry on doing this and he, he pointed out the higher success rates [of IVF/ICSI], so we went back and forth, you [to Sarah] were seething, weren't you, you were absolutely seething, seething, seething!"
Sarah Hampton (calmly): "Yeah."

None of the German families told me of similar pressures to use IVF *during* the DI treatment, but most families actually spoke rather negatively of their contact with fertility doctors in general. Criticisms centered on physicians being generally insensitive and particularly uninformed about donor insemination. The Feldmans even had had the experience of, after getting the information that the biopsy was not successful, being falsely told in the clinic where it was performed that DI was illegal in Germany.

Interviewee Philip Steger also expressed a criticism of not being presented with DI earlier as an alternative to other methods during their fertility treatment. His and his wife Melanie's reproductive history—although structurally quite different from all my other research partners' in that a genetic disease was the reason for the donor treatment—equally underlines the picture of DI as a *technology of last resort*, which has its place after all other means have been exploited. The Stegers, instead of using a genetically tested sperm donor from the start, travelled to Belgium for one round of pre-implantation genetic diagnosis (PGD) as this was then still fully illegal in Germany.[9] This was bound up with spending large amounts of money on the treatment, which produced only one embryo unaffected by the hereditary disease their first daughter had previously died from. After not falling pregnant following the single embryo transfer—and still affected by their daughter's death less than a year earlier—Melanie Steger had a break-down and went into fulltime treatment in a psychosomatic day care clinic for several months.

It was after this experience that the Stegers decided to not do another round of ICSI combined with genetic tests on the resulting embryos, but go for donor insemination after a further period of recovery instead. In the interview passages quoted below the Stegers told me about their

9 During PGD fertilization and subsequent genetic testing takes place in-vitro, *before* embryos would be transferred into the woman's womb. At the end of 2011 a new law has been passed in Germany (Präimplantationsgesetz 2011), which—in contrast to previous regulations—makes PGD legal in exceptional cases involving severe and potentially deadly genetic diseases. Under the new regulations the Stegers could have undergone PGD-IVF legally in Germany.

decision making process during that time. I would argue that this interaction exemplifies coming to know DI as a *technology of the last resort* as a knowledge-practice in itself. For the passages to be comprehensible I need to add that the couple had a longer history of fertility treatments—due to Philip Steger's low sperm count—reaching back to the time before the conception of their first-born and now deceased daughter.

Melanie Steger: "After travelling to Belgium for PGD, Philip had again had a spermiogram done, and then the lady in the lab said to him…"
Philip Steger: "-the lady in the lab said to me, because she knew our story: Well, why don't you try donor sperm? And I said: How? What does that mean, donor sperm? And she said: Well, a donor can be tested [for the double-recessive disorder their first daughter died from]. And I asked: Is that legal? [PGD was then illegal in Germany] She says: 'Of course, that's legal'. I didn't know that. I had not even thought of that before! That was when I also realized that from the beginning, we did not really take our time to think about artificial reproduction, just didn't take the time to think, what is important to us? How can one become a family? […] DI was never really presented as an alternative to us…"
Melanie Steger cuts in: "-of course, because we do not need it, your [spermiogram] results in themselves…"
Philip Steger: "-yes…"
Melanie Steger: "-were good."
Philip Steger: "Yes, but others [implying that he has met someone in the DI patient group with a different reproductive history] might have had the same situation to start with and still, they immediately decided against ICSI and for DI. The doctor did not even mention DI, or at least I don't recall that."
Melanie Steger: "Naw, they just said, your results are good, we can do IVF/ICSI with you. And it worked, it worked immediately. [She is referring to their first-born daughter]."

As becomes clear above, the clinic—at least as the Stegers recalled—did not inform them of donor insemination as a treatment option when conventional ICSI (instead of pre-implantation genetic diagnosis) was still an option for them while trying for their first daughter, nor did the Stegers subsequently know for a long time that sperm donation from a genetically tested donor was legal in Germany and an alternative to testing their embryos in-vitro. Only the lab personnel led Philip Steger to realize that this was actually a possible legal alternative.

In the interview itself, the couple situationally re-enacts how DI can be a *technology of the last resort*: Melanie repeatedly fails to engage with, or signal understanding of her partner's reflection that donor insemination might potentially have been an *earlier* option. She just repeatedly addresses that his lab results were "good enough for IVF", and thereby situationally dismisses that DI could be anything else than the last step of a succession of repro-technological interventions.

In summary, although critically interrogated in hindsight by some interviewees, during fertility treatment DI always seemed to "lose out" against the clinically more prestigious hope-technology IVF/ICSI presenting the opportunity of a genetically related child. In fact, HFEA statistics (e.g. 2011) show that declining DI rates are met with diametrically rising ICSI rates, suggesting a displacement of DI through IVF/ ICSI. The parents did not reflect long on why in the past a biologically related child had been important to them, but made hints at the joy of a corporeal continuity between lovers without going into longer reflections on genetics or heredity. The clinics, in information politics and pre-established treatment pathways, treated the assumed parental wish "to try" as the absolute unquestioned norm—thereby contributing to a retrospectively described sense of lost agency and lack of reflection among the families of my sample. Recent anthropological research (e.g. Lock and Kaufert 1998) has tended to focus on patients' agency and informed engagement with medical technologies, for good theoretical and empirical reasons. While I am not suggesting that my interviewees were not asserting agency throughout their reproductive histories, my research nevertheless shows how IVF/ ICSI in its socio-material enactment became a "machinery" (Silke Müller) with its own pervasive logic of practice.

When discussing with me the period of time *after* the failed attempts at IVF/ICSI, parents typically brought up two themes which had played a role in their decision to continue with DI: one entirely "social" (experiential knowledge of positive kin-relationships without genetic relatedness), and one entirely "genetic" (that donor insemination reduces "genetic unknowns" in opposition to adoption). Firstly, parents talked about their decision for DI as having been facilitated by their previous positive experiences, in their own family or social circle, with kin relationships without a so-called genetic tie. This included references to adopted or foster-child siblings, well-liked patchwork families among friends and family, and to other families-by-donation which my interviewees had met when first visiting concerned groups prior to the DI conception (also see section 6.2). German father Marc Schneider, as one example, brought up a particular experience during the long interview passages within which he and his wife Nadine recounted their decision for DI:

Marc Schneider: "The thing with the genetic kinship was not a problem, because I did my Master's project with another student who had just had a baby. That's my goddaughter. And I was with that kid every day for twelve hours, in the laboratory—and also during the writing-up phase, the little one was always there. I actually felt a little sorry for the father for a while, because I had more of a relationship with this child than him..."
Maren Klotz: "That's an interesting story... Because your colleague was still breastfeeding her child and you were working in a laboratory together, the child always had to be with you?"
Marc Schneider: "Yes, and I used to carry her around, or... Well, anything that needed to be done, changing diapers... We basically did the Master's thesis as a trio, over a period of nine months. And Lena, I love her like she was my own child. So I did not think that this wouldn't be the same when having a child this way [with DI]".

As captured in the example above, all parents brought up that they knew, through personal experience, that kinship "worked" even in the (known) absence of genetic relatedness.

During the reconstruction of the couple's reproductive history, they predominantly further also brought up why they had opted for DI *instead* of adoption. If they did not do this unprompted, I asked whether "at some point in time" they had "also considered adoption?" Before turning to an analysis of the theme of "the genetic unknown" as brought up in response to talking about adoption, I want to point out that I always made it very clear when talking about adoption to my interviewees that I did not perceive it as an "easy" or morally more high-ranking alternative to DI. (These were judgments that the families were often confronted with, as they told me, and I often heard this within my social circle when talking about my research topic). Very low upper age limits, highly complex criteria to qualify as adoptive parents, the extremely high invasion of privacy during control-visits of social workers, and the scarcity of younger children in national adoption programs generally makes kinship-by-adoption hard to achieve for many parents in the UK and Germany (e.g. see Hamra 2007). The high fees of international adoption agencies and controversies (potential incentive for kidnappings and forms of slave-trade, problems for developmental aid, celebrity "fashion", e.g. Wuttke & Terre des Hommes (1995–1996)) surrounding international adoption also contribute to it not being an easy alternative to DI.[10]

It was important to me to not reproduce the seeming hostility entailed in the apparently extremely common question for my research partners "why one doesn't *simply* adopt?" British mother Holly Greenwood, for instance, angrily remembered friends' comments towards her about "all the homeless children" they had seen in Brazil "as if these children were just readily and easily up for grabs!" Hence, I do not want to imply in this analysis that my interviewees chose DI over adoption *predominantly* for genetic reasons. Many told me how they had started looking into the process, but were put off by the age-limits for parents or by the high level of bureaucracy involved, for instance. Nevertheless, how my research parents related to biology also played a role, as became clear through typical references to DI as the option reducing "genetic unknowns" compared to adoption. These discussions entailed quite similar calculative language among German and British interviewees alike and in most interviews marked the first point at which my research partners touched upon notions of biology in some detail. German mother Berit Feldman, for example, laughingly recounted a playful calculation her husband and she had made:

> Berit Feldman: "We have always said that if you assume, pragmatically, that its 50 percent genetics, and 50 percent nurture, then we have 75 percent in check. And 25 percent, that's the black box, here. [Uli, her, and I break out laughing]. And with adoption, that's different. But you never know what we would have done had DI not worked out..."

Or, as another typical example, Nadine Schneider presented the following formula in favor of donor insemination:

> Nadine Schneider: "...with adoption we have two unknowns, with DI you have one unknown, in the genes, so to say".

Within such calculations, being genetically related is made analogous to knowing, while not being genetically related is linked to a potentially nega-

10 For excellent ethnographic discussions on kinship and transnational/transethnic adoption also see the works of Signe Howell (e.g. 2006) and Barbara Katz Rothman (e.g. 2005).

tive lack of knowledge and an associated potential loss of control or a sense of the uncanny (also see section 8.1 on resemblance). One can interpret these references as again touching upon the theme of corporeal continuity: the families were calculating, when comparing different means of assisted reproduction and wanted to ensure a high level of corporeal connections. These were however not only talked about as something physical (e.g. in a jointly experienced pregnancy), but also as something informational (when genetic relatedness was equated with knowledge). The decision for DI *after* ICSI and potentially *before* adoption could hence already be seen as a decision within a specific tactic in kinship knowledge-management to reduce perceived uncertainty.

All in all, analyzing my interview partners' reproductive histories brought forward more constrictions of how kinship-by-donation can be known and hence done than is apparent in the more flexible reflections on kinship analyzed in 4.1 above. However, my analysis of reproductive histories in this section also shows that there was not a simple learning process involved in why my research partners were addressing kinship as highly flexible and only marginally grounded in biology in the interviews, but in the past went through the extremely invasive process of IVF/ICSI-by-biopsy. My data have rather indicated how the reproductive histories of my interviewees took on a specific trajectory through an entanglement of wishes for a corporeal continuity as a couple and socio-material and informational pulls and pushes through the clinics. Donor insemination thereby emerged as a way of doing kinship only achievable at a specific point in a succession of reproductive interventions, making it a *technology of the last resort.*

5. Clinical Knowledge-Management and Beyond: How Kinship-by-Donation Becomes Constituted in Clinics

After providing a first glimpse of how kinship-by-donation became known within different parental knowledge-practices in the previous chapter, I now turn to my description and analysis of how it becomes constituted within the knowledge-practices in German and British clinics and associated regulatory institutions. Instead of too readily concentrating on a diagnosis of *naturalization* or *culturalization* (see 2.3), I shall instead foreground the more minute entanglements between substances, regulations, and individual actors' decisions in giving kinship differing figurations. I shall thereby take up Edward's (2009b) above discussed call to look closely and empirically at how kinship "matters" in different domains. Which information is collected (or not bothered about), with the help of which instruments and involvement of bodily substances? What is made durable within information infrastructures or tanks for cryopreservation, or instead ends up on discarded and shredded index cards or irretrievably deleted? And which ways-of-knowing are ultimately made accessible to children and parents and which are not?

This chapter is divided into three parts. Firstly I identify in detail regulatory demands (section 5.1) that I found to make an impact on knowledge-management in the clinical field sites. (Despite their influence, these demands were not necessarily, related to the juridical proceedings and regulations feeding into the current British and German anonymity/ non-anonymity regimes for gamete donation, as detailed in section 2.1). Secondly I focus on the clinical practices involved in constituting kinship by donation as apparent in my four clinical field sites (section 5.2). Thirdly I analyze what aspects of knowing clinically practiced kinship-by-donation were deemed to be of social relevance by making them accessible to concerned persons in the future (section

5.3). I have thus, for analytical reasons, divided the discussion of three intertwined aspects relevant to the clinical constitution of kinship-by-donation. I separately focus on the local influences of regulation, clinical routines, and the storage of information for donor-conceived children.

The first subchapter enhances the legibility of the analyses provided in the following subchapters through describing my clinical field sites and providing contextualizing information on the local rationales and wider regulations feeding into local practices. On the basis of my fieldwork materials I show how clinical practices in Germany were less embedded in regimes of "government at a distance" (e.g. Miller and Rose 2008) than in Britain and thus more idiosyncratic. At the British field site the HFEA was in contrast persistently invoked into practices on the shop floor. The analysis makes visible how kinship-by-donation in both countries was constituted within two differing modes of governance: a tight, yet processual approach strongly bound up with neoliberal "audit cultures" (Strathern 2000) in the UK and a "hands-off" minimal approach in Germany leaving much room for local negotiation.

The following subchapters focus on two different trajectories of knowledge, i.e. pathways of validation, storage, and distribution (see Barth 2002), involved in the clinical constitution of kinship-by-donation: the *medical trajectory* (section 5.2), and the *accessible clinical/institutional trajectory* (section 5.3). In section 5.2 I take the notion of constitutive knowledge literally and analyze how kinship is socio-materially constituted within the medical trajectory of knowing kinship-by-donation. I show how scientific standards, clinical information infrastructures, national regulations, laboratory equipment, biological substances and actual or anticipated parental knowledge-management are all part of this step-by-step constitutive process (see Latour 1999). Hence, these aspects become part of the relations arising out of the procreative process. I argue that it is one of the unique characteristics of kinship-by-donation how comprehensively it relates to clinical and institutional administration, infrastructures and scientific standards. This also means that clinical and parental knowledge-management becomes part of the physical constitution of the children born through the procedures: for instance through having specific blood groups.

When I analyze the accessible clinical/institutional trajectory in the last subchapter (5.3), I focus on which aspects of the clinical ways-of-knowing are made available to children and parents and thereby underlined as socially relevant. (In both Germany and Britain actual access requests of children were only expected to arise in the future during my fieldwork. The subchapter thus focuses on the preparations for potential access, not on what donor-conceived persons actually did). I demonstrate that the hybridity apparent in the medical trajectory becomes purified in the Latourian (1993) sense within the accessible trajectory: kinship takes more familiar shape again. This means that it becomes known as a biological tie of personal value and a connector among persons. Kinship-by-donation in the accessible trajectory nevertheless became interlinked with administrative rationales, as I will show. This section thus brings to the forefront how kinship-by-donation becomes entangled with particular modes of governance, but focuses on a more minute level of infrastructures and "paper technologies" (Levinson 2010, 163–188) than in the first subchapter.

Empirically, this chapter is mainly based on interviews, short periods of participant observation, and the analysis of various information materials, internal operating procedures and files at the HFEA and in three (or six—depending how one counts)[1] clinics: the German Sperm Bank Friedhausen, the German Sperm Bank and Fertility Clinic Luisenburg, and the British Largecity Fertility Hospital and Sperm Bank. This chapter demonstrates how kinship-by-donation is clinically constituted within practices reliant on diverse strands of legal, scientific, and administrative ways-of-knowing and therefore more diversely bound up with scientific-knowledge than originally entailed in Schneider's (1968, 23) assertion that Western kinship perceptions are generally always connected to what science might say about genetic relatedness, which mainly seems to take into focus

1 Economically and in terms of legal licensing not all three clinics were one unit: The Sperm Bank Friedhausen was one unit, only using cooperating clinics for the actual insemination; the Sperm Bank and Fertility Clinic Luisenburg consisted of two distinct economical and juridical units, with overlaps in personnel. The Largecity Fertility Hospital incorporated one sperm bank under its operating licenses, while the other operated under a separate license and still followed different work routines, because it had only recently been bought from different ownership. Six field sites can therefore be counted this way: 1) Sperm Bank Friedhausen, 2) Sperm Bank Luisenburg, 3) Fertility Clinic Luisenburg, 4) Largecity Fertility Hospital, 5) Largecity Fertility Hospital outsourced sperm bank 6) Largecity Fertility Hospital in-house sperm bank.

molecular biology. For kinship-by-donation as constituted in clinics and associated administration, what figures prominently in the forefront is not molecular biology, but rather such factors as WHO standards on sperm quality, nationally differing "transmission belts" which translate macro regulation into daily life, and administrative knowledge-management.

5.1 Local Fieldwork—Local Regulations

The clinical constitution of kinship-by-donation is embedded into two different modes of governance in Britain and in Germany: A "hands-off" minimal approach in Germany, and a tight, yet processual approach in Britain. Practices in Germany were more diverse, and bound up with local interpretations through privately contracted consultants and professional networks. At the British field site, in contrast, the HFEA was persistently invoked in practices on the shop floor. By introducing my clinical field sites and by providing background information on why practices were organized the way they were in the field, this section serves as prelude to the two longer and more empirically detailed chapters that follow.

My three clinical field sites had many structural similarities: location in big Western European cities with diverse populations (large homosexual communities and Muslim communities as potential clients/patients, for instance); opening in the early noughties; patients/clients who paid for treatment themselves (because sperm donation does not fall under the German national insurance coverage and because the British Largecity Fertility Hospital was a private clinic);[2] ISO 9001 accreditation (ensuring similarities in quality management protocols and—at least in theory—practices), similar numbers of active sperm donors (roughly around 150 for every clinic)[3]; and explicit targeting of lesbians by two (Sperm Bank

2 In Britain, gamete donation is both available from NHS clinics and from private clinics, with the extremely long NHS waiting lists in this sector and past difficulties for lesbians and single women to access (more below) producing a push towards private clinics.

3 Active sperm donors are those involved in clinical donation cycles (more about the detailed workings of sperm banks in section 5.2). 150 is only a rough estimate given that clinics monitored their stock differently, had sperm donors donate in different

Friedhausen in Germany and the British field site) of the three clinics. On the other hand, one stark contrast was of course that none of the German clinics were performing treatments with donated eggs, while the British clinic did. The numbers of personnel employed by the three clinics also varied considerably, as will become clear in the more detailed site-descriptions below.

The Sperm Bank Friedhausen was the first I visited for my research. It was the only sperm bank I came into contact with during fieldwork that was neither operationally nor economically associated with a classical, i.e. mostly gynecologically focused, fertility clinic. It was owned and managed by Dr. Dettmaringen, an endocrinologist with his practice next door. It could be found in one of the poorer districts of the large German city Großstadt, among shops selling car and motorbike components, Turkish fast-food joints, and small betting agencies. At the time of my fieldwork it was one of two larger sperm banks in the Großstadt area. Inseminations were not performed in Dr. Dettmaringen's endocrinology practice. Instead his sperm bank cooperated with gynecologists in Großstadt, but also throughout Germany, who were sent the sperm samples and performed the inseminations. Dr. Dettmaringen usually employed eight laboratory assistants and receptionists.

By selling sperm to them and providing information on cooperating gynecologists, it was notable that the Sperm Bank Friedhausen treated unmarried couples, lesbian couples (married or unmarried) and single women. This was the case even though the German Medical Association has always advised against such practices in their professional guidelines (Bundesärztekammer, 2006). A violation of these guidelines may in principle result in the associated State Chamber of Physicians revoking the treatment license, as already elaborated on in chapter 2. Dr. Dettmaringen however explained that there was an unofficial agreement with the Großstadt State Chamber of Physicians that they would not follow up breaches of the guidelines in that area. He also never failed to underline when being interviewed by my colleagues and me that according to his

frequencies, and stored the frozen sperm (resulting in many more donors than the 150 *active* donors being registered with the clinic). Semen quantity also varies between men and also between different ejaculations, leading to fluctuating numbers of actual frozen samples.

and his legal advisor's interpretation of the regulatory situation, he could not be prosecuted, because he was only *selling* sperm, not performing the inseminations.

During formal and informal interview situations, Dr. Dettmaringen frequently referred to his interpretation of legal rules supporting his practices, although these interpretations did not seem to be shared by most of his colleagues in the German fertility sector. He, for instance, invoked the fairly new German Antidiscrimination Law, to explain why he was not refusing any groups as donors (homosexuals as a so-called risk group) or clients (unmarried heterosexual couples, lesbians, singles)—although there was no precedent case suggesting that the law would apply to such areas. He also downplayed the importance of the EU Tissue directive with its longer documentation period for questions of non-anonymous or anonymous donation practices and—as mentioned in chapter 2—put forward his creative interpretation that the "right-to-know one's parentage" is guaranteed in the German constitution since 1949, which is not the case.

Operating since 2000, Dr. Dettmaringen had never been asked to give out identifying information on donors but interpreted the treating gynecologists as in charge of potentially making this data available (see 5.3), although also storing it himself. The non-binding guidelines of the small German professional association of sperm bank operators of which he was a member, however, state that the storage of identifying donor-data lies solely in the obligation of the sperm banks (Arbeitsgruppe Richtliniennovellierung 2006, 18). The guidelines of the German Medical Association in contrast locate this responsibility mainly with the gynecologist (Bundesärztekammer 2006, A1398).

My second German field site, the Sperm Bank Luisenburg, was associated with a gynecological surgery, the Luisenburg Fertility Clinic. It was located in a very expensive neighborhood close to Großstadt's tourist attractions. Sperm Bank and surgery were run by gynecologist Dr. Lindemann during the time of my fieldwork. He owned the gynecological unit together with a second physician and was the sole owner of the sperm bank. The overall clinic employed three senior biologists to manage the sperm bank and the IVF laboratory and a fluctuating number of around six laboratory assistants, plus additional physician's assistants and receptionists. The clinic was catering to a more upmarket clientele than the endocrinological practice of Dr. Dettmaringen, with far more capital invested in the glossy exteriors of the clinic and offering many more services not covered by insurance or covered only partly. It could also refer to more prestigious contacts, because Dr. Lindemann and his partner had both previously held senior positions in a well-known German university hospital.

The Sperm Bank Luisenburg had also treated lesbian couples for a short period of time in the past. Dr. Lindemann had interpreted the previous guidelines of the German Medical Association as outdated. However, the Luisenburg clinic stopped treating lesbians when the updated guidelines of the Medical Association continued to advise against the treatment of single women and lesbians. In contrast to Dr. Dettmaringen, the Luisenburg personnel did not seem to know of the consensus in the State Chamber of Physicians not to prosecute license-violations or found this information unreliable. The sperm bank manager at Luisenburg actually repeatedly expressed regret towards me about not being able to treat homosexual women. It did not fall into her scope of work to make decisions to simply ignore the Medical Association as was done by Dr. Dettmaringen at the other sperm bank. This would have been her boss' decision. Nevertheless, I was surprised that she did not even seem aware that Dr. Dettmaringen's sperm bank 3 kilometers away treated lesbians; she advised lesbians seeking assisted conception to travel abroad—while at the same time conveying how sad she found this. Furthermore, in contrast to Dr. Dettmaringen's judgment that it was the gynecologists in charge of securing donor-data for children-by-donation, which led him to give the parents sealed envelopes with identifying donor-data (see 5.3), the Sperm Bank Luisenburg instead expected that the clinic was in principle itself in charge of donor information. They had however not developed protocols on how to react to potential requests, although the vague German regulations on donor non-anonymity could actually be read to apply retrospectively and also to persons younger than 18. (In the absence of previous regulation, current German law does not actually clarify its status concerning children conceived *before* the 2007 regulations ended the de-facto anonymity, nor does it indeed clarify the legitimate age for accessing data (GewebeG 2007, §14(3)). The non-binding guidelines of the association of sperm bank operators also mention the possibility that access might be sought before turning 18 in "individual cases for the well-being of the child [my translation]" (Arbeitsgruppe Richtliniennovellierung 2006, 18)). This meant that theoretically requests could arise any day, as opposed to the British situation where the revocation of donor-anonymity only applied to subsequent donations.

My interpretation of why there were such pronounced differences between two clinics in the same German city was that the under-regulation of sperm donation in Germany made its clinical management highly idiosyncratic. The rules of what happened "on the shop floor of social life" (Griffiths 2003) were, much more than in Britain, determined by the physicians'—differing—interpretations (personally or through their local legal advisors or cooperating solicitors) of the legal grey areas within which their work took place and, more importantly, of which professional networks they were part. Dr. Dettmaringen, for instance was strongly involved with gay rights activists and their legal networks. He was openly advertising his services at local information meetings of a state funded gay rights association, which supports so-called rainbow-families. These networks, as he framed it to me, also extended into the Großstadt State Chamber of Physicians where many of its apparently large group of homosexual members were not fond of the guidelines put in place through its more conservative counterpart on the state level—or so I was told. The personnel of the Sperm Bank Luisenburg, on the other hand, seemed to be excluded from such informal ways-of-knowing and stressed that it was too high a professional risk to violate the guidelines.

My British field site, the Largecity Fertility Hospital (LFH) was operating two separate sperm banks: one in-house, and an external one under a separate HFEA license, in a separate building across the street. Quite similar to the second German field site, it was located in an upmarket neighborhood close to many of the tourist sites of Largecity. The second sperm bank had been bought by the large LFH enterprise less than a year before my fieldwork visits started and was only gradually synchronizing its workflows with the other clinic. In fact, at the time of my fieldwork it still had two different webpages online and they were not connected to or using the other sperm bank's comprehensive clinical data management software. The original staff from before the acquisition was still in place during my fieldwork. The overall clinic did not only offer DI and IVF/

ICSI to its patients/clients, but also IVF treatment with donated eggs in so-called egg share agreements. During egg-sharing, price discounts are offered to women in IVF treatment who donate some of their eggs to other women. The treatment practice has spurred controversial discussions in Britain (e.g. see Haimes et al. 2012), but is fully legal and covered in detail under the HFEA Code of practice (HFEA 2009a, Section 12).

The British field site was a private clinic, even more upmarket than the German Sperm Bank Luisenburg, with its flat screen-lined waiting room and two other units in other British cities. Having two additional branches in Britain, it could fall back on a much larger central administrative division than the two German clinics. It had staff solely in charge of public relations work, the publishing of their in-house magazine and the running of various PR events over the year. At the time of my fieldwork five senior embryologists and biologists were involved in running the laboratories with a large fluctuating number of assistants. The British field site also had a history and presence of celebrity clients, as one of the head nurses both secretively and proudly indicated to me. It explicitly targeted the lesbian community in Largecity and all over Britain, and had already done so from its establishment in 2003 onwards, when lesbians were still mostly excluded from NHS treatments (until 2008). The clinic cooperated with gay-rights groups, like Dr. Dettmaringen's sperm bank in Germany. It prided itself in running one of the biggest sperm banks in the country (the two units were newly advertised as one sperm bank to potential clients). Similar to the Sperm Bank Friedhausen in the German situation, the center benefited economically from the past discrimination of lesbians and single women through the NHS and its long waiting lists[4] and offered an attractive alternative.

According to British Olivia Montuschi, who was involved as an interest group manager, a DI policy expert, and a concerned mother as well (more on her work in 6.1), the Largecity Fertility Hospital, together with

4 Section 13 of the original British HFE Act of 1990 was interpreted by many NHS clinics to ban the treatment of single women or lesbian couples. It stated that securing the welfare of a child included "the need for a father". The amended HFE Act of 2008 (Part I, Section 24) instead speaks of "supportive parenting". The amended Act also introduces comprehensive new regulations on the legal status of lesbian partners of women undergoing treatment (Part II, Section 42–47). For an overview of the British regulatory proceedings in this field e.g. see Gamble and Ghevaert 2009.

one other big hospital in the North, was the only British clinic, which promptly reacted to the British changes to non-anonymity (see section 2.1) through changing their recruitment and administrative procedures. Nevertheless, the clinic was still forced to stop selling sperm to other clinics until 2011 in order to build up its own stock under the new regulations again. At the time of my fieldwork only the in-house sperm bank was actually working with clients/patients and performing so-called matchings. The outsourced sperm bank was only recruiting new donors and registering old donors under the new regulations.

Montuschi first brought to my attention the view that the widely reported sperm donor shortage in the UK soon after the move to non-anonymity (e.g. Woolf 2006), which the media and some clinics attributed to the legal change, should instead be attributed mainly to the clinics' own (mis-)management:

Olivia Montuschi: "The truth is that the vast majority of clinics *prior* to the ending of donor anonymity, started to run their services down, because they believed, without any research whatsoever, that they would not be able to recruit identifiable donors."

This, according to Montuschi, and supported by recent HFEA statistics, actually led many NHS units to lose the financial support of their local funders. Donors were put off by conflicting information about the legal situation being provided by the clinics themselves.[5] The owner and manager of my British field site, Dr. Steven O'Brien, had, like the leaders of the German Luisenburg Clinic, previously worked in a prestigious university hospital, and had not been supportive of the changes to non-anonymity. In fact, he had repeatedly appeared in the national press with public statements against the policy. He argued it was both clinically impracticable and potentially socially disruptive. Montuschi mildly critically mentioned that given Dr. O'Brien's public criticism of the change to non-anonymity, the quick adaptation of their services to the new situation was purely out of "commercial interests". (She thereby implied that the clinic

5 The HFEA (2011b) has recently released numbers, which seem to support Montuschi's view: they show that there has been no drop in sperm donor registrations after the move to non-anonymity; they actually have increased. This makes it likely that the purported British "sperm donor shortage" (e.g. Woolf 2006) has been a media hype and clinical delays were rather due to the reasons brought forward by Montuschi.

did not share the social/ethical concerns of the Donor Conception Network). Dr. O'Brien told me informally that he simply "got it wrong" at the time, shrugging his shoulders, and now seemed to be both economically satisfied with the regulatory situation and personally supportive of non-anonymity.[6]

In contrast to the highly diverse interpretation of regulation observable in the German field sites, all questions pertaining to why things were done the way they were in the two sperm banks and in the egg donation unit of my British Clinic led to one answer: because of the HFEA. The agency's meticulous Code of Practice (HFEA 2009a) actually lays down detailed interpretations of all legal rules and regulations applying to a sperm bank and fertility clinic. In fact, whenever I told the personnel at the British clinic, be it an embryologist, a sperm bank manager, an "ova coordination nurse" or a laboratory assistant, that I was eager to learn more about their workflows, they firstly handed over the Code of Practice as a thick almost 300 page print-out, signaling that, in their view, I could simply find everything I needed to know there.[7] This made highly diverse interpretations—not unthinkable—but less likely.

At the British field site the HFEA was a unit producing both shock and awe. Head-nurse and egg donation coordinator Maggy Riley, for instance, joked she did not want to be responsible for reports to the HFEA, because she "did not want to go to jail". Yet she subsequently also put forward that the detailed guidelines were sometimes very helpful. They "make things

6 The ideological currents at work in the different clinics are of course not easy to grasp and assess—and different motivations are also so entangled that it would not make sense to artificially "disentangle" them. It was my impression, for instance, that Dr. Dettmaringen's interests in homosexual clients was similarly commercially motivated just as much as a personal interest in gay-rights might also have played a role. What struck me equally about the British field site and Dr. Dettmaringen's clinic was that both clinic owners themselves seemed to like to downplay the commercial aspect of targeting the gay communities of Largecity and Großstadt and to instead underline the emancipatory aspects of this orientation.

7 I did not get the impression that this was done, because the personnel mistook me for an auditor whom they wanted to show that they were indeed only following the binding guidelines. Open criticism of the guidelines and the HFEA were common, as touched upon below. Further, I was told about delicate details of their work, such as gossip about colleagues, patients, and donors not to be repeated here, which the personnel probably would not have shared with someone perceived to be controlling regulatory compliance.

easier, because they lay it all out for one" and the contact to the HFEA inspectors was actually quite good. Largecity sperm bank manager Rose Daffyd said to me that it often seemed to her that the HFEA paperwork was not geared towards the practicalities of their everyday work, because it was set up by "civil servants, not scientists". However, she and a colleague later added that the HFEA was not "as daunting anymore as it used to be", that problems in the required workflows "seemed to iron themselves out" and the continuous close contact with the HFEA through the individually assigned inspectors helped to voice specific concerns. Failures in compliance were reported on the HFEA website and frequently reported on in the British press, including one incident pertaining to my British field site, where a mistake in certain testing procedures had been made. Repeated violations of the code would lead to the revocation of the treatment license. This was the reason why the Largecity Fertility Hospital management was actually happy to have one of the sperm banks running under separate license, as I was told by senior personnel. This was diverting "danger". In the medium term management was looking into establishing a separation between the gynecological patient-oriented unit and the one dealing with sperm donors and samples. Any mistakes made in the latter unit could not then fall back on the former, in terms of HFEA proceedings.

Every HFEA licensed unit also needed to appoint an HFEA reporter to make sure every client, donor, and treatment detail was registered with the watchdog organization and any future changes in guidelines carefully followed. For this, HFEA document templates needed to be used. Those were filled out and transmitted to the HFEA headquarters in London via Electronic Data Interchange (EDI), a standardized system for exchanging formatted messages and particularly widely used within international trade (more on the documents in section 5.2 and 5.3).

In the absence of any such tight regime in Germany, the EU Tissue Directive and its German implementation, the Tissue Law (German Government 2007), were able to develop into a powerful regulatory force at my German field sites (see section 2.1). In Britain the EU directive was viewed as "just another highly technical and expensive quality management system", along with ISO standards and the firm HFEA controls, as Dr. O'Brien commented to me. In Germany, the Tissue Directive's detailed laboratory and documentation protocols produced reactions similar to the ones I observed concerning the HFEA: disbelief and a calling-into-question of its applicability and usefulness to everyday workflows in the clinic, but also compliance. The lab assistants at Dr. Dettmaringen's Sperm Bank Friedhausen, for instance, joked about the new requirement to label the specimens they send out to gynecologists as "non-hazardous", because it would have made more sense to them that anything not labeled "hazardous", well, simply was not.

Since the EU Tissue Directive made the implementation of a quality management (QM) system mandatory, and the ISO 9001 standard was one of the industrial standards guaranteed to comply with the Directive, both of my German field sites combined the adjustments to the new legislation with getting ISO accredited. The British Largecity Fertility Hospital was accredited under the same standard (as the EU Tissue Directive also applies to Britain) as well as the British HFE Act, which requires treatment license holders to have a QM system in place. The HFEA Code of Practice in fact references the International Organization for Standardization (which accredits ISO) for further guidance (HFEA 2009a, section 23). The ISO-accreditation of the field sites led them to have similar protocols for documentation and internal audit procedures in place.

While the HFEA Code of Practice follows yet another standard, the "Clear English Standard" awarded by the "Plain Language Commission" (HFEA 2009a, 1) and thereby actually making a fairly straight-forward read (also for the German anthropologist), the situation was different in Germany. Both of my German field sites relied most heavily on privately contracted medical consultants to translate both the requirements of the new legislation and the ISO accreditation into understandable German and new idiosyncratic protocols. (I was told repeatedly by managing personnel holding PhDs that they were not able to understand the requirements). Additional interpretations of the new requirements of the Tissue Directive were provided through the medical professional associations, not only the German Medical Association, but also the smaller associations of specialists. However, the personnel of both clinics referred more often to the advice they got from their consultants than to that provided through the publications and newsletters of the associations.

Drawing this background-subchapter to a close and before turning to a more detailed analysis of clinical and institutional practices of knowledge-management in the next two subchapters, my above analysis has made visible how the clinical constitution of kinship-by-donation is embedded into two different modes of governance in Britain and in Germany: a minimal approach in Germany, and a tight approach in Britain. Practices in Germany were more idiosyncratic, and bound up with local interpretations through privately contracted consultants and professional networks. In contrast at the British field site the HFEA was persistently invoked into practices on the shop floor: through detailed existing guidelines, audits, and reviews within their framework of evidenced based policy-making (see 2.1). The agency served as "conveyor belt" between law and local practice and was thus part of what Miller and Rose (2008) have identified as "government at a distance", a mode of governance that is particularly acute in the UK. Miller and Rose's concept, which fuses perspectives from Foucault's (e.g. 2000) governmentality studies with Callon's (e.g. 1999) and Latour's (e.g. 2005) concept of mediated action within an effective actor network, underlines how governance in advanced neoliberal societies works through a diffusion of structures of accountability and calculation often falling outside the realm of classically conceived politics. (For ethnographic exploration of the thereby emerging "audit cultures" see Strathern (2000)). Their concept does not map onto my findings pertaining to the German field sites. The "hands-off" minimal approach to governance in Germany, marked by the absence of comparable audit measures or an agency similar to the HFEA, actually appeared more classically liberal: physicians were largely self-regulating (also see 2.1) and their privately contracted consultants were less clearly linked to governance. What became discernible was that both field sites were becoming part of a "global assemblage" (e.g. Collier 2006) of transnational standards and regulations, through ISO and the implementation of the EU Tissue Directive. The differing national modes of governance in both countries however meant that these aspects of transnationalization were becoming effectual quite differently. This subchapter has provided a first glimpse of how the clinical constitution of kinship-by-donation is actually interlinked with national modes of governance. This means that parts of these modes of governance, in the shape of administrative procedures and infrastructures, become part of the relations arising out of reproduction—as explored below.

5.2 The Medical Trajectory of Knowing Kinship-by-Donation: The WHO standard, Viruses, and Excel Sheets

Kinship-by-donation is unique in how comprehensively it relates to clinical infrastructures, and scientific standards. When analyzing its clinical constitution one also has to take into account viruses, freezing abilities of sperm, World Heath Organisation guidelines, eye-color classifications and Excel lists, to name only a few actors. Typically, those are neither considered part of kinship, nor are they made accessible to parents or children. However, I am going to show in this subchapter how scientific standards, information infrastructures, regulation, equipment, biological substances and an actual or anticipated parental knowledge-management are all part of the step-by-step socio-material constitution of kinship-by-donation. Hence, these aspects become part of the relations arising out of reproduction. And this also means, as I will demonstrate, that clinical and parental knowledge-management becomes part of the physical constitution of the children born through the procedures.

How these different aspects become part of kinship follows different logics during different working stages at the fertility clinics, as will be comprehensively analyzed in this chapter. Dominant logic at early working stages would for example be *inclusion* or *exclusion* of only certain donors and recipients on the basis of criteria ranging from whether sperm is materially configured in the way it copes with cryoconservation, to whether patients and donors are openly gay or not. Or, at other working stages, the logic to be found is one of *translation* (Callon 1999) of various *articulations* (Latour 2004) into clinical infrastructures, for instance when only certain classifications are made available to describe the appearance of the donor. And on the basis of such newly set-up ways of knowing, *connections* are made between donors and recipients, which means that quite diverse "matters" are in a sense entering the relations arising out of reproduction: for instance both the stolidity of an excel sheet enabling connections between donor and recipient only to be made in a certain way, and parental preferences for a certain hair-color, become physically incorporated in the children born.

To make this argument I will draw on Latour, who has described step-by-step processes of socio-material articulation within scientific practices as a "chain of transformations" (e.g. 1999, 70). The dynamic Latour describes is one of circulating reference from matter to form and vice versa (1999, 69). As mentioned in chapter 2, I am using the term *articulate* (Latour 2004) to analyze the interplay of "matters" in making knowledge, more precisely kinship knowledge. I am using the term *translation* inspired by Callon (1999) to refer to those appropriations, transformations, and reinterpretations taking place when such clinical articulations are put into new formats and relations within clinical documentation. Within the clinics I studied, such transformations form specific *trajectories of knowing* in Barth's (2002) sense, with kinship-by-donation "at each step losing some properties to gain others" and being made compatible with and thereby connected to what Latour calls "already-established centers of calculation", i.e. laboratories and their established practices (1999, 71–72). Because I was studying standard medical practices, instead of scientific research, the transformations taking place not only established connections and compatibility to laboratory practices, but also to centers of regulation and standardization, for example the HFEA in Britain or the WHO and their standards on sperm quality.

This section thus analyzes how only certain donors and certain patients/clients are accepted; how their bodies are articulated in specific ways, their procreative substances, too; how these articulations are translated into information infrastructures, thereby evidently transformed, and how these infrastructures are then used to assign a donor to a patient/client, following specific ideas—along with technical and material affordances—of how donor assignment should or could be done. I am going to call this first trajectory of knowledge practices *medical trajectory*. While discussing it I shall jump back and forth between a schematized typical version of this trajectory in a sperm bank, which traces the similarities between all different field sites, and a detailed discussion of the local, national, and egg donation-related specificities. I start with briefly describing how sperm banks typically work and which crucial working-stages they were following in their knowledge-management. I shall then move through a detailed analysis of each working stage.

As schematically depicted in figure 5.1, all sperm banks I came into contact with during my fieldwork more or less followed a similar routine, structured through what I classified as different working stages, following

Figure 5.1: How sperm banks work

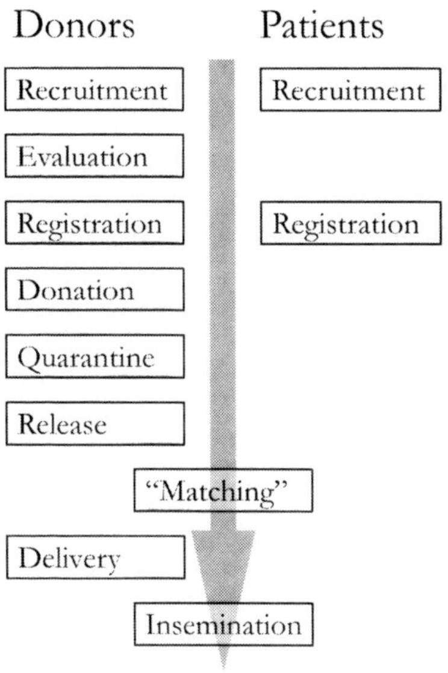

Donors | Patients

Recruitment | Recruitment

Evaluation

Registration | Registration

Donation

Quarantine

Release

"Matching"

Delivery

Insemination

different practical logics. Donors needed to be recruited and were then asked to come in for a first evaluation, during which a first trial-donation was made; if determined suitable, the prospective donor was asked to come back for further medical tests. If the donor was then accepted, he registered with the clinic. Then a round of donation started during which he typically donated once or twice a week for a specific amount of time, usually in intervals of several subsequent weeks. The sperm was cryoconserved, i.e. frozen to sub-zero temperatures, and stored in small vials in liquid nitrogen containers. Then it just sat there during a six month quarantine period. To release the samples from quarantine the donor was required to come back for tests again.

Patients/clients also needed to be attracted, accepted as clients and registered at the clinic. Then the so-called matching with recipients would be performed and the frozen sperm delivered to wherever the de-freezing and insemination would take place. As depicted in figure 5.2, what I came to call the medical trajectory of knowing kinship-by-donation was typically characterized through interlinked articulations at every working-stage of different socio-material aspects of donor and patient/client. At each temporal working-stage either new aspects were articulated or the documented outcomes of the last working-stage were used as basis for further articulations.

Figure 5.2: The typical medical trajectory of knowing kinship-by-donation in a sperm bank

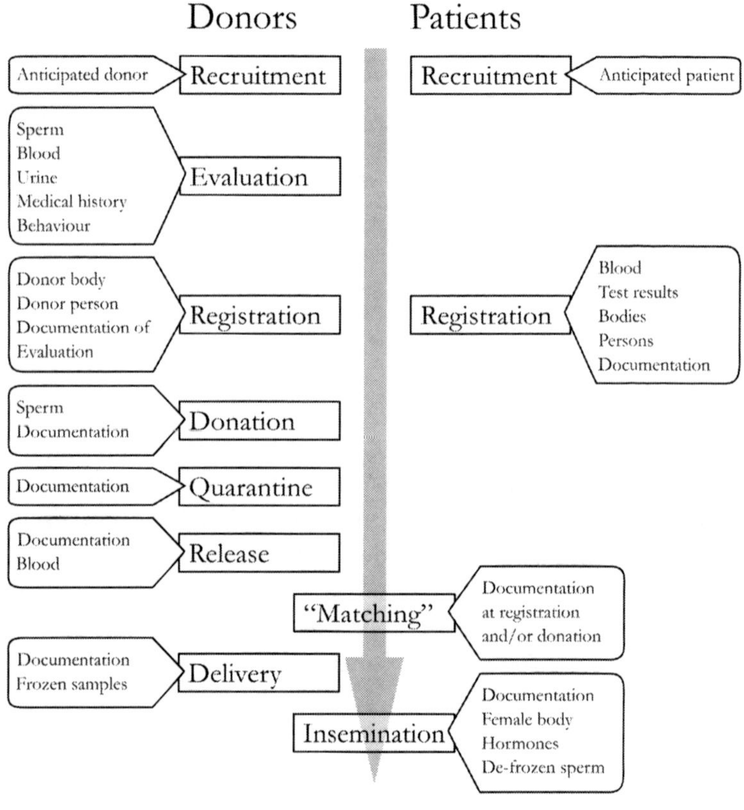

Recruitment Phase: Knowing Kinship through Prospective Donors and Patients/Clients

During the recruitment phase kinship-by-donation in the clinic was typically known through the prospective donor and (although slightly less in need of being actively sought for) the prospective patient/client: the target groups, so to speak. In this subsection I provide contextual information on why only certain donors and certain patients were targeted, while turning towards a more analytic discussion in the following subsections. I will argue that the recruitment phase determined who would actually present and/or be accepted at the clinic based on differing economic considerations, differing interpretations of what a risk-group is (e.g. homosexuals or the practitioners of unsafe sex), differing advertisement strategies, the marketing of DI as a "technology of the last resort" to heterosexual couples, and either specific targeting or exclusion of lesbian couples and single women from treatment.

At the two German field sites, the prospective donor was only a vague image: "fitness" was after all determined by various articulations during the subsequent evaluation phase. In both German sperm banks I was also told that they had no difficulties recruiting donors. This was probably because it is not illegal to pay for sperm donations in Germany. The sums rewarded, however, were not large in both clinics. And it was not "fast money" either, because part of the compensation was only paid after the donor had come back for his tests at the end of the quarantine phase. (At the Sperm Bank Friedhausen, for instance, a donor walked away with between 300–500 Euros of compensation for a round of six donations over six weeks when passing the six month quarantine phase successfully). The vague image of a prospective donor at both German clinics, as presented on their quite simple websites or relayed to me during fieldwork, was a young man (between 18 and 38 in Luisenburg and 18 and 40 in Friedhausen) with a healthy lifestyle (no drugs, no unsafe sex), no hereditary diseases, an interest in earning some money on the side, and a certain carelessness about legal uncertainties (because of his unclear legal connections to children born through these procedures).

Dr. Dettmaringen of the Sperm Bank Friedhausen did not follow any particularly planned or organized advertisement campaign to recruit these prospective donors: beyond the description on their website, Dr. Dettmaringen placed appeals for sperm donors within the classifieds section of Großstadt city magazines and newspapers. There was no reference to the prospective donor's sexual orientation in these appeals, and it was not asked about later. Dr. Lindemann of the Sperm Bank

Luisenburg had commissioned a small advertisement firm to place more risqué adverts in the subway and on Großstadt advertising columns, using the *double entendre* of the term "coming" (which exists in German just as in English). On his website, which briefly described the donors looked for, he explicitly stated that homosexual donors would be excluded along with other "so-called risk groups" (drug users and practitioners of unsafe sex). Dr. Lindemann said in an interview that he was aware that gay men found this discriminatory, but "as long as there was a higher incidence of AIDS among gay men", he would not change this recruitment strategy.

Altruism was not expected of the prospective donor in Germany, as both managers matter-of-factly stated. It was also not addressed in the advertisements. Asked to quantify if indeed all of his donors donated for financial reasons, Dr. Lindemann explained: "90 to 95 percent of the donors come for the money anyway. The last five percent have somehow come in contact with the topic of infertility and now want to help. They come for altruistic reasons". And Dr. Dettmaringen also said: "our donors come for financial reasons" (see chapter 7.1 for brief analysis of this from the parent's perspective).

At the time of my fieldwork — although this has subsequently changed[8]— sperm donations and egg donations were not paid for at all in Britain, because the HFE Act (e.g. in section 12(1)) outlawed this.[9] Not being able to draw on financial motivations for donor recruitment, the two sperm banks had to advertise quite heavily for donors. During my fieldwork they were looking to build-up their stock to start selling sperm again to other clinics, as they had done before the move to non-anonymity. By incorporating the additional recently bought sperm bank they were following an expansive goal and putting much weight on the recruitment of new donors and on previous donors coming back to clear their donations under the non-anonymous set-up. The prospective donors were specified on their website as having to be between 18 and 41,

8 After my fieldwork the HFEA has changed its guidance regarding donor compensation in autumn 2011 and is now allowing for higher and fixed compensations of 35 British Pounds per visit for sperm donors and 750 British Pounds per cycle for egg donors (HFEA 2011c), which comes quite close to the German payments.

9 Travel expenses and loss of earnings granted in the Largecity Fertility Hospital and its sperm banks were controlled by pay-slip and receipts, so not even small amounts of money were to be made.

"healthy", and not engaging in unprotected casual sex or drug use. Their large poster advertising campaign all over Largecity and their separate sperm-donor-only website tried to attract men by combining allusions to alleviating the suffering of infertile couples with allusions to male virility.[10] There was also a section advertising sperm donation to gay men as a possibility to have children. The website had been newly set-up and was far more professional looking (and sounding) than the quite simple looking HTML counterparts at my German field sites: this was using slick Flash animations and designs, and also short and informal explanations of the process of sperm donation. One of the donor recruitment managers told me that they were basically trying to raise as much awareness as possible through their large campaign and that they were hoping for not only students, but also businessmen to become donors. Their website and parts of their campaign were also alluding to a lack of sperm donors being a "British problem", non-existent in Europe or the USA. Hence, the anticipated donor at Largecity was expected to be altruistically motivated, but also someone captured through the allusions to virility and the nation.

Attracting patients/clients at all three field sites was not framed as a problem in interviews with me. The prospective patients/clients at the Sperm Bank Friedhausen in Großstadt and at the British Largecity clinic were characterized by an extreme inclusivity: single women, lesbians, heterosexual couples were all accommodated in the information materials available mainly on the clinic's websites and for Largecity also on glossy leaflets and magazines. The German Sperm Bank Luisenburg was more exclusive by anticipating only heterosexual married couples. At all field sites patients were expected to be affluent enough to pay for the treatment themselves. Roughly put (treatment options and plans were of course highly variable) patients/clients needed to pay 2,000 British Pounds for a three month treatment cycle in Britain, and about 3,000 Euros at the Fertility Clinic Luisenburg or roughly 2,600 Euros at Dr. Dettmaringen's Sperm Bank Friedhausen.

10 Of course, medically speaking, infertility and impotence (and the reverse: particularly good sperm quality—as needed for sperm donors—and potency) have no link. It is ironic that the campaigns to attract donors might be contributing to the perpetuation of this conflation, which is often experienced as quite problematic by affected men (see section 8.5).

One aspect of patient/client recruitment was striking for all three field sites: concerning the recruitment of *heterosexual* patients, kinship-by-donation was known through the anticipated patient/client who had explored *all other means* of repro-technological intervention. Hence, the framing of gamete donation as a "technology of the last resort"—as discussed in section 4.2—was also clearly visible in the clinics. The Largecity Fertility Hospital, for instance, only listed ICSI, *not* DI, on its website as the solution to "severe cases of male infertility". The gynecologists cooperating with the Sperm Bank Friedhausen, as another example, did not present DI as a potential alternative to IVF—but mostly listed unsuccessful IVF as the indication to try DI (see clipping 5.3 below).

Clipping 5.3: Indications for DI (Source: cooperating clinic's website)

Indikation und Eignung zur Samenspende:

- Mangel an Samenzellen beim eigenen Partner
- Erfolglosigkeit der künstlichen Befruchtung mit Samen des Partners
- Vorhandensein von Erbkrankheiten in der Familie des Partners

This clinic cooperating with the Sperm Bank Friedhausen lists on its website "lack of sperm cells of your own partner"; "failure of artificial conception with the semen of the partner"; and the "presence of hereditary diseases in the family of the partner" as indications for the "suitability for donor insemination".

In conclusion, the recruitment phase presented itself as the beginning of the clinical trajectory of knowing and thereby doing kinship-by-donation. Importantly, in Germany donors were paid, and this was expected to be their reasons for becoming donors. Pay for donation also meant that the clinics did not have to run large awareness campaigns to attract altruistic donors. In the UK finding donors was more complicated and more money went into attracting the anticipated altruistic men. None of my field sites presented detailed requirements (beyond being healthy, drug-free, and practicing safer sex) of a donor, except for his age range. Gay men, lesbian couples and single women were excluded from the prospective donors/patients in one German field site (Sperm Bank Friedhausen), while they were clearly part of the anticipations of the other two clinics. Heterosexual couples were not targeted as recipients before having "exhausted" IVF/ICSI. The recruitment phase thus figured as the entrance gate to who would become a donor or a patient/client in the first place.

Economic considerations, differing interpretations of what a risk-group is (e.g. homosexuals or the practitioners of unsafe sex), differing advertisement strategies, the marketing of DI as "technology of the last resort" to heterosexual couples, and either specific targeting or exclusion of lesbian couples and single women from treatment determined who would pass through this gate. It thus already determined a specific configuration of the starting point of the detailed chain of transformations set into motion in the subsequent evaluation phase.

Evaluation phase: Getting to Know Kinship-by-Donation through Sperm, Blood, Urine, Medical History, and Behavior

The evaluation phase began the moment that potential sperm donors first presented themselves at the clinics. Now quite detailed articulations of physical substances were brought into play, but also a few more informal and interactive judgments, to determine whether to accept and register a donor. I shall describe how during this working stage, kinship-by-donation typically became articulated through five different socio-material aspects: sperm, blood, urine, medical history, and behavior of the donor. The logic of these articulations was to a large extent binary: exclude or include on the basis of various internal and external, formal and informal criteria. The evaluation was generally performed in two steps: first sperm would be subjected to quality controls in the laboratory and if the quality was deemed acceptable, all other aspects came to figure —although samples of the different substances may have been taken on the same day. I am going to examine the diverging articulation of these aspects in some detail in the following passages.

For kinship-by-donation to become known via laboratory-driven articulations of sperm (quality), the donor needed to masturbate. Part of clinically *doing* kinship-by-donation was therefore providing a place for the masturbation. While the masturbation rooms were set up to cater to the donors' sexuality through a supply of pornographic materials, sexualized behavior outside of these rooms led to a negative evaluation (as elaborated on below). The sperm samples, ejaculated into labeled plastic cups, were either left in the cubicles or placed on a small counter to the laboratory. Now detached from the donor as a living-and-breathing person, they were analyzed in the laboratory. If the sperm did not meet the sperm bank's or clinic's criteria, the donor was excluded from the evaluation phase right away with none of the other aspects being articulated.

All of my field sites used the WHO (2010) guidelines on sperm quality to determine whether to accept a donor or not. They were required to do a quality test through the HFEA guidelines and the non-binding German professional guidelines. Furthermore, all clinics advertised to patients/clients that only particularly fertile men—according to international standards—were accepted onto their programs. That sperm quality always got reduced through freezing and de-freezing also produced the necessity to find donors with above average semen quality.

The WHO standards are controversial in both their clinical significance and in whether the thereby established threshold for "normal" sperm is too low or too high (e.g. Cooper and et al. 2009) within medical research. However, for the sperm banks the guidelines established an uncontested boundary for acceptance of a donor. The guidelines mainly classify sperm based on its motility, i.e. how it moves in a Petri-dish under the microscope; its morphology, i.e. how it looks in a Petri-dish under the microscope, and its concentration. This means that the laboratory personnel determined sperm quality, roughly summarized, through looking, counting, and comparing to the standard figures, using a microscope.

A second test performed in all field sites determined how the sperm (if it passed the WHO criteria) reacted to freezing and thawing. This was done, because, for reasons not fully understood, as I was told by the laboratory personnel, not all men's sperm tolerates cryoconservation. This meant that after de-freezing, the sperm cells were again counted and measured to protocol and the results compared with the pre-freezing values. How sperm reacts to being frozen to sub-zero temperatures is of course irrelevant for reproduction "in the wild", kinship-by-donation however could only include sperm tolerant to freezing. In other words: only men with sperm possessing this ability could become clinical sperm donors.

In all field sites, the percentage of men whose sperm was deemed to be acceptable after these tests was extremely low, particularly due to bad de-freezing results. At the Sperm Bank Luisenburg, the sperm bank manager Klara Bernisch estimated that it was significantly less than ten percent of all the men they saw who would be asked to come back. At the Sperm

Bank Friedhausen the laboratory assistant in charge of determining sperm quality said that it was "definitely less than twenty, often less than ten percent". In all field sites, the reporting back of exclusionary results from laboratory personnel to potential donors on the telephone always stressed that the combination of the "freezability question" and the high quality standards implied that even if a man was not suitable as a donor, he did not have a fertility problem.

Blood, as the classical substance through which kinship has often been known, also played a prominent role during the evaluation phase. At the clinics and during the specific working stage of donor evaluation, the blood samples were used to find out about the presence of bacteria, viruses, chromosomes, proteins, blood cells, enzymes and mutated genetic sequences—but not in the same way nor necessarily similarly comprehensive in all field sites. Since the blood samples were being analyzed anyhow, blood group and rhesus-factor were also determined, even though this would only become relevant information should a donor pass the evaluation phase.

At the Sperm Bank Friedhausen, genetic considerations—broadly speaking—did not feed into the articulation of the blood sample at all. The tests performed were only meant to find out about the presence of viruses (HIV, CMV, Hepatitis viruses and, if travel to regions with a high prevalence had occurred, also the HTL-viruses), bacteria (treponema pallidum, which causes syphilis) and—also only related to travel—the parasites causing malaria and chagas disease. (In this testing regime, the clinic quite idiosyncratically followed a mix of non-binding professional guidelines and their own considerations, for instance adding the test for parasites, but leaving out a recommended karyogram).

Only the presence of antibodies to the cytomegalovirus (CMV) was tolerated, i.e. documented and not used as grounds for exclusion, which also held for the other German clinic. A vast majority of women and men in the so-called Western world carry antibodies to this member of the herpes virus family, because they came into contact with it at some point, but most often suffered no symptoms (e.g. Elliott 2011). The virus tends to remain latent in the body. It could theoretically be transmitted during sperm or egg donation, although the risk is small and that of an infection breaking out and spreading to a potential embryo even smaller (e.g. Liesnard et al. 1998). Pregnant women with no antibodies themselves, can pass it on to the foetus, when contracting the virus. This can lead to congenital abnormalities, as is also known for rubella. Although all clinicians I spoke to found the risk of this happening absurdly small, my German research partners still followed the Medical Association's guidelines (Bundesärztekammer 2006, 1397) to base their matching procedures on the CMV antibody status of donor and recipient, as elaborated below. This had been a previous requirement in HFEA guidelines in Britain as well, but in the HFEA's dynamic and processual approach to regulation had been revoked again, as embryologist Keira Lorimer from my British field site told me.

The Sperm Bank Luisenburg mainly used blood to find out about possible infections but also performed a karyotype from a white blood cell. This cytogenetic articulation then did not articulate kinship-by-donation via blood as the material carrier of harmful organisms, but via chromosomes—which should be present in the right number and shape. Generally, no molecular genetic or blood-chemical options to make articulations about genetic diseases were used in the two German sperm banks, as would have been done to test for cystic fibrosis or thalassemia carrier status. And the German Working Party for Donor insemination actually states in its guidelines—without further explanation —that such articulations would "generally be not performed on donors" (Arbeitsgruppe Richtliniennovellierung 2006, 27, my translation), even though a couple would have the option to ask for additional tests.

However, at the British Largecity Fertility Hospital Sperm Bank, in addition to the same considerations of bacteria and viruses and chromosomes, blood was used as the first step in an interlinked trajectory to inquire into kinship-by-donation contributing to a genetic disease, although this is not mandatory according to HFEA guidelines. Every blood sample, or rather once again another substance being articulated via the blood sample (and interlinked techniques and materials such as Polymerase-Chain-Reaction and specific membranes)—DNA—was screened for some of the known and common genetic mutations on chromosome seven associated with cystic fibrosis. Other techniques not interrogating molecules but enzymes and blood cells were used to find out about thalassemia, sickle-cell anemia, and Tay Sachs, which are all recessive genetic disorders. However, this was only done if the sperm bank staff decided that it should be, based on what they had been taught about the correlation between ethnic groups (more discussion below) and certain diseases—such as the prevalence of Tay Sachs in Jewish communities of Eastern European origin.

Urine was the next aspect articulated during the evaluation phase: at all field sites urine was used to find out about the presence of chlamydia bacteria. Furthermore, there were also two more ambiguous socio-material aspects articulated to determine if a donor would be registered or not: the *donor's behavior* in informal interaction and his so-called *medical history.* When evaluating the suitability of the donor via his behavior, the laboratory personnel employed their own experiential knowledge of whether someone fit in. What the—mostly female—laboratory personnel of all field sites (embryologists, biologists, medical scientists and laboratory assistants) typically expected from a donor could be broadly summarized as reliability (making it to appointments, coming back for further tests etc., answering questions honestly, listening to their clarifications) and integration (into their workflows, but also into their individual regimes of dealing with the sometimes sexual nature of their jobs). When I asked Klara Bernisch, the manager of the Sperm Bank Friedhausen, how the donor evaluation worked by asking her to explain how someone becomes a donor, she—unprompted—added in the end:

> Klara Bernisch: "There is also... There is something of a common sense [Allgemeinerfahrung] in dealing with people. You can recognize if someone is completely out of it, we will not accept him then, no matter what he fills out in the forms, you know. There has to be a social qualification [soziale Eignung], but that you just assess through an indirect evaluation of the person. So not by concretely letting them prove something: But how does someone behave? How reliably does he stick to our appointment? I mean, can you even talk to him—or not... That already reduces the [options, we both laugh]".

Of course, these intuitions or, the sense of a donor's social qualifications as the manager Bernisch put it quite well, were not communicated back as exclusionary factors to the donor. Her boss elaborated in another interview:

> Dr. Lindemann: "If we find a donor particularly unpleasant, socially, we do not accept him, not because he is unpleasant, but we just say that the sperm quality

is not high enough. That's not really fair, but we just say, the quality is okay, but it is not what we are looking for."

However, it also became clear in the interviews, that this did not happen often and Dr. Lindemann was rather worried that if he applied *all* criteria that from his point of view were theoretically sensible, i.e. criteria concerning medical history *and* behavior (e.g. details of travel, quantification of sexual partners, how often unsafe sex was practiced), then he would be left with virtually no donors.

The personnel of the Sperm Bank Friedhausen did not as often stress unprompted and explicitly how they would not accept someone whom they did not find pleasant (Dr. Lindemann of the Sperm Bank Luisenburg in contrast: "We have our subjective criteria: Is he a nice person or will we only have trouble with him?"), but emphasized that they would not accept "sexualized" donors or donors who interrupted their work-routines. They told me of conversations where donors would go into detail about their sexual life or potency (One of the laboratory assistants, miming: "I always take very looong, and my girlfriend really likes that"), which led them to not further evaluate him. How long someone would take to perform the donation, in other words to ejaculate and leave the masturbation room, was important to them, too. The way they had organized the so called "donor rounds", keeping to a schedule which would stop the waiting room from getting busy and which enabled them to quickly perform all tests and the freezing, depended on a donor not occupying what they called the "men's room" or "masturbatorium" for long. During the donor rounds they booked the donors in one-hour slots for the paperwork and the donation, always accepting two at a time, because of the two masturbation rooms available. I did not get the impression that this approach generally tied in with the personnel being uncomfortable with the necessarily somewhat sexual nature of their job: donors were greeted in a friendly and open way, sometimes with a chat, and questions of a sexual nature were straightforwardly, often humorously asked—and answered. In interviews the personnel also typically stressed that they did not find dealing with the sexuality of the donors unpleasant or embarrassing. They instead stressed how they found the job in a sperm bank quite comfortable, because they had previously held clinical positions were they had more to do with infections, diseases, or excrement.

The personnel of the Largecity Fertility Hospital Sperm Bank was under more pressure than the personnel of the two German sperm banks to be successful in recruiting, given the clear goal of their employer to expand the Largecity Fertility Hospital Sperm Bank into a supplier for other clinics and the need to focus mainly on non-financial motives for donating, instead of being able to draw on either financial or non-financial motives possible in Germany. They were not as pre-emptive in rejecting donors who through their behavior possibly seemed unreliable. Instead, one of the assistants spent most of her time following-up on donors who had missed appointments or had not been in touch for a long time. Rather than making comments like the Friedhausen Sperm Bank manager that a donor should at least be able to "look her in the eyes", the personnel at the British clinic talked about how they were trying not to intimidate, in their view, the often very shy potential donors. Their recruitment officer also, instead of not accepting someone with seeming emotional issues, would send him to a counseling session at the clinic itself. The German clinics in contrast had no system or infrastructure in place to offer counseling to donors: behavior was either acceptable or unacceptable.

The Largecity Fertility Hospital Sperm Bank personnel, similar to the one in Friedhausen, also would not accept donors whose behavior appeared to be "sexualized". The manager of the outsourced Largecity Fertility Hospital Sperm Bank, Rose Daffyd, mentioned to me several times how it made her quite aggressive if donors seemed to be using the sperm bank as grounds for sexual adventures i.e. asking if they could bring girls in or if there would be girls around to "assist". This kind of sexualized behavior was seldom apparent with donors who had already come into the clinic personally, but quite common on the phone—with the demarcation line somewhat unclear between prank phone calls, molestation, and real, but clearly sexual interest in becoming a donor. Daffyd and her colleague in charge of donor-recruitment, quirky young women who laughed a lot in their office, either took it with mild humor when once again someone called and a young voice said that he had "a lot of sperm to offer"—or they more aggressively answered with lines such as "clearly you must have misunderstood what kind of business a sperm bank is". They hung up if they felt like the questions and advances where actually putting their work in line with sex-workers. Daffyd also told me that donors who were very young, only 18 or 19, sometimes—according to her "intuition"—did not "fully grasp what they are doing". But she also did not exclude these donors, as maybe the manager Bernisch at Luisenburg would have done on the grounds of a supposedly not well enough spermiogram; Daffyd would also send them to counseling. At my British field site counseling figured as the most common exclusionary factor for an otherwise acceptable donor. In other words: far lesser donors were discovered to be carriers of genetic diseases or infections and excluded than those excluded because they either did not show up for counseling or were excluded after a session. The personnel at the German field sites referred to unacceptable behavior informally—someone should look one in the eye, not behave strangely sexualized, be pleasant—and did not relate their exclusion of such behavior to heredity. At the British field site senior personnel described the exclusion of donors on the basis of a counseling session as being ambivalently related to inheritance: "if the counselor cannot exclude that there are mental health issues involved, the donor is excluded, who knows what would be passed on" (Dr. Keira Lorimer).

How kinship-by-donation via so-called *medical history* (with its blurred boundaries between someone's personal history of infections and diseases and a whole family's history of infections and diseases) was dealt with involves less translating back and forth between particular standards, regulations and substances than was the case with sperm, blood, and urine in my field sites. The HFEA guidelines specify that the medical history of a donor needs to be recorded in a questionnaire accompanied by a personal interview through a healthcare professional (HFEA 2009a, section 11 (T52a)) and the German Working Party for Donor Insemination states in their non-binding guidelines that to "minimize the risk of a genetic disease through donor insemination [my translation]" a doctor has to go over a potential donor's medical history with him and exclude donors who are carriers or sufferers of genetic diseases (Arbeitsgruppe Richtliniennovellierung 2006, 27). However, as extensively discussed in the critical literature on the "new language" of genetic risk and susceptibility (Rabinow and Rose 2006, 197), who is at risk of what and how is a highly ambiguous and context-dependent category (for further discussion see Featherstone 2006; Konrad 2005b; Novas and Rose 2000). Most common diseases are multifactorial and not monogenetic, after all. This ambiguity led to an articulation of medical history in the clinical setting which hardly ever contributed to the exclusion of a donor.

In the Sperm Bank Friedhausen I got the sense that the donors were not actually known and therefore evaluated and selected through the ambivalent category of medical history in any elaborate sense. It rather seemed to have the status of a legal disclaimer. In this vein, its owner Dr. Dettmaringen repeatedly stressed how one of several donor signatures in the recruitment contract marked that the donor had answered all questions about his medical history and possible hereditary diseases in his family to his best knowledge. Dr. Dettmaringen seemed to be particularly worried about the unclear legal situation concerning the donor evaluation and selection: could he somehow be held accountable if a donor-conceived child turned out to have a genetic disease? He told me that he was convinced that if a donor falsely told him that "his parents had nothing, were healthy—and then it turned out that actually everyone in the family died of lung cancer at 41", the donor—instead of him who would not have registered the donor in the first place had he known about the prevalence of lung cancer—could be held financially responsible when the child developed the same disease.[11] During the time spent in his sperm bank I got the impression from overhearing telephone conversations with potential donors and from what I was told (though I was not present at the actual consultations with a doctor) that donors were very clearly and repeatedly told that if they had knowledge of any diseases running in the family they should not consider becoming donors. This way it was already presumed during the evaluation stage that the donors were neither sufferers nor carriers of genetic diseases. This was asked about again by Dr. Dettmaringen when he saw the donors alone, but only in short and commonsensical seeming fashion, coming down to whether the donor knew of any diseases "clustered" in the family. The donor's answer was recorded by Dr. Dettmaringen in a small section (see clipping 5.4) on hereditary diseases in the donor file, which also recorded any other diseases, medication taken regularly and allergies (to be discussed in more detail below).

11 No such regulation or precedent case is in place in Germany. The British Human Fertilisation and Embryology Act of 1990 (e.g. section 35), however, explicitly makes legally possible such a scenario, because in such a case a donor's (temporary) anonymity could be revoked and the case then further tried under the Congenital Disabilities (Civil Liability) Act 1976.

Clipping 5.4: Medical History at the Sperm Bank Friedhausen (Source: Author/replica)

Medizinische Abklärung durch Befragung des Spenders durch den Arzt

1. Krankheiten: ______
2. Medikamente: ______
3. Allergien: ______
4. Erbkrankheiten: ______

(autosomal rezessive Gene)

This section of the Evaluation sheet states in somewhat wordy German: "Medical Evaluation through questioning of the donor by the physician". Then it lists "1. Diseases, 2. Medication, 3. Allergies, 4. Hereditary diseases (autosomal recessive genes)".

At the other German field site, the "posher" Sperm Bank and Fertility Centre Luisenburg, used a more elaborate questionnaire on medical history during the evaluation phase. The questionnaire also needed to be signed by the donor and therefore also functioned as a legal disclaimer. The form asked if the donor or a family member (specifying even family members up to third cousins) had suffered cancer, hepatitis, "severe" allergies, epilepsy, cystic fibrosis, Down Syndrome, hereditary muscle atrophy, STDs, asthma, rheumatism, mental diseases or mental developmental disorder and miscarriages or stillbirths. However, I was told no donor had ever not passed the evaluation phase just because of his medical history. (The same was the case at the other German field site). Luisenburg manager Bernisch told me that she did go over the medical history questionnaire with the donor. Clinic owner Dr. Lindemann also used the filled-out and signed form during his one-off consultation with the donors.

Usually ignorance of the particular diseases was interpreted as a good sign:

Klara Bernisch: "If someone is from a family with a prevalence of something, he will have more information on those diseases, he will know then, he will be familiar with it."

She also explained that the question about cancer was more a hindrance than leading to any clear evaluation, because "with people growing older and older nowadays" the incidence of cancer was high in any family. Only if several people had died from the same type of cancer, would she assume that there was "a genetic predisposition involved" on which grounds she would theoretically exclude a donor, but never has.

The positive interpretation of lack of knowledge on the donor's side about a particular hereditary disease was also shared among the personnel of the Largecity Fertility Hospital Sperm Bank. In fact, the "ovum donor medical history checklist" (more about the specifics of eggs donation below) given to a potential egg donor and to be signed by her and her GP stated that if a donor "has not heard of" the diseases mentioned, this was "usually a good indication that they do not apply to you."

The (differing) medical history questionnaires used for sperm and egg donors at the Largecity Fertility Hospital were by far more extensive than in the two German field sites. For sperm donors, the sections recording not only a personal history, but also an incidence in the family (thus presupposing a hereditary or parental link) asked about more than 40 dispositions from monogenetic diseases such as Huntington's, to autosomal recessive disorders such as thalassemia, to often gonosomally (i.e. for sperm donors on the Y-Chromosome) transmitted disorders such as hemophilia, to either highly ambiguous or multifactorial conditions and dispositions such as asthma, eczema, autism, hypertension, psychosis, coronary heart disease and speech anomalies. The questionnaire used for egg donors, (to be filled and signed not in the clinic but in the presence of the donor's GP, who also signed as a witness) was even split up according to specific heredity: "A. X-linked disorders, B. Recessive disorders, C. Dominant disorders, D. Genetic familial defect, E. Genetic familial disease", naming 40 dispositions without including infections or multifactorial diseases.

At the two sperm banks of the Largecity Fertility Hospital—in contrast to the practices with egg donors—the medical history evaluation of donors was done in-house. (This was the case because the clinic's egg-sharing scheme, as further discussed below, led to egg donors being highly compliant since they were awaiting treatment themselves, while sperm donors were more likely to "get lost on the way" if they would be sent to their GP to assess their medical history). Kate Clifton, in charge of donor recruitment at the outsourced Largecity Fertility Hospital Sperm Bank, told me that in the five months she had worked at the clinic, she had excluded one donor during the evaluation phase, because two of his closer family members had epilepsy. When the recruiter went over the form with potential donors I had to keep in the background of the surgery to give the donor privacy. I later asked the recruiter to recapitulate how she talked about it with the donors. She explained to me that "basically anything which was clearly hereditary" would be a "factor for exclusion". This also came down to a flagging of conditions strangely "clustered" in the donor's family.

Altogether, while knowing a donor through medical history was more tied into current genetic/genomic discourses in my British field site and in practice this led to a far more complex naming and discussion of potential dispositions than in the German field sites, in terms of actually including or excluding potential donors, a similarly commonsensical approach of simply looking for "unusual" disease clusters in the donor's family prevailed in my British field site just as in my German field sites. And of course the documentation of the consultation also served as a legal disclaimer in Britain, with the HFE Act having established the legal possibility of a disabled child or his parents suing for damages, as explained above.

In summary, during the evaluation-phase kinship-by-donation started to be known through sperm, blood, and urine. It also became known and evaluated through donor-behavior following local and informal criteria for reliability and integration. This meant that the donor's sexuality was only accepted if confined to the masturbation rooms. Kinship-by-donation further became known through the ambiguous genre of medical-history, which established links to genetic/genomic risk discourses more in Britain than in Germany. In all field sites, however, medical history alone was hardly used for exclusion practices. The practical logic dominating this phase was one of binary inclusion or exclusion: specified bacteria, viruses, sperm reacting adversely to cryoconservation or not conforming to the WHO standard, donors from a family with disease "clusters" or an inability to interact with the personnel and contain their sexuality appropriately were all banned from further entering the relations constituting kinship-by-donation—just as openly gay donors and patients/clients were banned at the Sperm Bank Luisenburg.

Registration Phase: Translation into Information-Infrastructures

The dominating logic during the registration phase was not one of inclusion or exclusion, but of *translation*: Now, the accepted donors—or rather various articulations of "him"—were all translated onto information infrastructures of practical and/or legal relevance in the clinics. This entailed setting up patient- and donor-files. Sometimes those files were only brought into being performatively, without any transformations, through simply allocating this status to the already documented articulations of the previous evaluation phase. Additionally, some new articulations took place and some of the documented articulations were used for further enquiry. Concerning the non-acceptable bacteria and viruses, for instance, only the recorded dates of the negative test remained of practical importance now and found their way into the donor-files, because they designated when the next round of tests six months later would have to follow and were needed for legal purposes. Other articulations, such as the cytomegalovirus antibody status, blood type, or rhesus factor of the donor were recorded in those parts of the files subsequently used for the so-called matching.

In all field sites, the label of patient- or donor-file lent a new durability to these ways-of-knowing. They now fell under the regulation for specific documentation.[12] In practice, however, "the files" were often diverse bodies of information, not stored in one single paper wallet or software folder, but in diverse formats and locations. In the Sperm Bank Friedhausen in Großstadt, for example, there were four main media and locations of storage onto which the different aspects relevant for registration became translated: firstly, a paper register, mainly used for legally relevant documentation purposes. Secondly, the donor Excel sheets, which were of major practical importance, because they were the basis for any ensuing matching practices. The Excel file held one spreadsheet for each blood group and then stated the donor's CMV antibody status, his rhesus factor, and some further articulations of the donor to be discussed below. Then there were the so-called donor-files, which were part of a comprehensive clinical management software package, used for bookkeeping, appoint-

12 The EU Tissue Directive makes it mandatory in all field sites that donor and patient records are to be kept for at least 30 years (Tissue and Cells Directive, 2004, Article 8) and storage periods for the HFEA have so-far not been clarified in terms of length and thus theoretically span an expected average life span.

ments, dates of donations, laboratory results regarding sperm quality for each donation given, etc. The donor-files were important during the everyday routines in the sperm bank. The last highly relevant media and location of storage was the so-called tank-register, another Excel file, which recorded the physical location of the stored sperm samples.

In Luisenburg, sperm bank manager Klara Bernisch was mainly working with three different media and places of storage onto which different aspects of knowing kinship-by-donation got translated: one classical paper filing system holding legally relevant information, one new, custom-made clinical filing and management software package, which operated on the basis of a databank, and an index card system—left over from pre-digital times—which additionally recorded all relevant information on an active donor. The clinical software package had been introduced to replace paper filing in Luisenburg, but turned out to be so unstable that instead several parallel filing systems were left running.

The British field site was in a process of restructuring during my research, which also influenced the media into which the articulations were further translated. In the newly acquired outsourced sperm bank, there were only two main filing systems in place: one was again a classic paper filing system, the other was linked to the HFEA, with further donor information electronically recorded and transmitted as an EDI document. What is important to point out in this context is that at the British field site, the registration phase was the point at which the medical trajectory of knowing kinship-by-donation and the accessible trajectory converged, because the information transmitted to the HFEA might later be made accessible to persons concerned (more in 5.3). The in-house sperm bank of the Largecity Fertility Hospital was of course also using the EDI system to register donors, but translated all the articulations made there into their own data management system. Their comprehensive and bespoke clinical data management software "Matchbook" clearly was the main storage medium used: it held most of the different articulations and was also most referred to during their routine practices, from matching to the tracking of sperm samples and laboratory materials.

During the registration phase, in addition to recording previous articulations onto the filing infrastructures described above, there were also two new aspects articulated in all the clinics visited. They were also documented right away, because of their practical relevance for the subsequent matching phase: kinship-by-donation became known via the donor's *body* (in the shape of articulations of his physiognomy), and via the donor as a *person* (in the shape of some recorded details of his life history, and in the British field site, even some of his personal opinions). In the German field sites these two aspects were articulated quite differently, because they only pertained to how practices were organized in the local clinics without direct links to national or transnational guidelines and regulations. In the UK the central registration of the donor with the Human Fertilisation and Embryology Authority now came into play, which meant that how the clinics came to know kinship-by-donation via the donor-body and the donor-person was also influenced by how the standardized HFEA format of knowledge-management allowed it to be. Furthermore, at my field sites, different, often implicit, rationales were used to explain why body and person needed to be first articulated and then translated in certain ways: ideas that the donor was supposed to resemble the father or parent (prevalent in different ways in all field sites); that there was a "patient demand" for these articulations, of which not all were actually needed for clinical practices (Sperm Bank Friedhausen); that clients needed this information so they could choose a donor themselves (Sperm Bank Luisenburg, and, to a more limited extent, Largecity Fertility Hospital Sperm Bank); or that a future child or its parents would benefit from accessing the documentation (only Largecity Fertility Hospital Sperm Bank). All of these rationales will be further discussed when turning to the matching phase.

I shall start with an analysis of how kinship-by-donation became known through the donor-body: all clinics documented his height, hair- and eye color, and at the British field site also his skin-color. Furthermore, in an articulation process ambivalently figured between translating the donor-body (in terms of his looks) or the donor-person (in terms of his or his family's life history) ethnicity was also recorded (more below). In Friedhausen the donor's body was articulated and then recorded on a paper-sheet within pre-defined categories before the one-off donor consultation with Dr. Dettmaringen. Or — more precisely put: The articulation took place through the distributed action of how the donor perceived his own appearance, with the available boxes on the donor registration sheet to tick, and, for instance, the advice asked of Dr.

Dettmaringen's assistant. To subsequently record his "build" (this was done by Dr. Dettmaringen himself in the consultation, still using the same paper-sheet), a dated typology was used: was the donor pyknic (i.e. stocky), athletic, or leptosomic (i.e thin)?[13] The paper-sheet with all those articulations (which would be stored separately, because it also held his signatures consenting to the donation process) was then used by one of the assistants to further translate the information into the donor Excel file.

At the other German field site, the Sperm Bank Luisenburg, the donor body was translated into clinical documentation quite differently to both Friedhausen and the British sites. The staff of Luisenburg used an additional medium of articulation and storage: photographs. The man's physical appearance (hair- and eye-color, height and weight) was translated onto open sections (instead of ticking boxes) filled in by the donor himself on the paper-registration sheet, while his "build" went unarticulated. This paper sheet was then further translated into the clinical management software used for matching and "stock monitoring" through one of the assistants. The digital photograph of the donor's face was most often taken by Dr. Lindemann during the single medical consultation with the donor during the registration phase. The photo was then saved in the database to be used during matching. Hence, while in Friedhausen (and in my British field site), the donor body was articulated through measurements (height, weight) and colors (hair-color, eye-color), during the registration in Luisenburg it was also articulated through a photographic depiction of his facial features.

In the two sperm banks of the Largecity Fertility Hospital, the HFEA donor registration form (called "Donor Information Form") and its classification system (less elaborate than in the Friedhausen clinic) was used as the entrance point for translations of the donor body into their documentation. Here blond, for instance, was not indicated along a six-point scale as at Friedhausen, but only as "blonde light" or "blonde dark". The most pronounced difference to both German field sites, however, was that the form had an additional section asking for "skin color" (see clipping 5.5).

---

13 This typology goes back to now entirely outdated seeming theories on the causal connection between body types and personality traits postulated through German psychiatrist Ernst Kretschmer in the 1920s. It is not commonly used in German language.

This specific articulation was always used at the Largecity Fertility Hospital sperm banks in relation to the donor's ethnicity during the subsequent matching phase: translating it into yet another new way of knowing the donor-body.

Clipping 5.5: Registration of the donor body at the Largecity Sperm Banks (and simultaneously with the HFEA) in 2010 (Source: HFEA)

10. Natural hair colour *	Black☐		Brown dark☐		Brown light☐
	Blonde light☐		Blonde dark☐		Red☐
11. Skin colour *	Light/Fair☐	Medium☐	Dark☐	Freckles☐	Olive☐

"Ethnicity" is unmistakably an ambivalent and highly politicized category. In a sperm bank, however it holds a particularly ambivalent status, because it is practically linked to questions of heredity. "Ethnicity" is not only implicated in the so-called matching of physical features, it might be linked to patient/client-demands to base matching procedures on markers such as religion, identity or nationality. Because of this ambivalence, the category and how it is put to use also squarely figures between what I summarized as donor-body and donor-person (e.g. hobbies, education, occupation, etc.). Not only the Largecity Fertility Hospital sperm banks, but also the two German sperm banks all had developed specific practices to translate such articulations into their documentation.

Other practices of documenting the donor as a person were also implicated with ethnicity. The Largecity Fertility Hospital sperm banks articulated ethnicity on the HFEA-form by referring to a coding-scheme similar to the ethnicity categories used in the UK census. The latter's perpetually changing choices for self-definition are influenced by the lobbying work of different communities (e.g. Aspinall 2009). In practice, one donor recruitment officer at the Largecity Fertility Hospital, Kate Clifton, asked the donor for his ethnic group, and his father's and mother's, and referred to the HFEA guidance notes (clipping 5.6 below) to find out which code to put in the donor information form. In contrast to Germany, most donors in Britain were accustomed to stating a "census conform" ethnicity, due to the prevalence of such usage in administrative routines there. Interestingly, when this articulation on the HFEA registration was translated into the database used for matching and stock taking purposes (at the in-house sperm bank), it was re-grouped and recorded in a way that one could also pull up the donor stock by US-American "race" categories: Caucasian, Asian, Black, Mixed. This enabled the staff on the one hand to firstly look for broad phenotypical resemblance according to this classical and of course also problematic classification system during the matching phase. Only subsequently, and also depending on the wishes of the parents-to-be, they took into account the more complex ethnicity category.

Clipping 5.6: Guidance notes on the HFEA "ethnicity codes" in 2010 (Source: HFEA)

HUMAN FERTILISATION & EMBRYOLOGY AUTHORITY

GUIDANCE NOTES ON COMPLETING HFEA FORMS
Donor Information Form
Version 2009/3

Appendix 1 – National Ethnicity codes

WHITE	**Category includes**
A White British	English, Scottish, Welsh, Cornish
B White Irish	
C Any other White background	Former USSR, Baltic States, Former Yugoslavia, Other European, White South African, American, Australian, New Zealander, Mixed White
CF Greek	
CG Greek Cypriot	
CH Turkish	
CI Mediterranean	Italian, Portuguese and Spanish
CJ Turkish Cypriot	
CN Jewish	
CY Other White European	
MIXED	
D White & Black Caribbean	
E White & Black African	

At the two German field sites, in contrast to the absent category "skin tone", ethnicity was articulated in the documentation, but without links to any standardized classification system, such as the UK census. At the Sperm Bank Luisenburg, in the registration form, which the donor had to fill out himself, one open field also asked him to note down his "origin/descent" ["Herkunft /Abstammung"]. This category only played a role for further documentation practices in the clinic, if a donor "really does not look like a normal Central European, like a 'Caucasian' (Dr. Lindemann makes a quotation mark gesture)". Only if the donor-body did not conform to this ambiguous norm, a note was made in the database—otherwise the information was not further recorded from paper into electronic formatting or used during the matching phase.

In the other field site, the Sperm Bank Friedhausen, ethnicity was articulated with the help of an unspecified page (i.e. no headline elaborated whether this actually asked for "ethnicity" or "appearance") in the registration paperwork. It was possible to record whether the donor appeared to be "Central-European", "Mediterranean" (with the sub-categories "Persian", "Turk", or "Spaniard/ Italian"), "Asian", "Japanese", "Arab" or "black" (clipping 5.7).

Clipping 5.7: Articulation and registration of ethnicity in the Sperm Bank Friedhausen (Source: Author/replica)

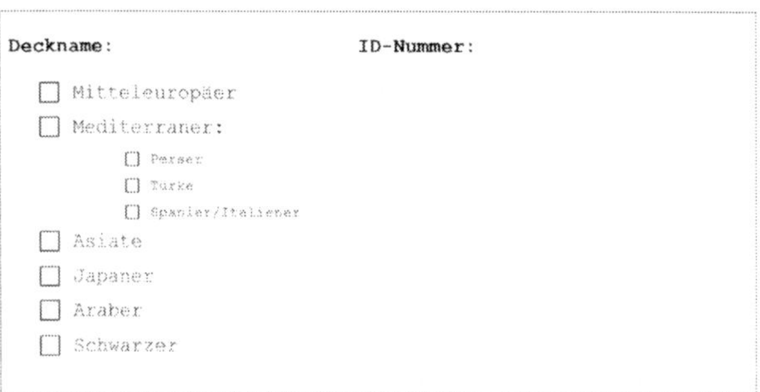

Deckname: **ID-Nummer:**

- ☐ Mitteleuropäer
- ☐ Mediterraner:
  - ☐ Perser
  - ☐ Türke
  - ☐ Spanier/Italiener
- ☐ Asiate
- ☐ Japaner
- ☐ Araber
- ☐ Schwarzer

This documentation practice, in its discursive racism and also in the way it randomly sways between referring to skin-color, contemporary nationalities or what would conventionally figure as ethnicity, almost seems like a parody of what Hall (1996) criticizes as the essentializing and ahistorical representation of black men: bluntly put, black is black, while everyone else is granted to be known via historical categories instead. It also once again points to the ambivalence of recording ethnicity in a sperm bank (which will be further discussed pertaining to the matching phase below). Similar to the practices in Luisenburg, only if the donor-body/person differed from a stereotypical German (i.e. white without very dark hair or complexion) appearance were the articulations on the paper-form in Friedhausen further translated into the Excel donor file for the matching phase in a column named "general remarks". The whole Excel spreadsheet row within which the donor was being registered through various articulations was then additionally marked red to alert the staff to his "other" looks.

The practical ambiguities in the recording of so-called ethnicity as apparent in the practices above—after all, was it skin-color, nationality, "race" or identification with a historical group of people that was being recorded here?— all field sites point to two further specific tensions around coming to know kinship-by-donation in a clinic: firstly, it points to the question if and how it is possible to clinically produce physical resemblance. (This will be discussed concerning the matching phase below and touched upon again in the families' experiences in section 7.1 and section 8.1). It secondly points to tensions in the field around concepts of heredity: is ethnicity passed on and in need of so-called matching—or only a broader "blackness" or "whiteness" as apparent in the re-grouping of the census categories at the British clinic? In practice, the staff in all field sites seemed to be mostly concerned with avoiding simple mix-ups pertaining to a child's phenotypical appearance during so-called matching, which would result to a "white" baby being born to "black" parents, or vice versa.[14] This concern was for instance apparent in the colorful labeling of the spreadsheet rows holding donors labeled to be different in one of the German sperm banks.

How the ambivalences and tensions lead to the perpetuation and situational reification of problematic classification practices for human physiognomic variation has been particularly analyzed for the US-American fertility sector and its strong emphasis on choice within capitalist market conditions (Mamo 2005; Thompson 2009; Tober 2001) but also pertaining to practices in Israel (Nahmann 2006) or Ecuador (Roberts 2011). I would like to tentatively put forward that in my own field sites, the more complex categorizations available in the British clinic reflect, in a broad sense, Britain's longer history in negotiating citizen diversity, as apparent in the politicized census categories used. However, they also reflect a "reinforcement of the outmoded discourse of race" (Price 1995, 184) in Britain, particularly when re-grouped again into simpler classifications. In Germany, both the long denial of the population's growing diversity and reluctance to categorize people in the aftermath of Nazism, have led to societal inexperience in addressing human difference (also see section 7.1). The randomness, implicit racism, and links back to dated typologies as apparent in the locally produced ethnicity and physique classifications used in Friedhausen (clipping 5.7) could be described as the counter-

14 There are a number of documented cases of this happening in fertility centers in the USA and in the UK, for a critical discussion e.g. see Tyler (2007).

productive result of such inexperience. (For a further discussion of "race" and resemblance see section 8.1. For a more comprehensive discussion of ethnicity and matching practices in European fertility clinics for example see Bergmann (2012a, 2012b) or Thompson (2009)).

In addition to the ambiguous documentation of ethnicity, kinship-by-donation during the registration-phase also became known through more translations of the donor's life story and opinions into clinical information infrastructures. At the German Sperm Bank Luisenburg information on his marital status, children, occupation, education, and interests was collected in the same paper form (using open questions) within which the donor recorded and signed his "medical history". The same questions were also asked at the Sperm Bank Friedhausen. The donor's "interests," however, were to be filled out by ticking applicable boxes: "technology, sport, natural science, humanities, music/art" (clipping 5.8).

Clipping 5.8: Sperm donor hobbies/interests as recorded at the Sperm Bank Friedhausen (Source: Author/replica)

Hobbys / Interessen

Technik	Sport	Naturwissenschaft	Geisteswissenschaft	Musik/Kunst

This category had been introduced only a few weeks before I started my more detailed fieldwork on the documentation practices there. It was being recorded into the Excel donor list (but only with newly registered donors)—and, interestingly, it was of no relevance for the matching practices in the clinic. I repeatedly asked why they had newly started recording the interests of the donor and I always got the somewhat vague answer it was used to "improve services". This probably meant that the category would potentially be used during the matching phase in the future and had been introduced out of market considerations and competitiveness since other sperm banks, including the Sperm Bank Luisenburg, were recording the category and actually using it during matching (more below).

At my British field sites, articulating and documenting kinship-by-donation via the donor-person also meant taking note of his (or her—the same form was used for egg donors) marital status, children, occupation, education, and interests, very similar to the practices particularly in

Luisenburg, where open questions were also used. But it also meant articulating additional characteristics, such as religion, skills, and the reasons for donating (see 5.9.).

Clipping 5.9: Registration of donor person at the Largecity Sperm Banks and the HFEA in 2010 (Source: HFEA)

HUMAN FERTILISATION & EMBRYOLOGY AUTHORITY

This page is to be completed by the donor
PLEASE WRITE CLEARLY IN BLACK INK USING BLOCK CAPITALS
Donor Information (Page 3) Centre: Form D

In the spaces below please supply a description of your:-

21. Religion or belief systems

22. Occupation

23. Interests:

24. Skills:

25. Reasons for donating:

What differed significantly from my German field sites was that these articulations not only marked the endpoint of the registration process, but also the starting point of the accessible clinical/institutional trajectory of knowing kinship-by-donation, as will be discussed in the next subchapter. The donor also had the option to leave a "goodwill-message to be shown to anyone born as a result of your donation" (as stated on the registration form) and an additional "description of yourself as a person". These articulations were not further used within the clinical processes but were saved (locally and with the HFEA) for future access by parents and children (see section 5.3).

It was not only the donor who in extremely heterogeneous articulations found its way into the medical trajectory of knowing kinship-by-donation during the registration phase: similar things happened with the person or couple seeking treatment. They, however, did not have to pass an evaluation phase (for orientation refer back to figure 5.2). All clinics, of course, registered their patients for practical and legal purposes, locally in Germany and Britain, and also centrally with the HFEA in Britain. Of practical relevance in all field sites (as shall become clear below) was for instance that all mothers-to-be's blood became articulated for its blood-group and rhesus factor and whether antibodies suggested contact with the cytomegalovirus. This was documented in a paper patient-file at the Sperm Bank Friedhausen, and in the electronic patient-files in the Sperm Bank Luisenburg and the in-house Largecity Fertility Hospital Sperm Bank.[15] Then the practices started to differ locally, but also between heterosexual couples, lesbian couples, and single women.

In the Sperm Bank Friedhausen, with a heterosexual couple presenting for treatment, kinship-by-donation became articulated through similar aspects as during donor-registration for *both* the recipient and the father: blood (blood group, rhesus factor, CMV), body (height, weight and the same scales for hair, eye-color, and build were used as with the donor) and person (education, hobbies, and ethnicity). This got translated onto the paper-sheet used for patient registration. Dr. Dettmaringen slightly dismissively noted that he had actually started the patient-registration process in his newly founded sperm bank *without* registering the appearance of the woman to be inseminated, only that of her partners—but that women always complained to him that they wanted to have their phenotype recorded as well. He made it sound as if this part of the patient-registration was only taking place to "appease" slightly irrational female patients ("you know how women are sometimes") and that this was of no relevance during the matching phase. (As further discussed below, I later realized that this was not entirely the case. Sometimes when for various reasons difficulties arose in matching physical features of father and donor, the sperm bank personnel did refer to the articulations of the mother-to-be's appearance. For instance when a certain unusual combination of physical features on the father's side was felt to be "overridden" by the mother's traits).

With lesbian couples Dr. Dettmaringen of the Sperm Bank Friedhausen asked whether they liked the partner to be recorded according to the same aspects used for heterosexual couples. Or they could, as done with single women, instead note down *wishes*. Hence, the section would then be used to articulate wishes on how the donor "should be like", which of course ambiguously overlapped with wishes on how a potential child "should be like." This introduced new ways-of-knowing kinship within

15 As mentioned in 5.1, the outsourced Largecity Fertility Hospital sperm bank was not registering patients at the time of my fieldwork.

clinical documentation. Women expressed wishes at the fault line between hereditary thinking and an intuition for entering into a diffuse social relationship with the donor (for further discussion see 7.1). Nevertheless, these wishes were confined to the articulations possible through the paper-sheet, yet again making use of the same typologies and scales (clipping 5.10): twelve possible ways to know hair-color, nine for eye-color, and so forth.

Clipping 5.10: Hair- and eye-color articulations at the Sperm Bank Friedhausen (Source: author/replica)

Haarfarbe	weiß-blond	hell-blond	blond	weiß-blond	hell-blond	blond
	dunkel-blond	aschblond	hell-braun	dunkel-blond	aschblond	hell-braun
	braun	dunkel-braun	schwarz	braun	dunkel-braun	schwarz
	rot-blond	rot	rot-braun	rot-blond	rot	rot-braun
Augenfarbe	eisblau	blau	blau-grau	eisblau	blau	blau-grau
	blau-grün	grün	grün-braun	blau-grün	grün	grün-braun
	braun	dunkel-braun	schwarz-braun	braun	dunkel-braun	schwarz-braun

The recipient's hair- (upper line) and eye-color (lower line) is articulated on the left side, the father's, co-mother's, or simply the wished for characteristics are articulated on the right side. The hair color options given in German translate to "white-blond, light-blond, blond, dark-blond, ash-blond, light-brown, brown, dark-brown, black, red-blond, red, red-brown". The eye-color options translate to "ice-blue, blue, blue-grey, blue-green, green, green-brown, brown, dark-brown, black-brown".

In my British field site—with its long history and specialization in lesbian clients—a practice of knowing during the patient-registration phase similar to that used in Friedhausen was in place, but for heterosexuals, lesbians, and single women alike. Instead of registering material and social aspects of the father- or mother-to-be and then using these details for matching, they let all couples or singles fill out a matching request form during the registration. In this form recipients and partners were asked to define "suitable margins" (e.g. a height between 1.80 and 1.90 meters) of a potential donor.[16] In the German Sperm Bank Luisenburg, where only heterosexual married couples were being treated, the matching of a donor's physical features with that of the father was taken extremely seriously (more below), the patient/client registration process concentrated on a thorough articulation of various aspects to do with the father-to-be. In the electronic patient file the mother's body and person was not articulated at all, only her blood to check the CMV and rhesus factor. Then the father's body and persona were articulated and documented according to the same open questions used for the donor. This was recorded in direct interaction with Dr. Lindemann, who—instead of having the father fill out the paper form as with the donors—noted down everything directly into the "partner section" of the electronic patient file during the consultation. The most important difference to the other field sites was once again the use of a camera: Dr. Lindemann took a photo of each father's face for further articulation of the body during the matching phase.

Apart from the mother-to-be's body subsequently also becoming articulated along the lines of hormonal cycles and within the gynecological insemination process, the registration phase established everything that fed into the trajectory of knowing kinship-by-donation in the clinical documentation from the patient/clients' side. No further articulations outside of the now established documentation-trail were needed to work kinship-by-donation until the intended outcome of a pregnancy.

For the donor, further articulations of substances (sperm during each donation, blood and urine for the release from the quarantine phase) would be still to come. These latter articulations would however be again following logics of inclusion/ exclusion and documentation for legal purposes. They would be less constitutively interlinked with other articulations during the working-stages leading up to the insemination, as will become clear below. Furthermore, for donors and patients alike the registration phase had established the articulation and documentation of several new socio-material aspects: the donor-body and donor-person at all field sites; the mother-to-be's body and persona (only at the Sperm Bank Friedhausen); father's or partner's body (both German sperm

16 When I returned for a last visit during the writing-up phase of this research, the British clinic had actually started to make available a catalogue online, which fully transferred matching choice to the parents.

banks); the more ambiguous wished-for-donor/child (Sperm Bank Friedhausen and the British field site). All of this was made durable for the first time within the information infrastructures.

The dominant practical logic during this working-stage was one of translation into these documentation infrastructures, heavily relying on various classifications to make this translation possible. In Germany, these classifications—some with an outmoded scientific legacy—were locally developed. In Britain centrally formatted and also more politically scrutinized classification categories were used, but also those operating with simple race classifications. An ambiguity in recording human physical variation for the purpose of "making resemblance" during the subsequent matching phase was apparent in all field sites: were only physiognomic appearances recorded—or more complex entanglements of a person's history, nationality, identity or religion, as might be seen to be implicated in ethnicity? Of course in a fertility clinic this practice marked a reification, not only through assigning categories to people or in marking bodies deviating from an implicit norm (the latter was only apparent in the German field sites), but also in thereby implicitly or explicitly acknowledging their supposed hereditary relevance. At the end of the registration phase, durable ways-of-knowing kinship-by-donation had been established, which were of high practical relevance particularly for the so-called matching. Into the relations arising out of reproduction, classifications, some of them quite problematic, as well as clinical infrastructures had now entered. The donor and the patient/client, as a living-and-breathing person presenting in the reception area of the clinic, were made only two of many relata in this process at this point, along with the interlinking articulations and documentations pertaining to substances, bodies, and personas.

Donation, Quarantine, and Release Phases: Articulations along Established Paths

During the donation, quarantine, and release phase—which will only be discussed briefly here—it was again a logic of inclusion or exclusion which dominated and which needed to be documented. On the sperm donor's side, during the actual donation phase, more translations into paper trails were taking place. Now that he was showing up weekly or biweekly to make donations, each sperm sample was again articulated and documented along the already established paths. This involved following the WHO guidelines for sperm quality (the sample was discarded in case of sudden failure to conform), checking for possible new acquaintances with bacteria, noting again how some of the sperm cells coped with being frozen and de-frozen, and documenting the laboratory materials used. All of this was, of course, stored; the actual sperm samples within liquid nitrogen canisters and the associated documentation in the information infrastructures of the clinic. This meant that kinship-by-donation now also became known through the *specific* quality of one sperm sample—filled into a batch of cryoconservation straws, stowed away in a nitrogen tank and found again through assigned codes. It also meant that during each donation there was another negotiation of the sperm donor's sexuality: it was required for the donation, but expected to not interfere with work routines or the personnel's wishes for a non-sexual behavior of the donor outside of the masturbation rooms.

During the subsequent quarantine phase no articulations took place. When walking past the nitrogen tanks labeled "quarantine" in the Sperm Bank Friedhausen, I caught myself thinking of the sperm samples themselves as being under quarantine: like animals waiting to potentially develop a disease. Instead, they were still linked to the donor and his blood. For them to pass the release phase, the donor's blood and urine needed to be articulated again concerning the presence of HIV and other viruses and bacteria. If no infections were detected through the donor's blood or urine after the quarantine phase, the samples got released into the daily work routines of the clinics again.

Matching phase: Anticipation and Material Incorporation of Parental Knowledge-management

Only after all those working stages—recruitment, evaluation, registration, donation, quarantine and release—were the now established ways-of-knowing kinship-by-donation used to decide which donor would be matched with which recipient. The practical logic dominating in this phase was one of connection, using all the now established file-trails for this process of allocation. It was not a living and breathing donor, as should now have become clear, and a living and breathing recipient who were being coupled here. But rather various material and informational aspects of them, intermingled with standards established locally and "elsewhere", classification systems, and the specific set-up of the clinical infrastructures. The donor himself might have long stopped donating at the sperm bank during the matching phase.

Which detailed practices and entangled rationales were actually followed to perform the matching differed significantly between the field sites, as already touched upon above. In the Sperm Bank Friedhausen, matching was mostly performed by the laboratory and physician's assistants, not by Dr. Dettmaringen, although he officially countersigned all decisions taken. The normal procedure there did not involve any choice on the side of the clients nor any information about the donor: the donor was simply picked for them. Dr. Dettmaringen signaled to me however that they were fairly flexible and had in the past—with demanding patients/clients—printed out parts of their donor lists so the patients could make the choice. The assistants normally agreed on about five suitable donors and chose a new one from this group for each donation cycle, with the idea that there might be "unknown parameters playing a role why a woman does or doesn't get pregnant from a certain donor".

While Dr. Dettmaringen always presented himself in interviews as rather a proponent of an open handling of the donation on the side of the parents-to-be, the design of the Excel spreadsheets that were used for the matching practices suggest that the start of the process was a blood group match. Thereafter the classical matching procedure to make potential parental secrecy water- or rather "bloodtight" was followed. In other words: since there were separate spreadsheets for each blood group, the starting point of choosing a donor always began by choosing the blood type. In the case of the heterosexual couples this meant looking up which had been recorded for the father during patient-registration and then starting the matching process with the corresponding spreadsheet. One of the assistants at Friedhausen then checked in the first columns that the donor's blood had been articulated to have the same rhesus factor as that registered for the recipient.[17] The CMV status of the mother was also checked, to not match a CMV negative recipient with a positive donor. She would do this with the patient *and* partner registration paper form (with the recorded articulations of appearance, person, and blood) in front of her. With the Excel spreadsheet on the screen, she would simply copy and paste each row conforming to those basic parameters into a new spreadsheet. (Ignoring those rows, labeled in red—as described above—in cases of "ethnic non-conformity" of the donor). In the new document the assistant would then keep checking and deleting donors (moving from similar eye, to hair-color, to height, to build) until she arrived at the desired number of about five, sometimes fewer, donors to be used successively.

As common within fertility clinics (e.g. see Bergmann's 2012a analysis of similar ambivalences in Spanish and Czech hospitals), who was being matched with whom, or what, remained ambivalent. Matching clearly was not a straight-forward substitution in Friedhausen, neither of the father being substituted by the donor, nor gametes standing in for each other. Renate Tolmin, for instance, explained:

> "As a rule of thumb, I always try to find five matching [passend] donors. [...] Sometimes—as an example—I might not find light brown hair as with the father, but a potential donor has dark blonde hair. Now then you always also check what the mother has. If she has blonde hair... -well, then it's not like it would exclude him."

Simply put, in Friedhausen *the couple* often was substituted by the donor in the rationales of the matching process. More precisely: the previously established articulations pertaining to the receiving couple were now being translated into very basic and mostly implicit hereditary probability calculations[18] concerning the appearance of a child-to-be. These probability calculations in turn determined what aspects of the donor were deemed acceptable. The outcome of this matching practice left it to the heterosexual parents to decide on a knowledge-management tactic: non-disclosure of

17 The rationale here is not to match a rhesus negative mother-to-be with a rhesus positive donor, because of the danger of the mother developing antibodies against a foetus who could be rhesus positive. This is a complex but treatable condition for mother and foetus, usually referred to as rhesus disease.

18 Hair and eye-color are complex traits which do not straight forwardly follow Mendelian patterns of heredity, nor could one for instance speak of "the gene for blue eyes" (see Moss—2003 e.g. 41–50—for an enlightening discussion of the latter).

the donation was not sufficiently adept to withstand challenge by *some* biological articulations, such as blood typing or assumed everyday informal recognitions of parental-child resemblance (see section 8.1) *or* disclosure of the donation. The infrastructural organization of donor data according to blood group (and, within Excel, no easy ways of reorganizing, as would have been possible within a complex data-base) suggested this practice, rather than parental decisions on knowledge-management being made prior to matching. More generally, I argue that the matching practices in place in a sperm bank and fertility clinic both anticipate and potentially foreclose parental tactics of kinship knowledge-management, not only on the discursive level (i.e. advice given or medical opinions), but evidently through the trajectories of knowing put in place through informational infrastructures. Clinical and parental knowledge-management (anticipated and/or practiced) are co-constitutive, so to speak—and within this they actually constitute children with specific bodies.

While Dr. Dettmaringen in Friedhausen strongly tapped into the right-to-know discourse, Dr. Lindemann of the Sperm Bank Luisenburg was far more ambivalent about the subject. In one interview, conducted in 2005, he quite frankly dismissed the suggestion of disclosure (as further discussed in section 6.1). In subsequent interviews he did not argue against disclosure in principle, but only warily acknowledged that non-anonymity seemed to matter to concerned persons quite often ("Well it *seems* to be important, let's put it that way."). Lindemann argued that a comprehensive physical matching was important for a child, his arguments somewhat ambivalently figuring between supporting parental non-disclosure and saving the child from *outside* confrontations regarding its physical appearance (also see section 8.1).

In Dr. Lindeman's sperm bank and clinic, the main difference in practices to both the other German clinic and my British field site during the matching phase were twofold: clients were given a *list* of donors to choose from and the clinical personnel made use of the previously taken *photographs.* In terms of the documented articulations used for choosing the donors to offer to parents, blood-group, CMV status, and rhesus factor were used just as at Friedhausen. Since they had translated this information into a comprehensive database, rather than Excel spreadsheets, the staff was not infrastructurally confined to start their searches with a blood group match as at Friedhausen, but mostly did so nonetheless. When a possible match had been performed, the photographs came into play. These steps were mainly performed by Dr. Lindemann himself, sometimes by the sperm bank manager Klara Bernisch. (None of the laboratory assistants were essentially performing the matching by themselves, as at Friedhausen). I got the impression that while matching was merely viewed as a necessity at Friedhausen (and also at my British field site)—with the pairing up of the various articulations definitely not viewed as a craft – there was more tacit knowledge and pride in the outcomes involved in Luisenburg. Dr. Lindemann, for instance, when asked whether parents were afraid of a lacking resemblance emphasized:

"Fortunately, we can say now, after several years of professional experience within this area, that our matching procedures yield good results. And this is crucial, that one reassures the couples: 'We have seen very many children conceived this way, this works out very well. Do not worry!'"

It was the usage of photographs as an additional medium of articulation to look for a potential resemblance between the donor's and the father's facial features which crucially contributed to a different figuration of the matching process in the Luisenburg field site. The photographs of the father-to-be and the potential donors were brought up on the computer screen and now neither discrete matches between previously done classification-work nor basic probabilities of heredity came into play, but a subjective overall impression of the face.

Klara Bernisch: "We do refer to our data. Hair-color and eye-color, for instance, you cannot really see that clearly on a photograph. But despite all of that, we get the photo and *that* is actually the first complete impression of appearance… And it is with the facial features that we then start comparing…"

Dr. Lindemann described that he was for instance comparing the sizes of different areas of the face or the space between individual features. Bernisch and Lindemann underlined that there was a subjective element to the choices made and that they were good in clinically "making resemblance". However, I shall argue in section 8.1 that the recognition of parent-child resemblance is not a straight-forward cognitive ability, but rather the enactment of a pervasive cultural script and corporeal continuity between family members. This implies that Bernisch's and Lindemann's presumed proficiency in establishing resemblance—or the matching practices of my other research partners in Friedhausen and Largecity—are not evaluated through simple feedback loops on how well this job was done. In section 8.1 I will show how for the families I worked with, resemblance was almost always positively noted, not called into question, even in the face of striking (to the eye of the ethnographer) differences in appearance.

In the Sperm Bank Luisenburg, the usage of the photographs of father-to-be and donor meant that the matching was being performed between those two, or rather between documented articulations of various aspects of father and donor. Simple calculations on the heredity of physical traits, thereby actually gearing matching at an imagined amalgamation of the couple as in the other German clinic, did not come into play. Since the photographs did not articulate discrete or already quantified characteristics like, for instance, an eye-color classification would have, they added a qualitative and interactive element to the matching phase absent in all the other field sites. This was—in its proclaimed subjectivity—a more prestigious and not merely laborious task: a craft to take pride in and a skill in Tim Ingold's (e.g. 2000, 312–322) sense: a technique dependent on tacit knowledge, context, observation, and embodiment—not on objective rules.

In the Sperm Bank Luisenburg photographs were not a present-absent way of knowing kinship-by-donation as for my parental interview partners. (The lack of photographs depicting the donor is discussed from the parents' point of view in section 7.1 below). In Luisenburg they were part of constituting kinship within the medical trajectory. The parents-to-be however were not given access to the images. The lists from which they got to choose their final match usually contained five donor options, presented in the form of a print-out generated with the help of the donor data-base, listing the articulations of the donor's hair- and eye-color, height, blood-group, profession, education, and interests. Usually, Dr. Lindemann had marked one or two of the donors on the donor list, indicating the closest match in facial features. This practice seemed to produce—at least this featured prominently in the interviews with Dr. Lindemann—situations for the parents within which they needed to balance their preferences for different articulations. The limited information on the donor body given to them, needed to be weighed up with Dr. Lindemann's already highlighted choice of the "visually closest" option and the personal relevance of other listed categories such as education and interests. The latter Dr. Lindemann often deliberately seemed to ignore within the matching practice. From what he said I got the impression that from the approximately 150 active donors registered with them, a match satisfying Dr. Lindemann's careful practice of photographic matching, plus a blood group match, plus the correlation of articulations of appearance *and* persona between father and donor often was impossible. Lindemann said a couple insisting on a matching according to interests and education, which he viewed as unnecessary anyhow, "should then not care about the [donor's] looks".

In effect and different to the clients of the Sperm Bank Friedhausen, this led to parents often making more explicit decisions on their own knowledge-management tactic *prior* to matching. Faced with a *choice* of donors (partially a result of the more flexible database), with some proclaimed to be a perfect physical match, and others which were perhaps deemed more amicable, the parents needed to enter into an explicit dialogue with each other and with the quite assertive Dr. Lindemann to come to a final decision (also see 7.1). Thus, in Friedhausen matching practices had more or less "in-built" a safeguarding of potential parental non-disclosure of the donation. In Luisenburg, in contrast, parental decisions on disclosure or non-disclosure were often part of the matching phase. Furthermore, matching operated with the complex practice of "making resemblance" between photographs. Outcome of the matching phase at the two German sperm banks thus was either the clinical anticipation of parental knowledge-management tactics or the parental tactics themselves being physically incorporated in the child-to-be.

In my British field sites matching was only performed by the in-house sperm bank during my time of observation and interview-visits. The matching system was mostly explained to me—rather than being able to watch how matches were performed—by the managing embryologist of the in-house bank, Keira Lorimer. Parents were presented with a donor-offer via e-mail or mail, which they needed to accept or refuse (see clipping 5.11). Three-quarters of the parents were happy to accept the first recommendation, according to Lorimer. The offers tried to meet the requirements for a potential donor, which the parents themselves had laid out on the matching request form as previously described for the registration phase.

Clipping 5.11: Matching offer form at Largecity Fertility Hospital (Source: author/replica)

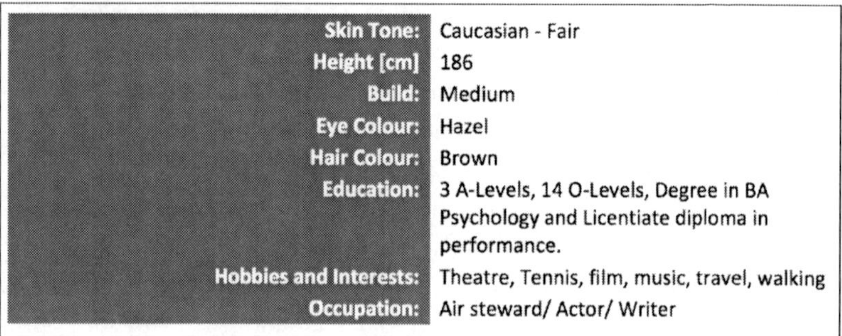

Skin Tone:	Caucasian - Fair
Height [cm]	186
Build:	Medium
Eye Colour:	Hazel
Hair Colour:	Brown
Education:	3 A-Levels, 14 O-Levels, Degree in BA Psychology and Licentiate diploma in performance.
Hobbies and Interests:	Theatre, Tennis, film, music, travel, walking
Occupation:	Air steward/ Actor/ Writer

Interestingly, the Largecity Fertility Hospital Sperm Bank had earlier computerized their matching system, but when I arrived for my fieldwork had changed it back to being done by a staff member. Their bespoke software "Matchbook", which—as previously mentioned—they used as a comprehensive clinical data management software, had initially been designed to relieve personnel of this task. But the clients were not happy with Matchbook, Lorimer told me. According to her, it was mainly the idea that a computer was making this important decision, rather than a person, which bothered them. Marre and Bestard (2009) have described the imaginations of adoptive parents associated with matching during transnational adoption, which attribute almost a magical note to it. Similarly (see 8.1) some of my interviewees were particularly happy with the idea that there was a doctor's expertise at work during matching. I suspect that because computerized matching in contrast lacked the aura of personal expertise, parents-to-be did not like it. The sperm bank staff also felt that Matchbook was not a great help. Although I did not get a sense that they took the same pride in matching as the personnel in the Sperm Bank Luisenburg, they nevertheless still felt they could do a better job than the software. Since they struggled with a limited donor stock, perfect matches were often hard to make. And this was where they thought Matchbook's algorithm failed —in the weighing up of different articulations against each other.

During the matching phase in the British clinic the parental knowledge-management tactic itself, not only its general clinical anticipation, also became incorporated in the physical constitution of the resulting child. In this the clinic was more similar to Luisenburg than Friedhausen. The temporality of when parental knowledge-management entered was, however, different because of the matching request form already filled out during the earlier registration phase. This had already created an imaginary third person, only known along clinical parameters and in that already (as discussed above) ambiguously figuring between delineating the ideal donor or rather the ideal child. This "third person" already contained the parental knowledge-management and was then correlated with the diverse articulations of the actual donors on Matchbook. What I found notable was the specific situation the parents found themselves in during the matching phase: not weighing up different donors, nor just accepting the "matching authority" of the clinic, as in Germany, but accepting a specific donor available at a specific time. Or, in contrast, not accepting this donor, but thereby potentially prolonging the treatment process.[19] The difficulty of making a choice in this situation of uncertainty led many parents, as embryologist Lorimer told me, to make informal inquiries about the donor before confirming him. (The parents needed to confirm via phone or e-mail and by making a payment). She had the tactic of always giving vague positive answers to these informal inquiries.

In summary, the dominating practical logic during the matching phase in all clinics was one of connection. It had the goal of allocating a particular sperm sample to a particular patient/client or couple. This allocation took place within the established trajectory of knowing kinship-by-donation and thereby made use of the diverse articulations already stored. In other words: there were not two everyday persons, donor and father, being matched here. There also was not a simple logic of substitution at work; who was matched with whom carried a certain ambivalence. At the Sperm Bank Friedhausen, the couple—or rather probability calcu-

19 The figure potentially at work here—do-we-go-for-this-donor-or-might-there-be-a-better-one-in-line?—seems analogous to the clichés (and associated realities) of late-modern dating practices, particularly online-dating. Mamo (2005, 247) draws similar analogies.

lations on their physiognomic amalgamation—was matched with what was known about the donor. Only the Sperm Bank Luisenburg used photographs for a qualitative matching of donor and father rather than following standardized ways-of-knowing. In the British sperm bank an imaginary third person was used for matching, because parents indicated wishes on the donor request form. At this point in clinically working kinship-by-donation not only the various clinical standards, classifications, and infrastructures entered into the reproductive relations. On top of this either anticipations of the parental knowledge-management, or that in itself (through choice or the donor-request-form) also entered into the constitutive process. Parental knowledge-management became physically incorporated in the children-to-be, for instance as a particular blood-group.

Delivery and Insemination Phase: Liquid Nitrogen Canisters and Hormonal Cycles

The practical logic relevant to the last two typical stages of working kinship-by-sperm-donation, delivery and insemination, was again connection. In contrast to the matching-phase this connection was however not only performed within the clinical information infrastructures: the samples needed to be physically delivered and the insemination itself performed. At both working stages I was not present. For that reason —but even more importantly because there were few new articulations entering the reproductive relations at these stages—my description of these phases will be brief.

The inseminations were never performed within the sperm bank itself in any of my field sites: Friedhausen only delivered to other clinics, Luisenburg delivered to their own clinic located on a different floor of the building—which was however operating under a separate license—and sold sperm, just as my British field site. The single entirely new addition to the medical trajectory during the delivery was the documentation of the delivery itself, which featured the information on the specific samples used, such as the reference-code for the particular charge, and the original articulations of sperm quality for possible comparison by the gynecologist performing the actual insemination. This evidently also entailed documenting that a sample had been sold and left the clinic within the clinical information infrastructures. In the Sperm Bank Friedhausen the delivery phase also marked the point of convergence between the medical and the accessible trajectory of knowing kinship-by-donation. As comprehensively discussed in section 5.3 below, the staff included a sealed envelope with identifying donor-information with the delivery. The envelope was to be stored by the treating gynecologist.

The last step in what I have called the clinical trajectory of knowing kinship-by-donation was the insemination itself. During this last step in the chain of transformations kinship-by-donation also became known through the female hormonal cycle. With the sperm, still frozen, delivered to the gynecologist, the recipient's blood needed to be articulated and an ultrasound performed to find out when she would be ovulating to perform the insemination at the right time. Or—as common in many fertility clinics—the hormonal cycle would be not only articulated, but medicinally intervened in, to make its temporality fit clinical routines and boost success rates. (See Knecht, Klotz et al. (2011) for a discussion of the temporal conflicts and synchronizations between clinical and familial practices and the female hormonal cycle during assisted conception). And this is where my analysis of the medical trajectory ends: with the potential conception of a child through a woman on a gynecological chair. The patients'/clients' accounts of this exact moment always underlined the technicality and perceived absurdity of that moment. (Sarah Hampton: "My mom and my first-born were there when I conceived my second child [laughs], they were in the waiting room, my partner was at work"). For all my familial research partners the practical logic of physical connection relevant at the last working stage had, much to their joy, worked out with a pregnancy, mostly, however, only after several repetitions of the previously described working stages.

Ova Donation and Treatment

It is useful to take a short contrastive look at how the medical trajectory differs between sperm and egg donation. Because egg donation is unlawful in Germany, I was only able to gain insights into its specific medical trajectory in my British field site. In this clinic, with only rare exceptions, as ova donation coordinator Maggy Riley told me, egg donation took place in egg share agreements. This meant that the female donors were also having treatment and were receiving price discounts on their IVF in exchange for donating some of their eggs. The Largecity Fertility Hospital benefitted from their tradition of treating lesbian couples. Many of their lesbian clients, as clinic owner Dr. O'Brien pointed out, opted for an IVF treatment with their partner's eggs. These clients were "the perfect egg sharers", because they were not affected by clinical infertility (Dr. O'Brien). In addition to such clients, women with medically diagnosed fertility problems also went for egg sharing to finance their IVF treatment, though these patients did not always produce enough eggs to enter the egg sharing program.[20]

In general, all regulations (registration with the HFEA, non-anonymity of the donors etc.) also applied to egg donation. British law in fact does not differentiate between female and male donation in most respects. This also contributed to the medical trajectory being similar—and the accessible trajectory alike (see 5.3). Nevertheless, egg donation and treatment with donated eggs, as is important to point out, are evidently in many ways highly different from sperm donation. There are significant dangers for the women donors and more invasive medical operations, and questions of commodification and exploitation pose themselves with more acuteness in this area, for instance, given increasing reproductive travelling, where women from more affluent and/or differently regulated countries buy eggs from poorer donors (for ethnographic analysis of such practices e.g. see Knoll 2012 or Nahman 2012). Treating male and female donations alike in the law could therefore also be viewed as a problematic practice, which eclipses some of the women-specific dangers of exploitation and suffering. I have for instance elsewhere critically pointed out that during the British move to non-anonymity the meaning of egg sharing for women with fertility problems has not been sufficiently explored (Klotz 2006, 2007), though this is a topic beyond the scope of this book. Instead, I shall only discuss the decisive differences between egg and sperm donation within what I have come to call the medical trajectory.

20 A women needed to produce more than ten eggs during one ovulation cycle to qualify for the program.

Figure 5.12: Typical working stages during egg sharing

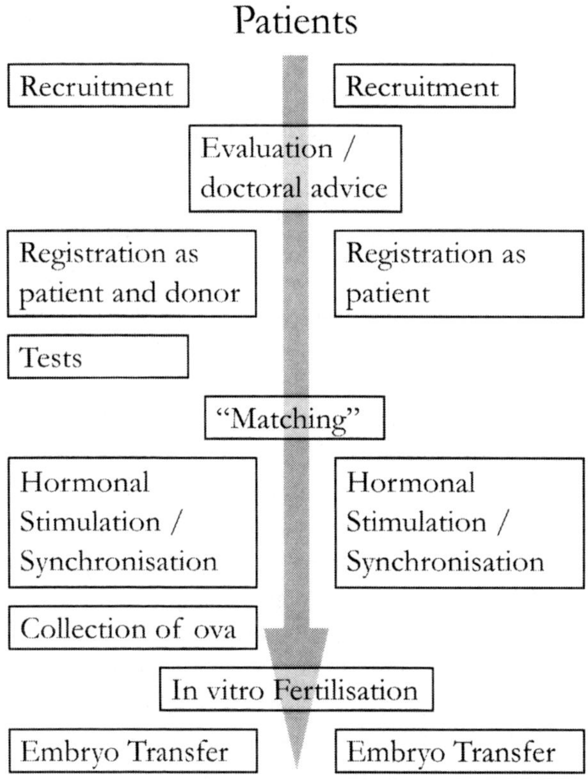

Figure 5.12 depicts the typical working stages involved in working kinship-by-egg-sharing as followed in the Largecity Fertility Hospital. The process can be summarized as follows: patients/ clients presenting at the clinic (if they had not decided for this option by themselves beforehand) were advised on the option of egg sharing, or the option of potentially still conceiving with donated eggs if the chances for conception through ordinary IVF/ICSI were deemed extremely low. After being registered as patients, the egg recipients had to wait: it usually took six months to get on the waiting list to be matched (which means donor and recipient often did not make first clinical contact at the same time). While there was no quarantine period similar to sperm donation, patient-donors

had to go for similar tests as the sperm donors before starting the cycle and again at the beginning of the cycle. During the latter, patient-donors' and recipients' hormonal cycles were synchronized through hormonal stimulation. Then eggs were collected from the patient-donor, and if there were enough available for sharing, half of the eggs were fertilized in the laboratory with the sperm of each woman's partner or chosen donor. The embryos were transferred back within the following days into the patient-donors' and the recipients' womb. This usually took place during the same day, with one woman coming in the morning, the other in the afternoon. The two women were kept anonymous to each other.

The aspects through which kinship-by-*egg* donation became known in my field site and how those were translated into clinical pathways of knowing were similar to those discussed above: for the patient-donors, for instance, blood was articulated for viruses and bacteria and for chromosome-numbers, enzymes, blood cells and molecules; the ambiguous genre of medical history was comprehensively discussed and recorded; and both women's blood was articulated for their hormone levels.

Two notable aspects of egg donation differed from sperm procedures: the absence of freezing and the scarcity of eggs. Firstly, because eggs to date cannot be frozen as successfully as sperm and the success rates of IVF involving frozen embryo transfers are also not as good as those of "fresh" ones, as Dr. O'Brien and Maggy Riley explained to me, the temporality of the whole process and many administrative steps were far more closely linked to the living and breathing bodies of patient-donors and recipients. While after release from quarantine, the frozen sperm samples were decoupled from the actual donor (with the documentation on his person remaining the only link), no such comprehensive decoupling took place during egg donation. The bodies of both women were synchronized hormonally and eggs transferred on the same day.[21] In other words: not only paper trails linked them to the eggs and each other, but they were in a sense also linked to them and to each other by what their bodies were doing (or being done to) at the same point in time. Because of this less comprehensive decoupling between bodies and gametes, there also was not a similar

21 "Spare" embryos which could not be transplanted due to the two to three embryo limit to prevent multiple births (HFEA 2009a, section 7) could be frozen and stored for a fee of 500 British Pounds per year.

quarantine phase: the eggs were simply never outside the patient-donors body long enough to check as comprehensively as during sperm donation whether a viral infection had taken place (e.g. by repeating the AIDS test after 6 months of donation to check whether the donor really had not been infected during the time of donation). Most recipients accepted the small risk associated with this practice.[22]

Secondly, it was not that there were so many fewer egg donors than sperm donors available to the clinic. Egg sharing had proven to be a successful business model. But from the approximately ten donations the clinic got per month, evidently less "reproductive substance" resulted than from a sperm donation. Additionally, egg sharers (or also egg donors) could not be asked to come back at all or at least not in the same intervals as sperm donors, due to the invasive nature of egg collection. The scarcity of eggs, in addition to the long waiting period, made the articulations considered during the matching phase far more basic. There also was no request form available. Head nurse and donation coordinator Maggy Riley told me that clients were matched by looking for very basic correlations of height, hair- and eye-color. She also added that "often not all details fit, but [the recipients receiving a matching offer similar to the one at the sperm bank] still agree". The only unbridgeable boundary seemed to be "race"/ethnicity, as became clear when Riley told me about their problems of finding a fitting patient-donor for a "black" recipient. This was also reflected in setting up the files used for the matching process in Excel spreadsheets separated by the American race categories. (The more complex ethnicity categories of the donor information form needed to be filled out as well, since the same form was used and transferred to the HFEA for egg and sperm donors. They played no practical role, however, during the clinical matching phase). Otherwise close physical matching seemed to be secondary. Whether this resulted only from the scarcity of eggs and the associated long waiting periods, with people more intent on physical matching potentially travelling abroad, remains unanswered. Additional factors might have been that egg donation is not associated with common notions of adultery and that it becomes more "corporeal" through the pregnancy, and thereby "making resemblance"

22 To date, there has been no documented case of a woman contracting the HIV virus this way (e.g. see Resolve 2011).

becomes less important to both clinical personnel and clients. The clinic's knowledge-management of egg donation was clearly less complex than the system used for sperm donation: Matchbook was not used, only basic Excel files. Complex matching procedures would not have been possible on the basis of the few documented articulations. No hereditary probability calculations took place, finding just a few correlations between donor and recipient was enough.

Hence, unlike sperm donation, clinical and parental knowledge-management tactics were less entangled in the case of egg sharing. In the absence of thorough physical matching down to the blood group, parents choosing to leave the donation a secret might potentially have to develop quite comprehensive "counter-tactics" in knowledge-management, such as not disclosing their blood groups to the child. What is apparent from the empirical descriptions above, is that neither parental knowledge-management tactics, nor their clinical anticipation, became part of the physical constitution of a resulting child for egg sharing. It was first and foremost clinical knowledge-management which was to become physically incorporated. This clinical knowled knowledge-management reflected the material (i.e. economic and biological) specificities of ova sharing. Clinical information infrastructures and scientific standards, classifications, and material articulations were, however, entering the relations arising out of reproduction quite analogous to the more detailed practices discussed above.

Recapitulation

To summarize, what I call the medical trajectory of knowing kinship-by-donation has been characterized by the differential and successive articulation and documentation of various aspects pertaining to the donor and the parents-to-be: blood, sperm, urine, antibodies, chromosomes, enzymes, bacteria, viruses, hormones, physical appearances, personal opinions, life- and medical-histories, among others. Cryoconservation machines; microscopes; Petri-dishes; computer programs; filing cabinets; classification systems; questionnaires; local, national, and international standards and regulations; plus rooms filled with pornography —a list without a claim on completeness—were part of making these articulations. The crucial point of my argument has, however, not been simply to point to hybridity in the processes analyzed above. Instead, I have shown how a Latourian chain of transformations was socio-materially constitutive in its consequences, so that clinical and parental knowledge-management became part of the physical constitution of the children-to-be. Part of the chain of transformations became diverse scientific classifications and legacies, regulations, economic considerations, and articulations of biological substances and historical details. Diverse actors and actants were thus put into relation.

Thompson, in her ethnographic analyses of how legitimate parents are brought into being in US fertility clinics (see section 2.3), has described similar practices as "ontological choreography" (e.g. Thompson 2005). Given my detailed focus on how the working-stages in my clinical field sites interconnect and which ways-of-knowing are drawn on at specific stages, I have remained with an adaptation of the Latourian notion of an interlinked chain of transformations to foreground how "the practices that produce information about a state of affairs" are brought into being through socio-material articulations which are then constitutively interlinked (Latour 1999, 24). The practices described for the clinics showed a consecutive decoupling of the donor or recipient as living-and-breathing-person from various materials and bits of information all once folded into this body and person—to make specific babies at the end of the chain. Taking the notion of constitutive knowledge quite literally, kinship was here socio-materially constituted within these complex (knowledge-) practices, letting WHO guidelines and Excel sheets become relata of kinship-by-donation. This I identified as unique, because it is neither to be found for kinship "in the wild", nor for adoption or IVF.[23]

Summarizing in more detail along the different field sites and along national boundaries, a nuanced picture emerges. At Friedhausen, kinship-by-donation became known through relatively inflexible infrastructures heavily constraining the further translations taking place (e.g. Excel spreadsheets arranged by blood-group used as the basis for matching

23 IVF/ICSI without donor gametes might seem analogous at first glance, but is not: its driving logic pertains to achieving pregnancy from a specific couple. Although scientific standards also play a role, they cannot become similarly constitutive, because practices are geared towards working with the couple's gametes.

or locally developed classification systems), and patient demand was sounded out through clinical anticipations, not choice. Kinship-by-donation did not become known through any practices aiming at the molecular level, in fact not even at the chromosomal level, of articulating so-called genetic diseases at all. Within this specific medical trajectory, kinship-by-donation was typically constituted without parental decisions on their own knowledge-management tactics. What rather became incorporated was, so it seemed, not an elaborate ideology of non-disclosure or the skillful clinical production of resemblance, but specifically configured clinical infrastructures.

At Luisenburg, more complex and flexible infrastructures that were heavily geared toward "making resemblance" were in place. Through offering the parents a choice in donors presented to them along very basic parameters (with other aspects only implicitly, from the parent's perspective, determining the configuration of the list) their own decisions also became part of the physical constitution of the child. The articulations made were slightly more interlinked with genetic considerations (e.g. through the realization of a karyogram) at Luisenburg than at Friedhausen.

At Largecity, what Bergmann (2012c) has summarized as the "Fordist" logic (i.e. towards accumulating stock) of sperm donation versus the "Toyotist" logic (i.e. flexible and personalized simultaneous processing in highly market-determined settings) of egg donation determined the differences in the knowledge-management involved. I argue that the different logics were largely attributable to the material specificities of sperm and eggs: their "freezability", how they got detached from human bodies, and their quantity. Articulations aiming for so-called genetic diseases or dispositions and connections to molecular-biologically informed risk discourses were part of making, or not making, specific children at Largecity. Parental wishes already became translated onto the matching request form used, often substituting what in the other clinics were articulations of actual living-and-breathing persons with articulations of wishes set at the fault line between articulations of the partner, hereditary probability calculations, and a wished for child. The infrastructures in place were on the one hand much more advanced in terms of digitalization, flexibility, and complexity in Largecity—but they were also docked with those of the regulatory institution HFEA: determining their shape through affordances, reaching from interoperability requirements to the detailed guidelines regarding medical practices laid out in the Code of Practice. This section thereby again showed a stronger interconnection between kinship-by-donation and governance in Britain, with its tight, yet processual approach of government at a distance, as described in 5.1. This meant that the HFEA's "paper technologies" (Levinson 2010, 163–188) extended into the medical trajectory. This was generally the most pronounced difference between Britain and Germany as discernible through the analysis of my fieldwork materials: the medical trajectories in Germany were far more diverse than those in Britain. The medical trajectory in the latter was also more closely connected to contemporary genetic/genomic scientific knowledge—while interactive and subjective criteria in evaluating the donors seemed to play a bigger role in Germany, along with the easier recruitment within the compensation-oriented regime.

5.3 The Accessible Clinical/Institutional Trajectory of Knowing Kinship-by-Donation: Sealed Envelopes, Donor Files, and a National Registry

After recounting how kinship-by-donation was constituted in the clinics I visited, I now turn to those parts of this trajectory, which actually become accessible to later children and their parents. The aspects made accessible are thereby officially recognized as of relevance for kinship-by-donation. These aspects also provide the only officially endorsed means (see 7.4 for subversive practices) for the donor-conceived to potentially make real-life contact to the donor. I will show how the locally and nationally different accessible clinical/institutional trajectories actually find their beginning, their starting point for a different chain of transformations, within the previously described medical trajectories. They are, as I demonstrate, however far more limited: purified in the Latourian (1993) sense, because the hybrid "mess" described in section 5.2 above is excluded. Viruses and WHO standards for sperm quality, for instance, are not known within this pathway, or at least not intended (through regulators and medical practitioners) to be known to children or parents concerned. I will demonstrate how within the accessible trajectory kinship takes more familiar shape again and becomes administratively recognized as a biological tie of personal value and a connector between persons. I will also demonstrate how the constitution of kinship-by-donation within the accessible trajectory entails that new administrative rationales and infrastructural affordances become part of the relations arising out of reproduction. This, as demonstrated below, links back to my analysis in section 5.1. In Germany, clinical preparation for access to donor-information was rudimentary and regulatory preparations non-existent, while the HFEA was building up a comprehensive accessible trajectory in Britain. Kinship-by-donation thus again becomes visible as linked to differing modes of governance, here discernible pertaining to its administrative shaping and recognition.

At the time of my fieldwork donor-conceived persons had not actually made use of the accessible trajectory themselves—although they were expected to do so in the future. Within the different working stages of the medical trajectory analyzed above, the accessible trajectory had differing starting points at the different clinics (see the schematic depiction in figure 5.13): while the accessible trajectory had its beginnings during the registration phase both at Luisenburg and at the British field sites, it started only during the delivery phase at Friedhausen.

The regulatory set-up that influences this trajectory has already been discussed in section 2.3 and in section 5.1, hence I add only a few sentences to recapitulate. In Britain gamete donation has been non-anonymous since 2005, with all donors recorded in a national registry (currently run by the HFEA) that children-by-donation can access when turning 18. In Germany the legal situation is unclear, with potential legal obligations between donor and child still in place. However, that German children-by-donation have a right to information on "their" donor has been underlined with the new Tissue Law of 2007, without any clear guidance about what this might mean in practice. Grown up children actually accessing this information in both countries cannot be ethnographically followed yet, because the legal changes only affected future children-by-donation;

Figure 5.13: Starting point of accessible trajectory within the medical trajectory

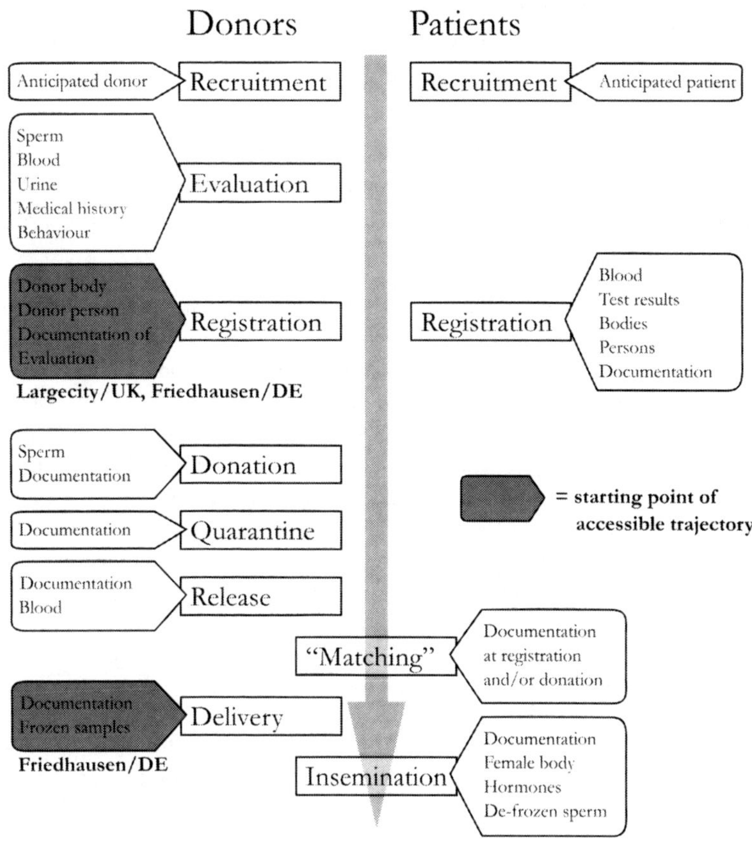

in the 2020s, when they begin to turn 18, they will be eligible to access the information.[24]

24 To be precise and as already elaborated on above: it is actually not entirely legally clear whether the German regulations only affect donations made after 2007. Nonetheless, the clinical actors in Germany interpreted them to do so, as shown below.

Sperm Bank and Fertility Centre Luisenburg

Due to the ambiguity of the German legal situation, the story about the accessible clinical/institutional trajectory in my German field sites is quickly told—at least in one sense: in Luisenburg, there was none. While principally aware that the regulatory situation had changed to a fragile non-anonymity, no specific preparations had been taken as to how to turn the medical trajectory of knowing kinship-by-donation into an accessible one. The only thing that was clear, was that in the future children-by-donation might access parts of the articulations stored in the registration phase. As sperm bank manager Klara Bernisch explained to me:

> Klara Bernisch: "I did not read this [the legal requirements] in a way that one needs to collect so much information. One has to be able to lay open the identity of the donor. That information. […] Identity means first and foremost: Name, first name, date of birth and one usually identifies the donor by is ID card number. That's all, I don't record more. We have not really thought about a more personal page or message or the like, that would be quite nice from the perspective of the child. And we are not working on that, yet. I know about the USA, that they sometimes even have sound recordings of what the donor wanted to say to a child. But that is also the point where we would put the donors in a situation, to really have to think about the children's situation. […] I don't know of such practices in other [German] sperm banks. […] I also don't know if it is really helpful. It is nice for the child. I look at it from my perspective: documentation… Then you would have to store up even more."

The sperm bank manager summarizes "identity" as the basic information saved on an ID card, and is thereby referring to the nationally established means for the task of securely identifying one unique person over time. Her statement that she does not "record more" shows how the in fact far more detailed recordings of the medical trajectory, in her opinion, are not to be seen as data a future child might want to access. In other words: the medical trajectory is not recognized to be of relevance to kinship. Bernisch's reluctance to encourage the donor to think about "the children's situation" I interpreted as touching upon the unclear German regulatory situation, where thinking too much about the consequences of sperm donation might discourage men from donating.

Bernisch's colleague Dr. Margret Hagedorn, who managed the associated IVF laboratory, also approached the subject of an accessible clinical/

institutional trajectory as highly hypothetical—and worryingly complicated:

Margret Hagedorn: "I actually think this is not so easy. Everything, really everything, has to be safeguarded so that the facts are correct. I mean, truly, you have to realize what you are confronting the donor with there... [...] Until now, no one ever came [to ask about a donor's identity]. I have actually never heard about this in Germany, that there is this wish, but the children are also not there [implying old enough for an enquiry] yet."
Maren Klotz: "They are still small, right? But there was a [grown up DI] child who's been in the media quite a bit. She also has a website. And I think she is suing "her" clinic."[25]
Margret Hagedorn: "But I think that at the time she was conceived, the clinic did not have this obligation [to keep and potentially lay open clinical records]."

Hagedorn, just as Bernisch, did not come across as ignorant of the social implications of her work in general, because both reflected on kinship, reproductive technologies, and changing moralities in Germany and other parts of the world quite extensively in interviews. Nevertheless, Hagedorn, like Bernisch, was also solely taking the donors' perspective when reflecting on a potential accessible trajectory. She also implied that there was no interest in non-anonymous donation practices discernible in Germany, which is not the case (e.g. see section 7.4 for the activities of German adult donor-conceived persons). As apparent in both women's statements, how they thought about a possible future accessible clinical/institutional trajectory mainly pertained to safeguarding that the donor as a living and breathing person could potentially be identified in the future through—minimal parts—of their clinical documentation.

Sperm Bank Friedhausen

At the Sperm Bank Friedhausen the personnel had already established an accessible way of knowing kinship-by-donation, rudimentary though it is if looked at in comparison to the British system. While owner Dr. Dettmaringen was a more outspoken advocate of non-anonymity and the "right-to-know" in interviews, he or his colleagues had not established any

25 As previously mentioned: The website is called www.DI-Kind.de. As an example for the extensive media coverage of the case see Haarhoff (2007).

specific measures, such as counseling, to accompany the children's potential future data access.[26] What they had established as a beginning of an accessible trajectory was to translate previous articulations onto further documentation during the delivery phase and send this to the inseminating gynecologist (along with the actual sperm sample). Some gynecologists insisted that the sperm bank should only send this documentation if a pregnancy occurred, so sometimes this translation only took place at a later stage. It was then the gynecologist's responsibility to ensure the durability of this documentation; I was told that some stored the sealed envelope in their practice, while others enlisted a notary to keep the document for a child, who might access it after turning 18. Similar basic information to that used at Luisenburg was put in the document: not the ID card number, but the donor name, address at point of registration and basic patient information (see clipping 5.14). They also put both the donor- and the patient-ID number into the document, which meant that they also provided the "key" for accessing the sperm bank's medical trajectory.

It struck me as absurd that the document, which might be stored for 20 years before being accessed was so carelessly drafted that a blatant grammatical error was printed both onto the document and onto its seal. Its contents were also nonsensical in parts: who is addressed here as "you" if only the child is supposed to open the sealed envelope? It is hard not to —even unwillingly—employ a morally charged tone here or to put too much weight on that possible situation of discovery (thereby reifying the personal importance of this information and event). What is important to note for analytical reasons, however, is that it is the comparison between the medical and the accessible trajectory and between the British and German system which contributes to my critical impulse in this context. Most of the documents comprising part of the medical trajectory actually get quality checked and reviewed in regular intervals as part of the QM system in all field sites, and (as shown below) the British HFEA already now streamlines how to answer any enquiries into the accessible trajectory. At Friedhausen exactly the document that could set into motion the *Gestalt*

26 The Working Party for Donor Insemination makes some vague references to sperm banks and inseminating gynecologists potentially ensuring that contact between donor and child takes places under "dignified circumstances [würdiger Rahmen]" and that the possibility of counseling should be mentioned, but does not specify any practical details (Arbeitsgruppe Richtliniennovellierung 2006, 18–19).

Clipping 5.14: Information provided for DI children through the Sperm Bank Friedhausen (Source: author/replica)

Persönlich/Vertraulich

Achtung!!!
Das mittels Fremdsperma gezeugte Kind ist die einzige Person, die nach Prüfung deren Identität, den versiegelten Umschlag von Ihnen ausgehändigt bekommen und öffnen darf, wenn es volljährig ist.

Patienten ID	Name der Patientin	Geburts-datum	ID-Deckname	Name des Spenders	Geburtsdatum	Anschrift	Tag der Auslieferung

The first line translates to "personal/confidential" and the second line simply states, "Attention!!!". The third and fourth line are convoluted and in incorrect grammar: "The child conceived by donor sperm is the only person, who after verification of those identity, is allowed to have handed over and open the sealed envelope from you, if it has reached majority" [majority is reached at age 18 in Germany]. The small table lists "patient ID, name of the patient, date of birth of the patient, ID-pseudonym, name of the donor, date of birth, address, date of delivery."

switch a sense of self can undergo due to the constitutive force of kinship knowledge seems to have fallen outside of any checks or deliberations by the clinic personnel. This shows how access through the donor-conceived and the accessible trajectory in general were subject only to marginal deliberations and planning at Friedhausen, although staff underlined their anti-anonymity and pro-disclosure stance in interviews.

Largecity Fertility Hospital and Sperm Bank

As is clear from my previous descriptions, the HFEA was directly involved in the working stages at the British field site. It contributed to the medical trajectory and established the accessible trajectory in interaction with clinical practices during the registration phase. At that point the comprehensive articulations made of the donor body and the person were also registered with the HFEA and were completely alike for sperm and egg donors. The registration form also held an optional section only designed for purposes of recording statements of the donor to be later accessed by the parents or the child (see clippings 5.15 and 5.16). In contrast to the rest of the form, which was transmitted to the HFEA using the EDI system, these last two pages were simply sent from the clinic by registered post. (They held not only the optional personal statements, but also the section on occupation, religion, interests, and skills—as depicted in clipping 5.9 above). At the HFEA the forms were scanned and saved on their registry, which meant that the donor's hand-writing was preserved and no mistakes in transcription could be made, as the HFEA officers explained when interviewed. Additional copies were kept in the paper donor files at the clinic.

Clipping 5.15: Optional goodwill message on HFEA donor registration sheet as used in 2010 (Source: HFEA)

HUMAN FERTILISATION & EMBRYOLOGY AUTHORITY

This page is to be completed by the donor
PLEASE WRITE CLEARLY IN BLACK INK USING BLOCK CAPITALS
Donor Information (Page 4) Centre: Form D

PLEASE COMPLETE ELECTRONICALLY OR HANDWRITE

27. The space below is provided for you to give a description of yourself as a person. The type of information that may be helpful could include your education, achievements, values, and life experiences. Try to imagine yourself as a donor-conceived person, and think about what you might wish to know.

Clipping 5.16: Optional donor self-description on HFEA donor registration sheet as used in 2010 (Source: HFEA)

Optional Additional Information

You may wish to provide in these sections a goodwill message and description of yourself. This information is not compulsory but it is recommended you complete these sections as the information you provide can help parents tell children about their origins and answer some questions a donor-conceived person may have.

Non-identifying information provided in the following sections can, upon request, be shared with patients requiring treatment with donor gametes/embryos, parents of children conceived using your donated gametes/embryos and children conceived using your donated gametes/embryos, once they reach the age of 16.
The full content of this form can be made available to donor-conceived people when they reach the age of 18.

I understand that by completing these sections I have consented to the information therein being shared with patients, parents and donor-conceived people, as outlined above. (Please tick to confirm)

26. You may wish to write a goodwill message to be shown to anyone born as a result of your donation.

The personal statements of the donors, which had no practical value for the medical trajectory, had an ambiguous regulatory status. Whether parents indeed were entitled to access them had been hotly debated during the review of the HFE Act in 2008 and again during policy reviews in 2009 and 2010 that the HFEA itself conducted, as patient group leader Montuschi and the HFEA managers told me (also see HFEA 2009b). After all, was this information not left for the children only? However, many clinics (including my British field site) were making this information available to parents. Montuschi explained to me that the parents' rationale for wanting to access this information was, in her view, to gear their own knowledge-management tactics towards the details the children could potentially find out later by accessing the records (see chapter 6).

On a discursive level, the notion that the donor should describe him- or herself "as a person" in their own words and in their own handwriting seemed like a policy-led holistic counterpoint to the medical trajectory, with its step-by-step transformations and heavy usage of classifications. However, during my clinical fieldwork I learned that only a minority of the donors at both sperm banks and in the egg donation program was actually filling out the two "holistic" boxes (the sections were optional) on the HFEA registration form. Recruitment officer Jones and sperm bank manager Daffyd explained to me that the donors often found it hard to "to devise something [to fill in the sections], just on the spot." They were giving the donors the form to take home, fill the sections out there, and bring them back. Not all returned them during subsequent visits to the clinic, although encouraged to do so by the personnel.

Human Fertilisation and Embryology Authority

At the time of my fieldwork, the way the accessible trajectory of knowing kinship-by-donation was further translated within the practices of the HFEA was characterized not by actual requests for access, but only by their anticipation through the HFEA (since the first requests by grown-up children-by-donation conceived in the non-anonymous legal situation in Britain cannot occur until 2023). What was more pressing was another temporal threshold: the first children conceived in the non-anonymous, but highly regulated setup in place between 1991 and 2004 had just turned 18 at the time of my fieldwork in August 2010. These children were now eligible to approach the HFEA with requests to "open up the register" (often shortened in HFEA terminology to "OTR request") for so called non-identifying donor-information, but none had done so yet.[27] Furthermore, the clinics were registering back still active donors as non-anonymous and, more importantly, the HFEA was also offering all past and present donors to become non-anonymous. These changes made it necessary for the HFEA officers to prepare for a scenario that someone potentially soon contacting the HFEA to access *non*-identifying information, would then be informed that their donor had chosen to become identifiable.

The practice of re-registering donors as non-anonymous was controversially received among parents-by-donation, as information manager Fern and policy manager Peterson told me.

Iris Fern: "From the patient perspective, not all patients want it, because they have brought up their children telling them that they're donor-conceived, but that the donor isn't identifiable. […] Some patient groups definitely would like it, but not all former patients."
Janine Peterson: "I've certainly had a lot of parents-by-donation say to me they don't believe in giving donors the right to retrospectively be registered. […] The other side of that argument is that given that we [the HFEA] think it is right that anonymity should be removed. And given that there are now in a sense unequal rights between donor-conceived people before [the change to non-anonymity] and after—but also given that we obviously cannot infringe on the [anonymously registered] donors' rights by just whipping anonymity away, we do give them the choice [to register back non-anonymously]."

One situation in which the HFEA itself would inform donors of this choice was when donors themselves were contacting the HFEA registry to find out how many children had been born with the help of their donation—a right that had been granted to them with the regulatory changes in 2004. The controversies surrounding the shape and the admission to the accessible clinical/institutional trajectory show that parents interpreted the ways-of-knowing within the trajectory to be crucial for their

27 During my last brief fact-checking visit to Britain in 2012 I learned through head-embryologist Keira Lorimer at the LFH Sperm Bank that by now the HFEA has had to deal with 400 access requests. This would provide fruitful follow-on research to this book.

own knowledge-management practices (also see section 7.1 and chapter 6). Having developed specific knowledge-management tactics in the face of one specific trajectory of access (to non-identifying information) and within a specific regulatory set-up, the possibility of the donor suddenly becoming identifiable was not welcomed by all parents.

In addition to contact scenarios likely to arise in the near future (donors asking for the number of children conceived with their donation; requests by children conceived in the early 1990s) there were two more possibilities of how an "OTR request" would reach the information department of the HFEA: firstly, as part of a newly set up contact option for adult donor-siblings, "sibling link", which enabled mutually consenting brothers and sisters to contact each other (also see section 7.4); and secondly, when parents accessing non-identifying information stored on the donor learned of the option, as discussed above. HFEA information manager Fern had composed an internal manual holding the standard operation procedures HFEA officers had to follow for such requests. The manual included minute instructions on phrasing to use within telephonic or written contact, software operations to perform in order to obtain the requested information from the HFEA database, and successive documentation steps to be taken. The novelty of the requests, the complicated data retrieval entailed in answering them, the high level of bureaucracy and audit measures characteristic of HFEA work culture make it very likely that differences to actual practices were not pronounced.

To access the registry, donors, parents, and donor-conceived persons could approach the HFEA directly through a web interface. However, post, e-mail, or telephone requests were also anticipated. All personnel of the HFEA information department potentially dealing with requests had received basic counseling training. Information manager Fern explained to me:

Iris Fern: "We're a regulator, we cannot provide [professional and longstanding] counseling, we don't have the funding for that, but we are trying to make sure that people consider the implications [of making an OTR request]. Mostly people are just very happy to receive information. But then, once or twice, there might be somebody really in shock when they receive it. It is my number that's at the bottom [of the letter], and they have my name. They can call through and anybody [in the HFEA] whose name is at the bottom of an answer letter will have had training of dealing with people in emotional situations."

The knowledge-management practices in place at the HFEA hence anticipated that the kinship knowledge they would be dealing with had a personal impact on people. In other words, within formal administrative procedures they tried to actively manage the constitutive force of the information they were dealing with. This thus marked a convergence between regulatory and constitutive information as discussed through Strathern (see 2.2): the regulator itself was trying here to attend to the differing character that kinship-information assumes when accessed by personally affected individuals. The internal standard operating procedures of the HFEA, which I was not allowed to depict in detailed clippings, for instance lay out standard wordings to use on the phone when talking to affected persons. Callers who wanted the receive information from the HFEA register were for example to be told through the officers:

"Obtaining information from the HFEA Register may raise some unexpected emotions and you may wish to talk the decision through with someone before submitting a formal application. You may also wish to seek professional counseling or similar support services, on the implications of accessing information from the HFEA." (HFEA standard internal operating procedures 2010)

The slight surrealism of such detailed internal operating procedures, in my view, is produced through the friction between the highly formal administrative measures and the simultaneous anticipation of emotionality. This combination, however, epitomizes the specific kinship knowledge-management strategy of the HFEA. One could say that the agency was trying to anticipate kinship knowledge as constitutive information in Strathern's (1999) sense. At the same time the agency was trying to manage this "constitutivity" with the classic means of a liberal administration and the implicated notion of the autonomous subject capable of making informed choices—an idea absent from the original concept Strathern proposes (1999, e.g. 80). In other words, the HFEA's knowledge-management strategy brought the notion of choice back, by suggesting that the autonomous individual should consider the implications of accessing the HFEA register beforehand, and if need be supported by counseling.

When an applicant, after being told through HFEA officers "to consider the implications," would still go ahead with the access request, the officers would first confirm the person's ID via post. A case had to be generated within the administrative software used and that then automatically generated a case number and a monitored time frame within which to respond to the request. A case had to be closed after 20 working days, for instance, otherwise the software kept sending reminders. It also automatically deleted the saved scans of ID materials after a longer period.

The work of HFEA managers responding to requests, a process of data-retrieval, confirmation, and cross-checking, surprised me in its complexity and its potential for human error—even though all requests were also double-checked through a second officer. When, for instance, a donor applied for information, no list of his donor-children could be automatically generated on the computer screen, as I had naively imagined. Instead the officers only saw at which center he was registered and then needed to check the "donor usage report" of these centers on pregnancies related to that donor, which then needed to be further followed in a "pregnancy outcome form" that in turn showed whether there had actually been a live-birth. Parents were linked to a donor via their patient files and then the "pregnancy outcome form", then a "treatment form" listing the donor details, then the "donor usage report" to find out about siblings, and the actual donor information form (the document generated in the clinic as depicted and discussed above). Requests by donor-conceived persons were to be treated in a similar fashion, implying they needed to provide their mother's name at the time of conception, plus her date and place of birth. There had been various past changes within the different forms used, sometimes making all sorts of work-around and cross-checking procedures necessary.

Nor was the accessed information just printed or sent out but was instead translated into new templates for this purpose. Such templates, similar for correspondence with donor-conceived persons and for answering parental requests, were part of the internal operating procedures of the agency. Part of such letter-templates always was to include a table, which would hold donor-information, such as height, ethnicity, eye color and hair color. (During my time of fieldwork, no standard template for giving out *identifying* donor information existed yet). Part of the template also was a section giving the number and gender of "donor-conceived genetic siblings" an applicant had according to the HFEA register. Put more analytically, at the HFEA the remnants of the medical trajectory were further "cut off" by translating the clinical articulations into administrative formats. Within these transformations, kinship-knowledge started to take a more familiar shape again, through the anticipation of it being of personal value and effect and as a connector between persons. However, within these translations some of the clinical articulations of the donor-body (height, eye color, and hair color) and the more ambivalent articulations of ethnicity were also used.

The actual practices which would potentially unfold when a donor-conceived adult accessed this trajectory in Britain will, as pointed out before, only be possible to research in the future. In its anticipatory set-up during the time of my fieldwork, the British accessible trajectory presented itself as a selective translation of the articulations made during the medical trajectory into administrative formats. Kinship-by-donation here became known as pertaining to the donor as a person, but making use of selective aspects of the medical trajectory. It also became known as being of personal/emotional value and the potential basis for making connections between persons. The existent socio-material infrastructures and paper technologies became part of the relations arising out of reproduction here as well: for example through the software intervening in communicative processes, because it automatically generated a processing time for cases, or through the detailed development of standard operating procedures. The hybridity of the constitutive ways-of-knowing kinship-by-donation in the clinic was thus in a sense exchanged for a different form of hybridity: administrative affordances now became incorporated.

Recapitulation

I have shown how clinical practices relevant to the constitution of kinship-by-donation were in Britain embedded in regimes of tight, yet distributed "government at a distance", while those in Germany were more diverse. I demonstrated that for the clinical constitution of kinship-by-donation, two different trajectories of knowledge figured in my field: the *medical* and the *accessible trajectory*. Within these trajectories of validation, storage, and distribution (Barth 2002), knowledge-practices took on a specific path-dependence, following what Latour calls a chain of transformations from matter to form and vice versa (1999, 69). Within these pathways kinship became constituted in different figurations.

Within the medical trajectory, kinship was constituted out of interlinking *articulations* of biological substances; scientific, regulative, and industrial standards and guidelines; *translations* onto clinical information infrastructures; and parental knowledge-management. I argued that such a combination of links to scientific standards and regulation is one of the unique characteristics of kinship-by-donation. It also means that clinical and parental knowledge-management becomes part of the physical constitution of the children born through gamete donation.

Within the accessible trajectory, information was prepared for the potential later access by the donor-conceived. It mostly had its starting point within the medical trajectory, but drawing on and making available only selected parts of it. Kinship here became known as both a connector between persons and of personal significance. Such trajectory was much more comprehensively developed in Britain than in Germany. There, only small parts of the clinical information were anticipated to be accessible: basically only the address and name of the donor. Occupying fairly autonomous positions in the identified "hands-off" mode of governance, German clinical actors did not foreground the social relevance of kinship-information in general and donor-information in particular and in interviews often took on the perspective of their donors. The medical trajectory was not perceived to be of relevance for the accessible trajectory and was kept clearly separate in a more generally unclear regulatory situation.

In Britain parts of the accessible trajectory were comprised of articulations set up during the clinical trajectory, though of no practical relevance to it, as in the more "holistic" sections on the donor information form. The questions asked in these sections suggested that kinship-knowledge was mainly about the donor as a real-life person. The sections figured as an attempt of translating parts of this real-life person into the documentation, instead of only storing ID-information as in Germany. The HFEA officers also anticipated the personal relevance, the "constitutivity", the accessed information would hold. To manage this they underwent basic counseling training and put in place detailed operating procedures for communication. The configuration of the accessible trajectory in Britain thus particularly underlined that kinship was expected to be of identitary significance. The applicants were treated to access an important "truth" about themselves. The way the HFEA became involved in the accessible trajectory marked a convergence between conceptualizations of [k]information analogous to Strathern's (1999) notion of constitutive kinship information *and* conceptualizations incorporating the notion of an autonomous individual being able to make informed choices on [k]information. This chapter demonstrates how kinship-by-donation became clinically constituted within practices connected not primarily to the molecular-biological, but to more diverse strands of authoritative knowledge—for example techniques of administration and governance, or industry and medical standards. This insight guides me to the next chapter, where I analyze how the so-called psy-sciences are gaining currency in the constitution of kinship-by-donation in the domain of patient-group work.

6. Familial Knowledge-Management: Emerging Canons and Parental Reflections

Knowledge-management in the realm of kinship-by-donation is not only a practical policy problem and a clinical and regulatory area of responsibility and parental practice, it is evidently also laden with implicit and explicit normative assumptions. Who has a right to which knowledge? Who speaks for whom? And—as often used as a pun in articles dealing with the implications of donor conception—"what shall we tell the children" (e.g. O'Donovan 1990)? Or, maybe more importantly, what happens when they start talking (for) themselves? All of these questions are addressed throughout this book. Indeed, how—within these differing configurations—kinship becomes known in different ways is at the heart of my research interest. However, what I want to foreground within this chapter is that although openly acknowledging gamete donation and talking to children about it is a recent phenomenon, practices of disclosure do not take place within a normative vacuum. In this chapter I analyze how medical practitioners, psychosocial scholarship, and most importantly, new advocacy groups in both countries have contributed to emergent canons of knowledge-management, reinforced through authoritative advice literature and practices.

In section 6.1 I explore the tensions over parental disclosure or non-disclosure to children. I sketch clinicians' historical and still prevalent support (particularly in Germany) of parental non-disclosure and then analyze interest group activism and associated counseling practices in both countries. I examine in detail the most advocated tools for parental knowledge-management, such as children's books. I will argue that the canon of parental knowledge-management in both countries is characterized by an imperative of early disclosure of the donation to the child. I further put forward that the disclosure decision within the data analyzed for this chapter is predominantly framed as a moral question on equal sharing of information, not as a question either of the necessity or of right to knowledge about genetic relatedness.

Section 6.2 focuses on my familial interviewees' experiences with interest group activism and shows the advice they gleaned from these activities for their own tactics of knowledge-management. It analyses the kinds of value judgments about knowledge-management the parents make. Similar to the analysis in 6.1, disclosure, among my interviewees, again emerges as a moral imperative to be pursued early. Particularly the German parents expressed ambivalence regarding a potential later interest of their children in the donation and the donor, a situation I interpret as linked to the uncertain German regulatory situation.

This chapter thus sets the stage for a better understanding of the parental practices described above in chapter 4, and—even more importantly—of those described in the following chapters 7 and 8: showing these practices to be not only individual tactics, but also implicit or explicit standings in the face of historically derived and changing normative assumptions about discussing gamete donation. These assumptions are connected to strands of knowledge stemming from the "psy-sciences", particularly counselling and psychology more generally. Empirically, the chapter draws on my clinical fieldwork, of course; on the advice materials, publications and discernible web activities of advocacy groups; and on interviews with two influential interest group activists in Germany and Britain, as well as on my research with parents and adult donor-conceived individuals who are active in these advocacy groups of concerned people.

6.1 Normative Canons of Knowledge-Management

Medical interest in insemination practices in the Western world started to rise in the second half of the 19th century, although already sporadically contemplated or practiced within earlier veterinary and medical practices. In both Germany and the UK artificial insemination has been practiced for more than a hundred years. Reports of the first cases of insemination-by-*husband* were published in 1880 in the UK and in 1909 in Germany, and the first case of insemination-by-*donor* was published in the US in

1909—a case which reportedly took place in 1884 in Philadelphia (e.g. Katzorke 2008). When exactly the practice of insemination-by-donor was introduced to Germany and the UK is difficult to tell. In fact, considering that in the American case neither the mother nor the father initially were informed about the procedure, and given the longstanding "culture of secrecy" (e.g. Hargreaves 2006, 264; Thorn et al. 2008, 2419) associated with DI, there is a possibility that cases where the husband was reported to be the donor might actually have been cases of DI. In the medical world and in the wider public, the procedure caused controversy both in early 1940s Britain and in post-war Germany. Debate focused on DI as repulsive, e.g. by associating it with animal breeding, and on the illegitimate status of the resulting child. Egg donation of course became possible only about a hundred years after the first published cases of insemination-by-donor, facilitated by the advancement of IVF technologies in the 1980s. (For historical accounts and documentation of cases e.g. see Bateman Novaes 1998; Cook 1999, 122–123; Daniels and Haimes 1998, 2; Haimes 1998, 53–62; Katzorke 2008; Knecht 2010; Strathern 1992, 40).

Changing cultures of clinical and psychological advice have had a major impact on normative conceptualizations of the parental disclosure decision. Conceptualizations of parental disclosure differ among clinicians and counselors. Instances in which my familial interviewees had encountered advice *not* to disclose were more common among my German research partners. Historically, until the more detailed policy deliberations and changes surrounding donor anonymity emerged in the noughties, the culture of secrecy surrounding donation practices clearly dominated in both Germany and the UK—and actually the Western World in general. As Haimes (1998) traces for the UK, the few early official reports on donor insemination in the first four decades after World War II (in the UK coming out of church, medical and state institutions—whereas in Germany the controversies remained mainly within the medical profession) framed as problematic the issues of the resulting children's legitimacy, the kinship connection to the donor, and the disturbing effect that disclosure would presumably have on a child.[1] The reports however did not actually make a clear-cut argument for non-disclosure *per se*. In practice however,

1 The history of sperm donation in Germany and normative conceptualisations of the disclosure decision is not as comprehensively researched as for the UK. However, see

and separate from the occasional social and ethical debates on the topic, DI both in Germany and in the UK was practiced in a climate where non-disclosure was the unquestioned norm (e.g. Blyth 2008; Daniels and Thorn 2001).

With the birth of the first IVF-baby, Louise Brown, in 1978 in Britain and the later deliberations of the Warnock committee, reproductive technologies started to become an issue of concern in the industrial West. Haimes pointedly summarizes for this period in the UK:

> "By the late 1970s-early 1980s, three views were apparent on what the 'DI child' needed to know about his/her conception: first, the dominant view, propounded particularly by clinicians, was that s/he should be told absolutely nothing about the means of conception, let alone about the donor; a second view emerging from some adoption professionals was to tell the 'child' about the means of conception but nothing about the donor; a third view, from other adoption writers, was to be completely open to the 'child' about the means of conception and about the identity of the donor." (Haimes 1998, 60)

It would be beyond the scope of this work to trace in detail the institutional and individual practices in both Germany and the UK within which this dominant view on the necessity of non-disclosure stayed so tenable for several decades of medical DI practices. It may be suspected, however, that this view—in addition to dominant perceptions of the family and of legitimate and illegitimate sexualities—is deeply entwined with far more general questions regarding the changing relationship between physician and patient. On a more pragmatic level, prescribing secrecy probably relieved many clinicians from having to justify their work within a broader societal context, where DI was viewed as a dubious practice, and thus ensured a smooth everyday running of their routines of donor recruitment.[2]

Little is known about how kinship-by-donation was known *familially* during the times when non-disclosure was still the unquestioned norm. The occasionally emerging stories which seem to reconstruct these ways-of-knowing in the popular press or within research and also the views expressed in the interviews I conducted with adult donor-conceived per-

---

Katzorke (2008) and Knecht et al. (2010, particularly 6–29) for insightful historical discussions.

2 This was also underlined by German DI expert Petra Thorn when interviewed by myself. Thorn's role for the German canon of parental knowledge-management will be discussed in detail below.

sons frequently dwell on the sense of shock and betrayal produced by finding out, often accidentally, late in life. Such accounts dwell on the perception that there were things strange, lingering yet unnamable, going on in their family, which only started to make sense in retrospect, after disclosure (e.g. DI Kind 2007; Haimes 1998, 66–68). Hence, these stories are often structured by a retrospectively (re-)constructed sense of the uncanny that "things were not as they seemed".

Cultures of Secrecy and the Clinical Endorsement of Non-Disclosure

Today, parental non-disclosure *still* seems to remain the norm, although this might surprise since it seems like the culture of secrecy is not in place to the same extent anymore, and official advice is leaning more towards disclosure (for a highly critical commentary on this see Walker and Broderick 1999). In fact, although there is little research on the subject given its evidently private—and secretive—nature, the number of parents not telling is very high. Wallbank (2004, 259) argues, summarizing assorted pre-2002 research on parental disclosure, that almost three quarters of parents-by-donation participating in the different studies were not disclosing the donor conception. When I asked German and British clinicians and counselors to estimate the percentage of (heterosexual) non-disclosers, they typically estimated between 70 and 90 percent. Blake et al. (2010, 2527), summarizing post-2000 research, argue there is a discernible trend, however, that more parents disclose the donor conception to their children. Clinical psychologist Diane Ehrensaft is cited affirmatively in a brochure of the British advocacy group DC Network as summarizing the changes in normative clinical and psychological *cultures of advice* as follows:

> "...the social tides have changed. As they have changed, experts have done a 180-degree turn in their thinking about disclosure. Twenty years ago people thought disclosure would be traumatic for the child, humiliating to the parent, and disruptive of the parent-child bond. Now it is believed to be a violation of the child's rights, a denial of reality, and a threat to the integrity of the family not to tell a child the truth about his or her birth history." (Montuschi 2006a, 2)

DI experts Ken Daniels and Petra Thorn argue similarly:

> "From a culture of semen-provider anonymity and parent and professional secrecy, there has been a significant move to a more 'open' approach in which information concerning DI is being practiced by an increasing number of professionals, parents and semen providers." (Daniels and Thorn 2001, 1795)

As already touched in chapter 2's discussion of transparency, the trend toward disclosure could be seen as part of a wider cultural shift in which secrecy and not-knowing have become increasingly undesirable socially. In the role of interest group activists, as further traced in this chapter, parents certainly have been part of this shift. Yet the fact that in general most parents presently still choose *not* to tell their children also shows that there is a large group of parents with a different approach to knowledge-management, whose voices are not being heard.

Non-disclosure is most likely akin to other practices of secrecy in families, which are by definition not characterized by explicitly or publicly negotiated knowledge-tactics among family members. Smart (2011, 550) argues that family secrets perform a "governance by silence in which no clear responsibility can be attributed to specific family members because control over knowledge is acquired through intangible inaction and unremarkable acquiescence". Of the few psycho-social studies within which the topic of disclosure is interrogated, either the normal development of DI children is stressed irrespective whether the parents disclosed or not (Golombok et al. 2002; Golombok et al. 2004), or the studies show that less internal quarrelling seem to be discernible within disclosing families-by-donation in comparison to non-disclosing ones (Lycett et al. 2004; as discussed through Thorn 2008a, 101). In contemporary family therapy literature and most counseling literature in general, family-secrets are conceptualized as disruptive to family relationships, but also as an inherent and negotiable part of family life (e.g. Imber-Black 1993).

An autoethnographic side-note further illuminates the issue of family secrets. I subscribe to a project where the plea for transparency is explored as a cultural phenomenon (as for instance done by Edwards 2009a; Smart 2009, 2011; Strathern 1999), rather than simply classified as a further step in enlightenment. Nonetheless, I find it difficult affectively to relate to the parental or clinical past and present culture of secrecy surrounding kinship-by-donation. Indeed, Iain Walker and Pia Broderick (1999, 39) caution us that speaking of "secrecy" introduces an "emotionally laden and strongly pejorative word." (They propose the subject could just as well be explored by referring to "privacy" or "confidentiality"). Autoethnographically, I can report on experiences of non-secrecy. Being a child of what in Germany is called the *sixty-eighter generation*, referring to the politically active baby boomer generation participating in social movements in the late sixties and seventies, I was brought up with very few taboos surrounding conception stories. In fact, most of my childhood friends and I knew where we were conceived, because our parents told us: on the holiday in Greece or in a Volkswagen van visiting friends in the GDR or in the bed we were playing on, which almost took on mythical proportions for us as children, because it was also the bed this friend had been born in during a home birth. Walker and Broderick (1999, 40), maybe because of age difference or a potentially more prudish Anglo-Australian culture, simply discard the mere possibility of such conception-knowledge existing when they argue that "it is probably safe to suggest that most of us know nothing of our own conception". I remember playground-talk among my friends when we were still in kindergarten or had barely started elementary school about quite delicate reproductive issues. I learned from the twins next door, for instance, that they were adopted, and along with this I learned what adoption and infertility were in the first place. These personal experiences, I want to suggest, are already bound up with a West-German permutation of the cultural shift towards transparency, a cultural shift within which children were supposed to be brought up in a climate perceived to be less repressive concerning sexuality and reproduction. These experiences are also bound up with the *sixty-eighters* being the first generation of women "on the pill", which shifted conception towards often, not always, being straightforwardly intentional in a way that it never was before. Being told about—some—details of one's conception thus is to be seen as a knowledge-practice rooted in the so-called sexual revolution, within which the wantedness of a child was or is acknowledged. Politically, this parental openness can be linked to the *sixty-eighters*' endorsement of transparency as a key symbol in coming to terms with the country's Nazi past and their own parents' endorsement of secrecy regarding this past.[3]

Thus, the idea of bringing up a child *without* talking about the previous experience of infertility and how it was subsequently overcome does not come naturally to me, although the labeling of not-telling as "lying", as further analyzed below, also affectively strikes me as problematic. Given this personal "bias" and that the families I managed to recruit were all disclosers, I started my clinical fieldwork without further reflection assuming that hardly any remnants of the previous so-called culture of secrecy would be discernible. That assumption was wrong, especially given the only recent change to non-anonymous donation in the UK and its unclear status in Germany. In fact, among clinicians (in contrast to counselors, interest groups, or policymakers) anonymous donation regimes have often been stressed as the preferred and more practical set-up.[4] It was particularly in Germany (as already discernible from my analysis in chapter 5) that my colleagues of the kinship cultures project and I still encountered fragments of a yet distinct culture of secrecy. (Thorn and Daniels 2000, 205 also underline that German clinicians tend to recommend non-disclosure). This was more pronounced in what parents told me about the advice they got from clinicians than within statements physicians made to me. Dr. Lindemann of the Sperm Bank and Fertility Centre Luisenburg was the only clinician who straightforwardly dismissed disclosure in interviews.

3 See Sperling (2011) for an ethnographic exploration into differing conceptualizations of transparency in East- and West-Germany and the renegotiation of such conceptualizations after the German reunification.

4 The International Federation of Fertility Societies, which is first and foremost a body of physicians, for example still recommended non-disclosure in their 2001 consensus on reproductive medicine (as reported through Thorn and Daniels 2006, 50) on the grounds of this being more clinically practicable. In their 2010 surveillance the Federation makes a link between the drop of donor numbers in the UK and the change to non-anonymous donations. Such links—implicitly suggesting that anonymous donation regimes are more clinically sustainable—have been exposed as resting on media hype and local problems in clinical administration in the UK, and are not responsible for the drop in donor recruitments (e.g. HFEA 2011b) already touched upon in chapter 5. Prominent UK physicians appeared widely in the national press with statements criticising the move to non-anonymity at that time (e.g. British Fertility Society 2004).

The passages below are taken from an interview my colleague Sabine Hess conducted with him in 2005:

Sabine Hess: "Do you think families get stigmatized if they lay open that they used sperm donation?"
Dr. Lindemann: "It is hard to say, because I think most people won't tell that they have had this treatment or want to have this treatment. And I don't see any reason why they should do this differently. Why? What the neighbors, the child and the grandparents do not know, does not cause conflicts. And as long as the child still looks like Herr and Frau Müller, I guess everything is all right."
Sabine Hess: "So you are recommending being secretive?"
Dr. Lindemann: "Yes, and if at some point something should show up, because maybe the optical resemblance between donor and husband/partner did not come through as desired and the kid becomes suspicious at some point, or checks his blood group in biology class, and then comes home and ask questions… Of course the couple needs a plan for this case. But I think, not from the outset, how does that serve the child, how? Does a child understand when it is eight, nine, or ten years old?—Nope!"
Sabine Hess: "Maybe…"
Dr. Lindemann: "The child will just get more confused, the world is confusing enough in itself."

In an interview two years later Dr. Lindemann had however started to engage with arguments against non-disclosure. He acknowledged that "one can only refer to people who can judge these things, family therapists, psychologists, child psychologists, and it *seems* to be important to many people to be able to find out who the biological father is". His lasting emphasis on a "thorough" physical matching as analyzed in chapter 5 nonetheless suggests that he was still working not to make "the kid suspicious at some point".

The German parents I interviewed offered striking examples of clinicians arguing against disclosure. German father Philip Steger for instance recounted what he had heard from other DI parents:

"There are doctors who actually recommend to destroy all contracts, all copies, anything pointing to it [the donor insemination] so that the child does not see it and whatever happens, 'do not tell the child'… I don't think that's right".

When German mother Berit Feldman told her fertility doctor that she was planning to disclose the donation he—as she re-enacted for me—stressed not to tell, because "'this is how we have been running this clinic for 30 years'". Feldman quite incredulously recounted how the gynecologist apparently told her about a couple who had successfully undergone DI treatment at his practice and then completely forgot about having had the treatment in the first place:

Berit Feldman: "And then the doctor said that after three years they wanted another child and just tried for it the 'normal' way. Only after one year they noticed again: 'Ooh, we actually cannot have children, back then we actually had to go to the clinic'. They supposedly had totally forgotten [that they had gone for DI earlier]".

When Berit and Uli Feldman had asked the same doctor what would happen if he would be asked to make available the donor information, he said he would never give out any data: "He said: 'If necessary, there would be a fire or something like that [implying the records would be destroyed]' and that's what he had promised the donors" (Berit Feldman). When the Feldmans reacted with anger and confusion, the doctor looked at his records and told them that things were different for their donor, because this was a "Yes-donor". This information left the couple further confused. After our first interview, Berit Feldman contacted the clinic again by e-mail to enquire about the status of "Yes-donors". After she had written several unanswered e-mails over a period of some months, she finally got a reply. It turned out that her gynecologist merely seemed to be referring to his more recently recruited donors as "Yes-donors", probably in the light of the regulatory changes towards the—vague—non-anonymous donation regime in Germany. In other words: A "Yes-donor" simply seemed to be a donor whom the doctor had *not* told that the filing cabinet would burn down should someone come asking for his files.

As further explored in section 7.3 my familial research partners in their knowledge-management embraced the practice of compiling informal kinship-archives, of which treatment contracts or other clinical papers were frequently part. In the parental accounts of clinics favoring non-disclosure in Germany, contracts also figured quite heavily. For the clinicians, contracts seemed to be the material and informational remnants of the donation, and parents were advised to "burn them or throw them away" [the Feldmans, the Schneiders, and the Stegers by hearsay in their interest group]. German father Marc Schneider told me that in light of this practice their clinic at first did not even want to give his wife and him a copy of their treatment contract to take home. After he protested, he received a copy. Berit and Uli Feldman later realized that their contract actually did not mention the DI treatment at all, only that they had come for "fertility treatment". Thus, whereas the disclosing families were actively building informal kinship-archives, a preferred practice of knowledge-management on the side of "pro-secrecy" German clinics seemed to be to actively eliminate all evidence through destroying the material and informational remnants of the donation.

The story told to Berit Feldman of parents who not only had kept the treatment secret but supposedly had entirely forgotten the donation provides a glimpse of how the so-called culture of secrecy was locally constituted in clinics. Regardless of whether the incident really happened or was only a moral tale by the gynecologist, what the clinician apparently wanted to bring across to the Feldmans was his understanding that non-disclosure was possible without secrecy. Invoking his "30 years of experience" the doctor had seemingly advocated to the Feldmans that non-disclosure not only was the best knowledge-management strategy for parents, but that alongside non-disclosure, they could erase the experience of DI from their own memories. Given how impregnated German culture or rather Western culture in general has become with psychoanalytical thinking, this attitude on knowledge-management surprised me. Still, in this local stance on non-disclosure it was not seen as synonymous with secrecy. "Forgetting", in this case, was believed to leave no traces.

My British fieldwork materials did not provide similarly striking accounts of clinical advice not to disclose or similarly dubious statements or practices regarding contracts and clinical data management. The few accounts I gathered directly from clinical personnel or in parental accounts that did not concur with the British policy and counseling canon of being pro-disclosure and favoring non-anonymous donation practices, as further explored below, mostly called into question the move to non-anonymity, not parental non-disclosure. Dr. O'Brien at the Largecity Fertility Hospital for instance told me that in the past he had been highly critical of the move to non-anonymity. However, this criticism, like many other public statements by clinicians, mostly centered on the suspected impossibility of recruiting donors in this setup, not on more general questions of disclosure (also see Thorn et al. 2008, 2416). In my fieldwork materials it thus appeared that the so-called culture of secrecy was reigning less powerfully in Britain than in Germany. This was most likely enforced through the central role the HFEA takes up as regulator and registrar in Britain (see 2.1 and 5). Burning donor files, for instance, would not be an option for alternative tactics of clinical knowledge-management in Britain.

Given the central regulation of donation practices since the HFE Act in 1990 along with, firstly, the official introduction of anonymity and then, secondly, its removal, it might be no surprise that clinicians were rather interrogating questions of non-anonymity than complete secrecy. British mother Holly Greenwood told about her first cycles of insemination at an NHS clinic (she later changed to the Largecity hospital to avoid further waiting periods) during the transition period to non-anonymous donations:

> Holly Greenwood: "We had a consultation with the doctor and then one with the manager of the laboratory and that was the time when the legal situation in Britain was changing… So this was the year when one could decide if one wanted an anonymous donor or not. And the laboratory manager was really pushing us in one direction: 'well, we have a lot of donors who are still anonymous. It would be much better if you simply take an anonymous one. It will fit totally well. We will find a donor who looks just like your husband'. Maybe that wasn't exactly how he said it, but that was the route he was going down. And then we started to have the feeling that they only had one or two non-anonymous donors available anyhow. And we did not learn anything about the donors and it was all just really… really strange! It was actually an extremely odd situation…"

Hence, in my British data, discussions of parental disclosure/ non-disclosure were displaced by discussions of anonymity/ non-anonymity. There were only two accounts in the British fieldwork materials where clinical personnel recently advocated non-disclosure, and these were more ambivalent than the German cases discussed above. The first account came from 26-year-old British donor-conceived adult Bonnie Smith, whose father had developed a disease suspected to have a hereditary component when Smith was already a young adult. She, however, only found out accidentally that she was a DI child quite some time after her father got ill by comparing their blood groups. This is how Smith reconstructed a conversation she had with her mother *after* the discovery of her donor conception:

Bonnie Smith: "My mom said: 'When your dad got ill, we discussed telling you with the doctor at the hospital, and that doctor said not to'. So I think the original doctor they saw at the fertility clinic was like, 'you don't have to tell'. And then definitely our doctor at the hospital when my dad got ill also said to them 'you don't have to tell her. It'll be all right. She'll go for a test to see if she's got the gene, it'll come back negative and then there's nothing to worry about'. Except it wasn't that straightforward, I had to go and have [these scans], and I had to go every year, because it's not a conclusive test."

Bonnie Smith's case lights up like the burning records hint in Germany. Sending her into a monitoring regime for a disease she could not have carried underlines the disruptiveness attributed by the advising doctor to disclosing DI conception. However, from the way Bonnie Smith recounted the incident, I would not want to exclude the possibility that her mother used the doctor's supposed statement to justify her own decision not to tell her daughter about the donor conception.

I recorded another ambivalent British account when discussing parental knowledge-management with a counselor at the Largecity Hospital who stressed that he would not advise parents to tell, but that it was "only the parents' choice". (This approach is of course in line with a general professional commitment to neutrality in counseling in both Germany and Britain. Nonetheless, the guidelines for fertility counseling in both countries contain passages that seem subtly to suggest that parental non-disclosure would be the preferred counseling-outcome).[5] The counselor, who was also trained as a social worker, was very critical

5 This connotation is particularly discernible in the German guidelines for fertility counseling. An example of the arguments there is shown in the following passage: "the autonomy to take decisions lies with the parents, even if nowadays early disclosure towards the child is considered to be sensible for developmental-psychological and family-dynamic reasons" (BKid 2008, 3–my translation). It is also argued that, should parents choose non-disclosure, it would be "helpful to examine if this decision is compatible with the system of values of the parents, for instance the values of openness and honesty in a family" (BKid 2008, 4–my translation). In the British guidelines the phrasing is yet more subtle, but counselors are for instance advised to explore with clients how to take into account the welfare of donor-conceived children in relation to the disclosure decision and to also inform parents of the advancing usage and accessibility of genetic testing (BICA 2007, 5–6). There are voices in the international academic discussions around fertility counseling, which criticize the apparent tendency to implicitly or explicitly favor non-disclosure as counseling outcome (e.g. see Klock 1997 or Walker and Broderick, 1998).

of the DC Network and of its pro-disclosure stance. Given the Network's close work and association with the counseling sector in Britain, I had not expected this.[6] This particular fertility counselor, however, argued that the Network's clear position against non-disclosure was "in no way representative for all the families-by-donation in the country" and was "not useful" advice to take. He had a problem with the group's claiming to act on behalf of families-by-donation within policymaking "while they only have about 1,600 members and there are probably about 12,000 families out there". But most clearly he implied the Network was inappropriately pressuring parents to tell. This would make the parents so nervous that instead of telling they would be in need of further counseling, as he framed it. The only advice he would give to non-disclosing parents was not to tell anyone else, "so that there are actually no secrets around to be told". Thus, the counselor's statements revealed yet a different conceptualization of non-disclosure: a secret was negative, but was only brought into being interactively through unequal communication practices. Here, non-disclosure was, similar to the German case discussed above, not expected to have social effects in itself.

Canons of Knowledge-Management among Interest Groups

In recent decades, groups for families-by-donation have formed in Germany and Britain and were establishing specific national and transnational canons of knowledge-management at the time of my fieldwork. In Britain the Donor Conception Network appeared as an influential actor in the realm of gamete donation. Instigated by an initiative to publish a children's book on donor insemination (more about its content below) in the late 1980s, the DC Network was founded in 1993. Dr. Sheila Cooke, who began to set up the sperm donor conception unit at Jessop Hospital in Sheffield in 1982, began to engage closely with the few parents who told her they were thinking about disclosure and who were interested in what this might mean practically. Among them was Jane Offord, the later

6 Some of the most active members of the DC Network, as their manager Oliva Montuschi told me, were in fact persons concerned who also had a professional background in counseling, psychotherapy or social-work. Members of these professions also regularly appear in DC Network events as speakers or discussion conveners.

author of the first British children's book on donor conception (Offord et al. 1991). Cooke, as cited on the DC Network website, recounts their meeting as follows:

"Jane talked about writing a story and so the idea of writing a story that would help others to be open and honest, but couldn't find the words, became an exciting possibility" (DCN 2012).

Cooke, Jane Offord and her husband, an additional concerned couple, and an artist friend conceptualized the book together and saw to its private publication in 1991, after attempts at finding a publisher failed. When, to promote the book, Cooke mentioned its existence to a journalist, an article appeared in *The Times* in 1992. More disclosing parents, among them the DC Network's current manager Oliva Montuschi, whom I also interviewed, began contacting Cooke to be put in touch with each other. A first meeting among the original "book team" and newly interested parents took place, with further media coverage leading to the official founding of the DC Network. Thus, in Britain the children's book did not figure as end-product of parental networking, but at the center of what Michel Callon and Vololona Rabeharisoa, have identified as the "problematization process" (Callon and Rabeharisoa 2008, 237) crucial for the initial emergence of interest groups; their engagement with knowledge production and the associated public construction of specific identities and matters of concern.

At the time of my fieldwork the DC Network held yearly members' meetings and conferences, ran workshops on disclosure in different British cities and (probably most importantly concerning the canon of knowledge-management explored here) put out not only children's books, but also a vast array of advice materials. This was done both through its comprehensive website and as a mail-order service maintained through the website.[7] The DC Network had approximately 1,600 members, comprised of both homosexual and heterosexual parents-by-sperm/egg/embryo-donation and their children, some of them already grown up. As discussed with the DC Network's manager Montuschi and with other members, one of the group's tasks was to offer parents a direct personal connection by welcoming new members through an email from

7 See www.donor-conception-network.org

an older member and offering a personal telephone call to interested parents. The DC Network was financing itself through membership fees and project-oriented governmental grants. It was active in British policymaking, with Montuschi regularly being invited to give evidence or serve as a committee member when questions surrounding gamete donation were explored through the HFEA, the Department of Health, or the Nuffield Council of Bioethics.

Montuschi (who has a professional background in parenting-education and counseling) also networked closely with national and international infertility counseling organizations, regularly attending their meetings. This was how she met Petra Thorn, a German fertility counselor and interest group convener (more below), whom she kept close contact with and who could be described as her German counterpart. In fact, Montuschi and Thorn—as they both confirmed to me in interviews—have had various knowledge transfers: the concept for the workshops on parental disclosure the DC Network was regularly offering, for instance, has initially been developed by Petra Thorn and DI expert Ken Daniels for Thorn's German practice (for an analysis of the group work see Thorn and Daniels 2006). In turn, Thorn has used the DC Network children's books as inspiration to develop the first such German language book on donor insemination (Thorn and Rinaldi 2006), and cites some of Montuschi's advice from the British Network booklets in her own German language guide for families-by-donation (Thorn 2008b).

The children's books on donor conception were not only key to the initial formation of the DC Network, but also to their currently advocated knowledge-management strategies. They were frequently mentioned in the advice brochures on "talking and telling", published by the Network (e.g. Montuschi 2006a, 4, 10). These four brochures (see clippings 6.1 and 6.2) on disclosure tactics were available for a small fee on the Network's website. The brochures are split up according to age ranges, both incorporating questions on how to talk continuously to one's children about donor conception and how to first disclose to children of different age ranges.

Use of the children's books is tied with what I identify as the discursive core of the British interest group canon on knowledge-management, namely the ideal of early disclosure with the goal of making the child "know all

Clipping 6.1: DC Network Brochure for parental kinship knowledge-management with very young children (Source: Montuschi 2006a)

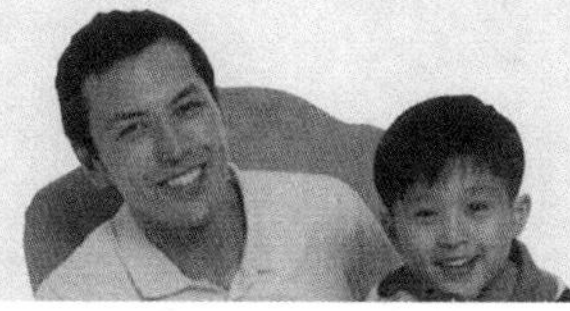
Telling and Talking
'Telling' and Talking about Donor Conception
with 0 - 7 year olds
A Guide for Parents

along". In an interview, DC Network manager Montuschi summarized this approach to knowledge-management as trying to achieve that "there's never a time when children didn't know about it at some level or another". The approach is also captured in the following quote from the DC Network advice booklet pictured in clipping 6.1:

> "By starting to sow the seeds of information early it is likely that your child or children will not remember a time when they did not know about how they came to be part of your family or that donor conception is anything other than (an ordinary) part of their story." (Montuschi 2006a, 4)

The frequent use of children's books as a tool for knowledge-management within families-by-donation has also been described in the more applied psycho-social and social scientific literature (for a short summary see Blake et al. 2010, 2528) and is further explored for my research partners in sections 7.3 and 8.6. The strategy is backed up by some smaller studies out of the educational sciences suggesting that parents experience it as least conflict bearing (e.g. Rumball and Adair 1999) and that children benefit most from the donation being talked about as a part of the family history, not as something marking the child as "special" (Daniels and Thorn 2001).

Clipping 6.2: DC Network Brochure for parental kinship knowledge-management with older children (Source: Montuschi 2006b)

Telling and Talking

'Telling' and Talking about Donor Conception
with 8 - 11 year olds
A Guide for Parents

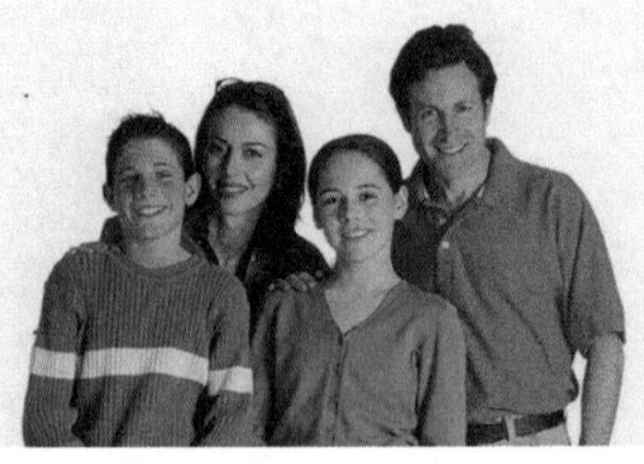

The few studies available on the topic convey that parents on average disclose when their children are between 4 and 5 years old (as summarised through Blake et al. 2010, 2527). Generally, the DC Network advises to either follow this method of active disclosure or follow a more passive approach, where the parents would start telling once their children start asking their very first questions about reproduction during kindergarten age (e.g. Montuschi 2006a, 6). As analyzed in section 6.2 below, my parental interview partners also typically used one of these two approaches to knowledge-management.

The formation of interest groups in Germany and their canon of knowledge-management has followed a rather similar trajectory. Although in Germany interest group activism was even more strongly entangled with counseling than in Britain. Social worker Petra Thorn was both the most influential counselor on questions surrounding gamete donation and an initiator to whom all interest group initiatives I encountered had a foundational link, for example, through personal encounters at one of her group workshops.

At the time of my fieldwork Thorn, however, unlike Montuschi, was not the head of an interest group herself. Although she had personally experienced a period of unwanted childlessness and had gone into patient activism after that, Thorn did not have children through DI like Montuschi. There were, nonetheless, striking similarities between the two. As previously mentioned, Thorn is also the author of the only two available German children's book on the subject (Thorn and Herrmann-Green 2009; Thorn and Rinaldi 2006). Just as the usage of the books is recommended through the DC Network advice literature authored by Montuschi, Thorn also recommends its usage in her advice book for DI families, the only one available in German (Thorn 2008b, 92). Thorn was also running workshops for couples considering DI and for already established families-by-donation. She is the founder of the German association for infertility counseling (BKid) and member in numerous German and European associations dealing with infertility and reproductive technologies, both in the patient group sector and in the sector of professional organizations for this field of work.

Both Thorn and Montuschi were regularly referred to by name, often forename, by my familial research partners, but also by the policy experts and physicians I engaged with. The parents had mostly met them at workshops, very clearly accepting them as authorities and simultaneously as familiars. Montuschi and Thorn are typical examples, I want to argue, of a new type of expert emerging out of the interest group sector and influential in introducing new modes of knowledge-production and power-relations in the health sector (also see Polat 2012). They are powerful through their ability to mobilize expert medical knowledge and—often more relevant—*psy*-knowledge, and the affective and experiential knowledge of DI parents/infertile persons. In other words: in contrast to the new modes of co-producing scientific knowledge via the engagement of concerned groups described through other scholars (e.g. see Callon and Rabeharisoa 2008; Epstein 1995, 1996; Rabeharisoa and Callon 2002), the new (lay-)expert knowledge emerging from interest groups in the domain of gamete donation concentrates more on the sector of psychology and counseling. This has the effect that instead of a *co-production* of knowledge on a new disease, new expert actors such as Thorn or Montuschi rather challenge some of the clinically maintained knowledge practices through their new expert status. They add additionally relevant and authoritative ways-of-knowing to the expert discourse, which, however, do not draw on the same scientific disciplinary roots as those of the clinicians they encounter. To illustrate the distinction, the AIDS activists described by Epstein (Epstein 1995, 1996) became experts on clinical AIDS research itself—experts such as Thorn and Montuschi in contrast introduce additional *psy-knowledge*.

The two interest groups specifically focusing on DI and active in Germany during the time of my fieldwork—*Spendersamenkinder*[8] and *DI-Familie*[9]—were much smaller than the DC Network and less professionally organized. They did not have an official membership system or group structure. Research partner Berit Feldman who was active in both groups in 2009 estimated that Spendersamenkinder was probably comprised of 40 to 50 active families. Later, in 2012, she mentioned the task to quantify this any further being inherently hard because of the unofficial grass root character of the networking. The administrator of the website of "DI Familie" told me via email that he estimated the site networking approximately 200 families. Hence, in 2012 there were circa 250 families-by-donation organized in emergent interest groups in Germany specifically focusing on gamete donation. In comparison to Britain, the groups did not have similarly comprehensive websites or self-published advice materials available. They did, however, provide comprehensive links both to Thorn's publications and to the DC Network's materials.

The two groups shared two significant characteristics: They were "internet-based" and they were founded by people who met at one of Petra Thorn's group counseling workshops on DI. In this case "internet-based" does not mean the groups did not meet face-to-face. In fact most of their web profiles served the purpose of enabling informal personal meetings. What it implies is that their basic websites, and the work involved in maintaining them, were the group's main organizational structure and their main tool for reaching other persons concerned. There were no lobbying activities and no meetings with a more formal character,

8 www.spendersamenkinder.de
9 www.di-familie.de

such as the conference-like annual DC Network event in London.[10] The main official purpose of the German groups lay in the informal sharing of experiences and in the exchange on strategies of knowledge-management. The DI Familie website, www.di-familie.de, for instance, states:

"After one of Petra Thorn's group-workshops, the couples of our group decided to keep meeting on a regular basis (as in the past the IDI-Group www.spendersamenkinder.de). In the beginning we mainly had exchanges about individual fertility clinics, their advantages, legal issues, notary contracts, but also about our own feelings, our fears and hopes. Now that we have children, our topics have evidently changed. Today we focus on how to disclose DI to our children, on reactions from our social circle, on openness among friends, neighbors, but also on our present thoughts about DI." [my translation]

During my fieldwork, I witnessed the networking endeavors of DI-Familie growing rapidly, while Spendersamenkinder did not accommodate new members. The latter did not want to outgrow by number their possibility of having their already traditional bi-annual meetings in a youth-hostel. Founding members of DI-Familie, of whom two had a background in IT, put up a simple tool on the website depicting regional groups or people interested in founding regional groups through flags on a map of Germany (see clipping 6.3).

One could click on the flags, sending a message to a person who had volunteered for that region to answer e-mails. This enabled both highly informal and highly effective networking, as it only needed one person to become aware of the website and then volunteer to answer emails and coordinate local meetings. Between the set-up of the site in 2009 and 2012 I could see approximately 20 more flags appearing, signaling that networking was in full flow.

During my research, the German groups were predominantly heterosexual and bi-parental, while the DC Network had a large section for homosexual families and single mothers, which manager Montuschi seemed proud to refer to as being part of the growing Network "right from the beginning". In Germany a representative of rainbow-families in a large

10 As this book is going into print in late 2013, German DI parents have set up a registered society: DI-Netz, translating to DI-Network (www.di-netz.de). The activities of DI-Netz are more formal and show more similarity to the activities of the British DCN. Unfortunately, these developments took place after the writing of this book was completed and could therefore not become part of the analysis presented here.

Clipping 6.3: Regional groups of the grass-roots interest group DI-Familie, as depicted on their website in 2012 (Source: website www.di-familie.de)

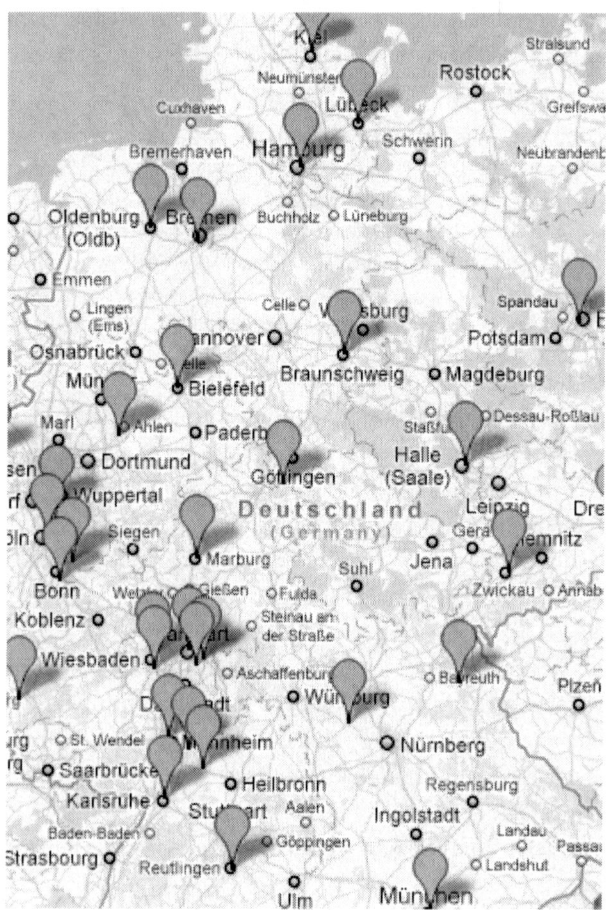

German gay rights' organization outlined to me that networking among homosexual parents in Germany had a different angle. Teaching their children that there could be families with two mothers or two fathers seemed to be at the forefront for many lesbians and gays, rather than gamete donation as an issue in itself. This was reflected in the local meetings of rainbow-families in Großstadt. These get-togethers were similarly geared to the informal sharing of experiences and to shared leisure activities resembling those of the predominantly heterosexual German groups. There was, however, no specific focus on questions of disclosure. In contrast to the heterosexual groups, the rainbow-families were also occasionally involved with political activism (pertaining to access rights of lesbians to reproductive medicine or more general questions surrounding the legal status of homosexual families—not to other more general questions on donor conception). During my time of fieldwork there was no specific German group available for single mothers, as my interview partner Maria Lieb noted unhappily. She had been interested in networking through the research of my colleagues and myself, but I could not put her in touch with other local single mothers. In fact, after I had sent an interview request to one of the "flags" depicted in clipping 6.3, a member of DI-Familie based in the same city as Lieb anonymously attacked me via e-mail for publishing on single-mothers-by-choice and thereby contributing to a "negative image of DI in Germany". I was retrospectively relieved I had not recommended to Lieb to simply contact the other bi-parental initiatives for families-by-donation. In Germany, interest group formation thus seemed to be more related to issues pertaining to family *form*, whereas in Britain the group identity was articulated around the method of conception.

While the idea that early disclosure, meaning during kindergarten age, was best for children dominated in the German interest group and counseling canon just as much as in the British (e.g. BKiD 2008, 3; Thorn 2008b, 83–96), the concept of an early *active* disclosure by talking to toddlers and young children about gamete donation was not as dominant in the German discourse. As she elaborated in an interview, Thorn in her seminars and in counseling practice advised parents to tell their young children about the donation the moment they started asking questions about reproduction. Thorn takes the same stance in her advice book for families-by-donation (Thorn 2008b, 87), nonetheless also citing the story of one of her clients who already started talking to his new born son about DI to "practice" (2008b, 87). The German interest groups generally alluded to their pro-disclosure stance on their websites without further details. Hence, an early passive disclosure seemed to be typical for the emerging German interest group and associated counseling canon of knowledge-management, although not as elaborated as the stance on active disclosure in Britain.

Children's Books on Gamete Donation as Part of the Interest Group Canon

Children's books explaining gamete donation were key to how the canonical idea of (passive or active) early disclosure was facilitated through the groups of parents (and children) involved with DI. The centrality of such publications (also see 7.3 and 8.6) has led to the emergence of books for all kinds of gamete donation families—particularly in the UK, with its seemingly high level of networking among the concerned, the legality of many different donation techniques, and their accessibility to both homosexuals and heterosexuals. There are for instance volumes available on sperm donation (Offord et al. 1991) and egg donation (Baxter and DCN 2002d), double or embryo donation (Baxter and DCN 2002c), others for lesbian families (Baxter and DCN 2002a) and for single-mothers-by-choice (Baxter and DCN 2002b). In Germany Thorn's first children's book on heterosexual families-by-sperm donation (Thorn and Rinaldi 2006) was followed by an altered version of the book for lesbian families (Thorn and Herrmann-Green 2009). Five of the children's book covers are depicted below.

All of the books portray the coming-into-being of kinship-by-donation in very basic form: there is little text in them, normally one simple sentence per page accompanied by a picture. Because all of the books were developed out of or inspired by the original British "My Story" book, the storylines are extremely similar. There are one or two parents who would really like to have a child; children are normally conceived by egg and sperm; there is a difficulty with this because of reason X; but then the parents—or a doctor—have an idea; the parents get help; "you" are born. The books usually close with a page where one can attach photographs of the child, and the parental happiness of now having a child is stressed. (Also see clippings 6.5 and 6.6 for an example of the similarities between the German and the British book on sperm donation). All of the children's books impart detailed information on procreative substances and biological reproduction (see clippings 6.11 and 6.12), but leave out further details of heredity, sexuality, genitalia, or masturbation. The donor is depicted as someone "very kind" who gives away sperm or eggs, because the doctor asked. Sperm donor sexuality is hence eclipsed. In German the term "schenken" is used, which translates both to "to make a gift" and to "to donate".

Clipping 6.4: The first German language children's book on sperm donation (Source: Thorn and Rinaldi 2006)

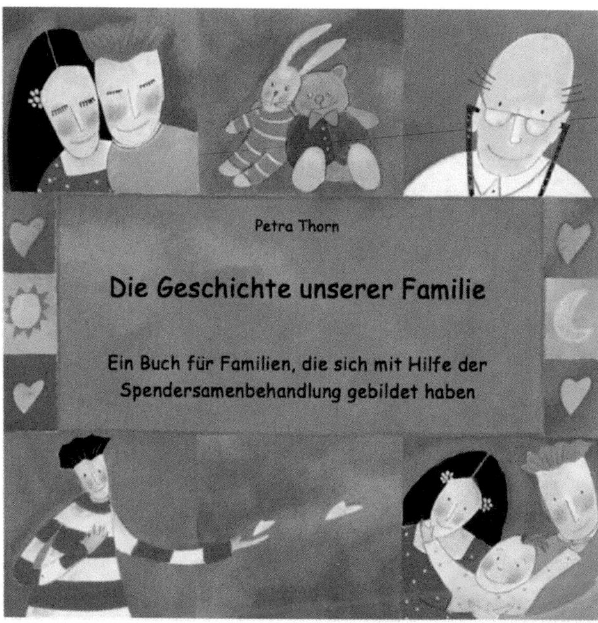
Petra Thorn
Die Geschichte unserer Familie
Ein Buch für Familien, die sich mit Hilfe der Spendersamenbehandlung gebildet haben

The German book title translates to "The story of our family: A book for families that were formed with the help of donor-sperm-treatment". It has been inspired by, and is in parts highly similar to the "My Story" book depicted in clipping 6.5 below.

All of my familial research partners had used or were planning to use children's books for disclosure (see 7.3). Below, I shall explore the symbolic universe of the books, without however implying that parents were not changing the meaning conveyed through the books during their own familial usage of them, let alone that the children just passively took in the books' messages (see 8.6). Kinship-by-donation is typically made known symbolically in the children's books through underlining three central themes: love, biological reproduction, and assistance. Firstly, parents in the books are depicted as loving each other intensely and longing for a child, which they then also excitedly welcome and love. (In the book for single women the theme rests upon love and longing for a child alone).

Clipping 6.5: The first German language children's book on lesbian families-by-sperm-donation (Source: Thorn and Herrmann-Green 2009)

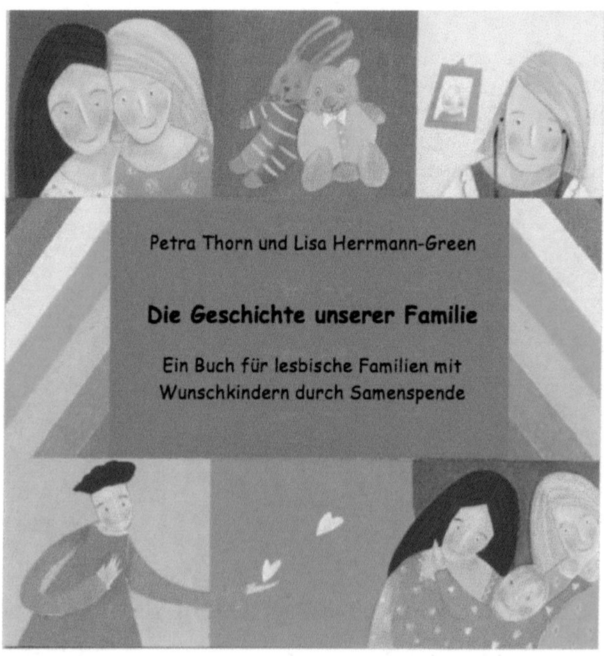

The German book title translates to "The story of our family: A book for lesbian families with wished for children [Wunschkinder] conceived through sperm donation. The term "Wunschkind" which would literally mean "Wish-Child", refers to a planned child, but has a less technical connotation.

This makes love a generative symbol within the books, driving forward the parental endeavors to become pregnant.

Secondly, the books depict becoming a family as bound up with biological substances that create a child. And thirdly, the publications convey that doctors and donors are capable and willing to assist when these biological substances are not available for various reasons. In chapter 4's analysis I have shown that in the interviews my familial research partners defined kinship as characterized through three tensions surrounding the themes of choice, (corporeal) continuity, and love. In the books only the latter theme is apparent, because neither solidarity nor heredity are touched upon.

Clipping 6.6: The first British children's book on sperm donation (Source: Offord et al. 1991)

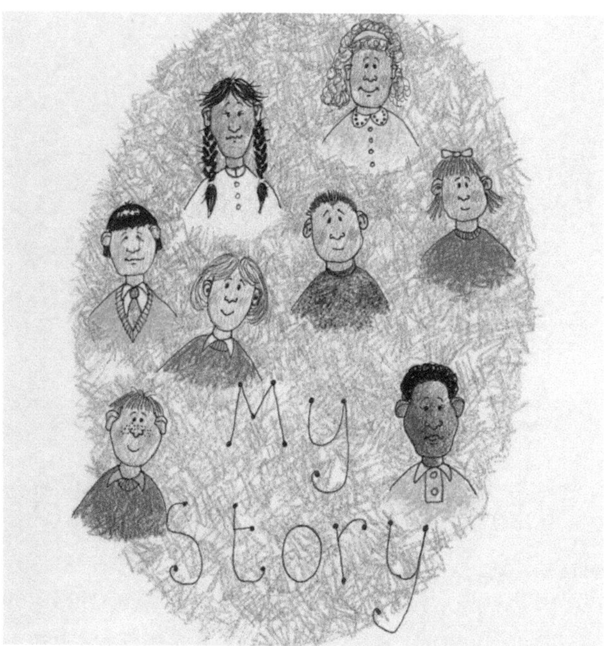

The work on the first version of "My Story" by concerned parents marked the beginnings of the DC Network in the late 1980s.

Love, as generative core-symbol of kinship is a contested notion. It has been postulated and analyzed in the U.S. by Schneider, who proclaims, "Love is what American kinship is all about" (1968, 40), and continues:

"The symbol of love bridges two culturally distinguished domains, first, the domain of kinship as a relationship of substance, and second, the domain of kinship as a code for conduct." (Schneider 1968, 52)

Crucial to Schneider's symbolic analysis of American kinship is the notion of heterosexual intercourse as unification, as potentially procreative act of "conjugal love" through which one shares physical substances, thereby begetting children to whom one is then bound through "cognatic love" (1968, 40). Many scholars in the new kinship studies have questioned Schneider's emphasis on the centrality of heterosexual intercourse as core-

Clipping 6.7: DC Network children's book on kinship-by-embryo-donation (Source: Baxter and DCN 2002c)

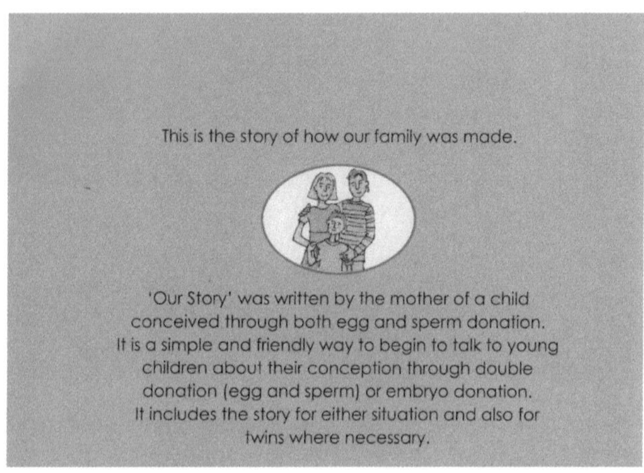

symbol for Western kinship, for instance through analyzing homosexual kin formation (Weston 1991, 35) or the imagined anonymous kinship arising between egg donors and recipients (Konrad 1998, 651). Other scholars out of the new kinship studies are, however, still using Schneider's assertions to analyze the ambivalences in actors' conceptualizations of reproductive technologies as partly resulting from the symbolic centrality of heterosexual intercourse for kinship ideologies being threatened through the technologies (Ragoné 2004, 350).

In the children's book analyzed, the symbolic nexus between love, sexual intercourse, biological substance, and procreation certainly is not given. In the German and the British books, kinship-by-donation is made known in ways both yielding to the societal taboos surrounding children and sexuality, through bracketing off themes such as parental intercourse, sperm donor masturbation or the depiction of genitalia—but also to the very material realities of assisted conception, where intercourse indeed is not part of reproduction. The books also simultaneously underline the notion of a rooting of kinship in Western scientific understandings of biology by introducing quite detailed explanations on biological substances, but they actually exclude the central kinship notion of shared substance/heredity. Kath Weston has argued in her beautiful ethnography of 1980s San Francisco gay culture that "no models or code for conduct applied to

Clipping 6.8: DC Network children's book on sperm donation for single women (Source: Baxter and DCN 2002b)

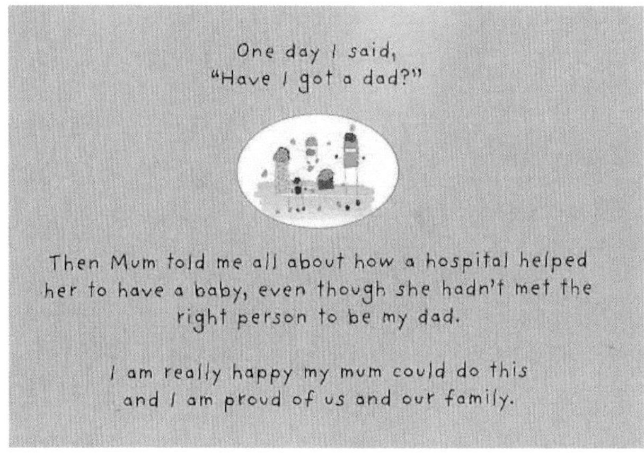

gay families (aside from love)" (1991, 191) and that "families we choose do not rest directly upon a genealogical referent" (1991, 193). I found that within both the heterosexual and homosexual versions of the children's books, such a separation between love and genealogical reference was not possible. Through the depiction of love as generative core-symbol in the books, love itself became genealogical referent. In other words: love, stripped of sexuality, remained the generative core-symbol for enrolling biological substances and helpers to create a child in the worlds within "My Story" et al. Yet this enrolling of biological substances did not entail parental intercourse, but consultation with a doctor instead. Thus, symbolically, the books leave intact some traditional aspects of Western kinship (e.g. love, procreative substances) while excluding others (e.g. sexuality and heredity).

The Conceptualisation of Non-Disclosure as Lying

Both the German and the British interest group canon of knowledge-management shared an underlying normative conceptualization of non-disclosure as "secrecy" or often even "lying", to be analyzed in this section. For myself, *secrecy* is an emic expression for non-disclosure and I needed to be alerted to the term's negative connotations, as suggested by

Clipping 6.9: Mourning infertility as depicted in "My Story" (Source: Offord et al. 1991, 5–6)

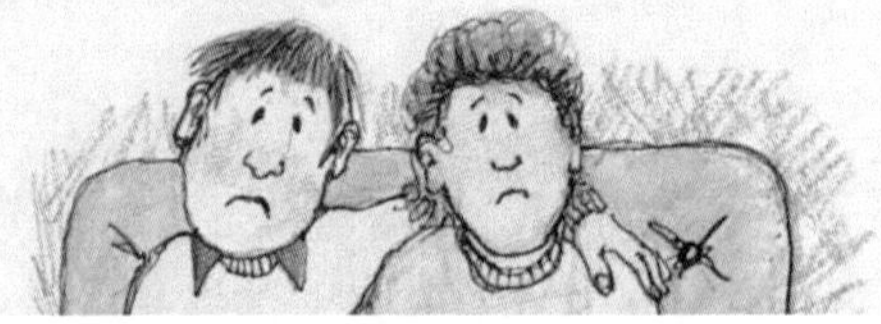
Mummy and Daddy tried for a long time to
have a baby and they were very sad when no
baby began to grow.

Walker (1999, 39), cited above. *Lying*, however, is obviously an even more morally laden term, although—as also discussed above—I can affectively relate to this conceptualization of non-disclosure. In the British DC Network brochure on telling young children about DI (Montuschi, 2006), for example, many such equations between non-disclosure and lying are made. The brochure is comprised of general advice (linked to experiences of Network members and academic research within psychology or social work) and individual accounts of experiences and opinions. The booklet is empathetic in tone, straightforward and occasionally humorous in language. That non-disclosure is *morally* wrong is clearly communicated. For instance, when a mother-by-donation is quoted with the sentence "'In essence, if you are not telling you are lying" (Montuschi 2006a, 1) or when a father-by-donation is quoted as saying "How could I spend the rest of my life lying to my children, my wife and myself?" (2006a, 25). It is further argued, for example:

> "Telling your child about donor conception definitely means that some other people need to know as well, and telling these people early means not having to get tangled up in a web of avoidance or lies." (Montuschi 2006a, 15)

Whether similar moral framings of the disclosure decision existed in the German interest group canon of knowledge-management was harder to research empirically in the absence of an organization similarly productive of written accounts as the DC Network. In the more limited German

Clipping 6.10: Mourning infertility as depicted in the German book for heterosexual families-by-sperm-donation (Source: Thorn and Rinaldi 2006, 14)

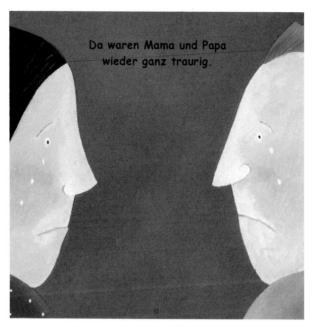

The German text reads "So Mommy and Daddy were very sad again". (They had already been "sad" earlier, because the mother did not get pregnant. Now they are shown as unhappy, because the doctor has told them about the father's infertility).

discourse I nonetheless encountered similar moralizations of disclosure. Thorn, although mostly arguing in a more neutral style, has made the equation between non-disclosure and lying in at least one of her academic publications (Thorn and Daniels 2000, 204). In her popular advice book for German parents a similarly moral tone to that of the DC Network cited above is adopted:

"Some parents also stress that openness and honesty are fundamental values to them in the upbringing of their children and that they cannot expect such values from their children if they are not living them as well. DI father Timo: 'We want to bring up our children in a way that they turn out to be honest people, that one can rely on them. Hence it is important that we are a living example of such

Clipping 6.11: The Facts of Nature as depicted in "My Story" (Source: Offord et al. 1991, 3–4)

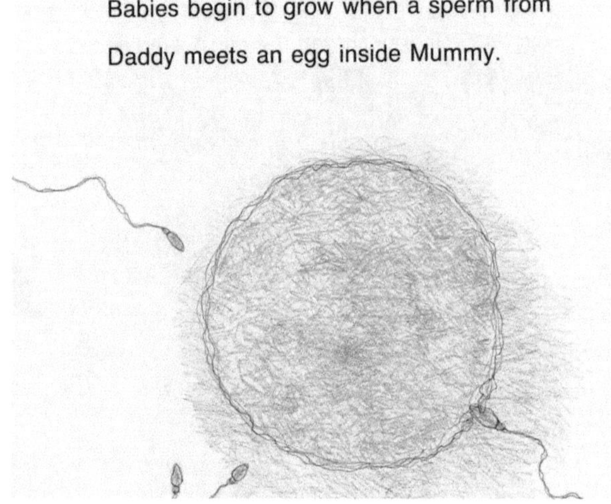
Babies begin to grow when a sperm from
Daddy meets an egg inside Mummy.

values. That's why it was out of the question that we would lie to them and not tell them that they were conceived through donor sperm. We cannot expect openness and honesty from them, but then lie to them ourselves.'" (Thorn 2008b, 85, my translation)

The international English language advice book for families-by-donation by Daniels (2004), which is advertised through the DC Network and which some of my German research partners had also read because Thorn recommends and sells it through her website, takes a similar stance. It is apparent in this quote from the chapter on "secrecy and Donor Insemination—an unhealthy partnership":

"With regard to secrecy, I feel there is no need to even discuss its morality (the rightness or the wrongness of such action) because I have never read or heard an argument that supports the stance that it is morally right to lie to children about their family history and their genetic heritage. It is not an argument parents would support either." (Daniels 2004, 71)

What distinguishes this passage from the other interest group conceptualizations of non-disclosure as lying is that Daniels also brings in the theme of the importance of genetics, a theme I did not encounter as

Clipping 6.12: The Facts of Nature as depicted in its German counterpart (Source: Thorn and Herrmann-Green 2009, 9)

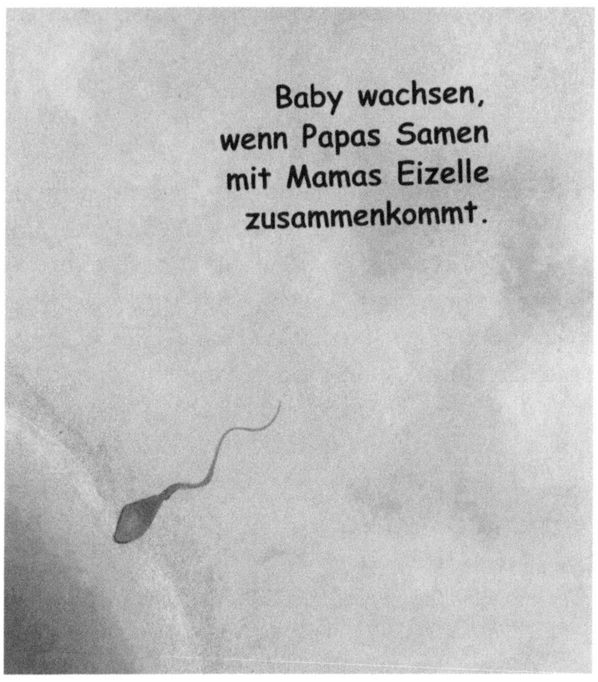

Baby wachsen,
wenn Papas Samen
mit Mamas Eizelle
zusammenkommt.

The German text reads "Babies grow when Daddy's sperm meets Mommy's egg cell".

pronouncedly in Thorn (although see the joint publication Daniels and Thorn 2001, 1794) and also not by the statements of the DC Network. My German and British interview partners involved in interest group work—as further explored below—also frequently made references to non-disclosure being "plainly a lie" (Philip Steger) or a "grand delusion [Lebenslüge = literally "life-lie"]" (Marc Schneider)—however without attaching this to a specific value associated with genetics.

Recapitulation

In conclusion, fieldwork data on the work of affected groups in both countries (compiled from secondary literature, interviews with advocacy group activists and parents, and a discursive analysis of websites, advice literature and children's books) conveys a broad shift in how kinship-by-donation became known in concerned publics in Germany and Britain. A historical swing occurred away from silent families and authoritatively knowing clinicians (who took the power to prescribe non-disclosure on now rather outdated moral grounds pertaining to illegitimacy and sexuality)—toward counselors and policy experts standing as advocates for families-by-donation and often stressing the "right to know" along with the importance of this knowledge on psychological and medical, or more precisely genetic grounds. The historical shift subsequently turns to a yet different form of moralization of knowledge-management by the organized representatives of families-by-donation *themselves*. As part of this shift, the question of disclosure is removed from being first and foremost a question of hereditary, identitary, medical, or legal importance, to being first and foremost a question of specific *family values* stemming from the psy-sciences. The equal sharing of (kinship) knowledge thus has become a moral obligation in itself, dislodged from biology and made a moral imperative.

Through this analytic lens, the shift to openness in gamete donation practices would not necessarily point to forms of geneticization (as one could imagine (e.g. see Finkler 2001), but instead to changing ideals and practices of knowing and thereby doing kinship: inequalities in knowledge distribution are not explicitly or implicitly viewed as a self-evident component to family life anymore, but something to be avoided. Children's books, in which a discursive universe of non-sexual love is the generative core-symbol, are the tools for practices of kinship knowledge-management through which the effort is made to overcome these inequalities (also see 7.3). This is advertised and practiced both through the large and highly professionalized interest group DC Network in Britain with its ideal knowledge-management strategy of *making known all along* and within the smaller and more informal German groups associated with Petra Thorn's work. Questions of identity, medical needs and heredity, which have featured in the historical and recent policy debates on gamete donation (as discussed to some extent above, but for a more comprehensive analysis e.g. see Haimes 1998; Klotz 2006, 2007), have been displaced in the interest group canons on knowledge-management.

The sociologist Carol Smart has argued that "there seems, in the UK at least, to be an urgency around revealing or exposing personal truths which was not prevalent fifty or more years ago" (2009, 2). She tries to analyze this shift concerning family secrets of different shades with a neutral attitude, which she herself nevertheless discusses as hard to maintain because "…it becomes increasingly difficult to imagine, let alone support, the idea of keeping secrets in families and relations. Axiomatically such behavior is deemed to be at best selfishly retentive and at worst harmful" (Smart 2011, 3). This links into my own previously described autoethnographic experience of being raised in a climate where laying open intimate conception knowledge to one's children was the norm, making the described *culture of secrecy* surrounding gamete donation hard to relate to as a scholar. In some of the statements and accounts cited above however, it became clear that German clinicians did not necessarily equate non-disclosure with secrecy, seemingly not sharing the *sixty-eighter* ideals on "openness" or more Freudian conceptualizations of suppression/forgetting. And in Britain I also encountered the idea that secrecy came into being only interactively if the parents talked to others about DI, without talking about it with their children. Keeping family secrets, Smart puts forward, could also be looked at as an inherent part of sustaining kinship, a practice through which power relations in the family, but also normative state and societal interventions are negotiated, and also through which certain relationships are privileged over others so that cultural imaginations are incorporated into family narratives (Smart 2011, 540–541). However, for what I called the interest group canon of knowledge-management in Britain and Germany the idea of personal relationships being deeply compromised through unequal access to knowledge prevailed. Thereby, it turned the ways-of-knowing kinship-by-donation into a personal and societal question of morality and a "struggle over the place of truth in family relationships" (Smart 2009, 4).

6.2 Familial Moralities of Knowledge-Management

How did my familial research partners position their knowledge-management in the face of these emergent normative canons? Concrete practices and experienced confrontations will be the subject of chapters 7 and 8 to come. However, within my family interviews and occasional less formal conversations during meals, walks or playground sessions there also emerged long reflections on "how to get everything right" while raising a donor-conceived child. We also talked a lot about my research partners' experiences with interest group work and discussed how this had played a role—or not—in arriving at their own convictions regarding disclosure. Such reflective conversations are the focus of this section. They give insight in the families' own moralities concerning knowledge-management. I shall firstly discuss how my parental interviewees had typically decided to disclose the donation and how they had experienced contact to interest groups. I shall then turn to discussing their conceptualizations of non-disclosure and close with an analysis of the fears and underlying rationales with which my interviewees reflectively broached the subject of knowledge-management.

Except for the Tönschs, who simply never felt the need to do so, all of my research partners had come into contact with the interest group work described above.[11] The families I engaged with separated into two groups in their overall approach to talking to their children about donor conception: those I typologize as *active disclosers*, following the idea of "making known all along" (Schneiders, Feldmans, Hamptons, Taylors, Greenwoods, Lieb), and those I typologize as *passive disclosers*, who had decided to wait for their children to start asking questions about reproduction (Tönschs, Müllers, Stegers, Kings, Nakamura). The Dünke and the Arnulf rainbow-family did not clearly fall into either typology of disclosure, given that they did not bring up disclosure as a clear-cut theme, but more generally discussed how to raise children in a heteronormative society. They were, however, also using children's books and interest group contact.

For arriving at their specific disclosure strategy, the families often underlined the importance of the exchange with other people concerned and with interest group publications. British mother Holly Greenwood for instance said to me:

11 This should not be interpreted as indicative of general levels of interest group organisation for families-by-donation in Germany and Britain, but rather was related to my sampling strategy for research partners (see chapter 3).

Holly Greenwood: "The DC Network has a local group in this area, and we regularly went in the past. They also organize this large picnic in the park with all the children once a year. Through those activities we got quite a lot of advice and found out that there are these books and workshops [on disclosure]. They have so much information. That was already very useful during the treatment itself, because that was a very difficult time for us. It was really good having people to talk to."

Greenwood thus expressed a sense of relief that through the group work she was able to simultaneously connect to forms of expert knowledge and meet other people in a similar situation. This was typical for my research partners' accounts of how they formulated their own knowledge-management strategies in interchange with the interest group activities and advice. German mother Berit Feldman, as another example, enthusiastically described her first group workshop with Thorn and Daniels as providing all the medical, legal, and psychological information she needed as well as offering a comforting and safe space to talk to other people in a similar situation: "It was brilliant, just brilliant". Another German mother, Nadine Schneider, particularly stressed how emotionally comforting she found her first interest group meeting: "I simply felt in good hands, understood. I realized—wow!—I am not alone with some of my abstruse worries". And British DI father Tim Hampton said to me that although he had already looked at the DC Network's publications on disclosure, he still found their additional workshop beneficial:

Tim Hampton: "I got two things out of that telling and talking workshop. First was that I met a Canadian bloke who lived around the corner and who, like me, was infertile. He and I got along immediately very well. He and his wife have now gone back to Canada, which is unfortunate. We have gone out for drinks a couple of times; we just spent a lot of time talking. That actually was a good thing, a really good thing. I've got that and you know what: the other thing that I got from that workshop, I remember getting it in the last ten minutes.... She [Olivia Montuschi] did all these exercises and I went in there expecting to come away with a script in my head of what to say and actually I didn't come out with that, but what I came away with was the clear knowledge that the only important thing was, however you tell your kids, to do it with confidence and not shame. You need to be telling the story honestly.—That's the one thing I took away from it: to be natural about it, to be honest about it."

Thus, Tim Hampton emphasized the positive (and typical) combination of both (lay-) expert advice and personal encounters.

British single-mother-by-egg-donation Shoko Nakamura used the workshops to convince her son's father and donor John Blake, with whom she was not co-habiting, but who regularly saw their son Ochi, that disclosing the egg donation was the right strategy:

Shoko Nakamura: "John does not know much about it [gamete donation] and he was sort of dragged into the project. He was so fast to say: 'oh, we shouldn't tell, we don't need to tell Ochi'. So I had to take him to go to the DC Network to a workshop. In the workshop we learned that it's no good… -that secrecy is quite a bad thing. Taking him to the workshop was really good".

Hence, Nakamura was using the DC Network as a resource for guidance on how to raise a donor conceived son. Instead of only discussing disclosure or non-disclosure of the egg donation with sperm donor and father John alone, she took him to a workshop so he would also come to know the DC Network's canon on knowledge-management.

Also highly important to most parents in my sample, heterosexual and homosexual alike, was that their children would grow up in contact with other donor-conceived children, or in contact with other rainbow-families. It was viewed as essential that through this networking the children would come to know kinship-by-donation and and/or rainbow-families as actually "quite normal" (Svenja Arnulf) and that there would be other parents and children around to talk to once the children "grow older and start asking new questions" (Holly Greenwood). The interest groups and their emergent canon of knowledge-management thus provided the families with a sense of normality and relieved them of having to establish pioneering strategies of knowledge-management (also see 7.3). This is also captured in the three interview passages quoted above. In a situation of insecurity for the parents on whether to use gamete donation or not, and later, how to raise their children, the interest groups provided validation for specific strategies of knowledge-management and the comfort of a community.

Criticism of the interest group networking or advice available was extremely rare. The German-Brazilian Tönsch family had no interest in networking with other families-by-donation during the time of my fieldwork, but they were nonetheless reading Thorn's advice literature and did not criticize interest group networking in principle. However, for them, the question of how to manage the potential bi-lingual upbringing of their two DI children seemed to be a more important subject of parental deliberations.

None of my interview partners explicitly questioned the canon of knowledge-management they had come into contact with through the group work, but rather appeared to be very comfortable with it. There was some awareness and criticism, however, among the German couples of group activities predominantly taking the shape of self-help meetings. This I did not encounter from my British interview partners, potentially because the DC network offered so many different genres of interaction, e.g. the "great annual conferences, where they have so many experts and also panels with donor-conceived children discussing their views" (Holly Greenwood) along with local groups focusing either on joint activities or on self-help meetings, or both. Berit Feldman reflected on the self-help character of the group she was participating in:

> Berit Feldman: "Only a certain type of people will join such communities: I mean, you need to be capable of speaking in front of a group, you actually have to enjoy psychologizing a bit, for sure… You got to have the nerve to cry in front of other folks and stuff like that. That's not everyone's cup of tea!"

German father Marcel Müller, in his lively and humorous ways, made it quite clear in the interview with me that this was certainly true for him:

> Marcel Müller: "I won't sit down in this round of sandal wearers and go: My name is Marcel, this is my problem, 'thanks for sharing that, Marcel', not for me! I am a very open kind of guy, but only in a relaxed kind of crowd, maybe over a drink or so."

During his one and only interest group meeting, as he told me, he had organized with some of the guys to get a case of beer and hang out more informally. That part of the meeting he had enjoyed and positively stressed the experience of meeting other men in a similar situation. Interest group activities, particularly where they took the character of self-help meetings, thus required a certain habitus of participants: a willingness to share intimate experiences and the eloquence and confidence to do so in front of a group of people. Nonetheless, as Marcel Müller's case shows, interviewees were also able to intervene in this genre if they did not feel comfortable with it.

The Framing of Non-Disclosure as Lying through Parents

The conceptualization that non-disclosure was *lying* and therefore morally wrong was not only prevalent in the interest group canon, but also in my familial research partners' reflections. In addition to those parental statements already cited above, German mother Silke Müller for instance said to me:

Silke Müller: "I think the betrayal of trust, if you have been lying to your child, you can never make up for. That's impossible."

The different stances on non-disclosure analyzed above, where non-disclosure sometimes did not equal secrecy—and even forgetting or suppressing knowledge was imagined without social effects—were not to be found among my parental interviewees. The Hampton parents interactively and eloquently shared their conviction with me that non-disclosure would always lead to negative consequences for those involved:

Tim Hampton: "No matter how difficult [disclosure is], it can't be worse than not telling your children. I couldn't have carried that around with me. There is no way of carrying that around with me."
Sarah Hampton: "I try to think what it must feel like for people who chose to do that!"
Tim: Hampton "-it must…"
Sarah Hampton: "-how would it feel like with your own family?"
Tim Hampton: "They must just put it away in a dark place and never think about it."
Sarah Hampton: "Hmm…"
Tim Hampton: "But of course—the things you put in a dark place they come out when you can't sleep at night. Or they make you not sleep at night."

Thus, while I indicated earlier my surprise about concepts of secrecy ignoring any effects of suppressed knowledge—as expressed through clinicians apparent in my data—my familial interviewees were much closer to the understandings of secrecy with which I was raised. This included the expectation that things not said or thought about could still have a social life. The Feldmans, who also stressed the "general disruptiveness of family secrets" (Berit Feldman) remarked:

Uli Linde-Feldman: "You don't need to study psychology to realize that if you hear about it [the donor conception] late and in a row, you will suddenly go: 'Oh I never really felt like you were my Dad' or stories like that. That's just obviously fucked up. So I guess, if you just talk about it in a relaxed way and on a regular basis, it should work out."

To be rejected as a *Dad*, as evoked in the quote above, was the single most voiced fear of my heterosexual interview partners surrounding DI and emerged as the worst-case scenario of what could happen if one got knowledge-management "wrong". (Egg donation did not seem to produce the corresponding anxiety. The two British egg donation mothers I interviewed did not address fear about their maternal status, most likely because they had given birth and were therefore also conforming to parts of the traditional definition of being a mother).

Interest group publications address the fear of rejected fatherhood differently. The British ones argue that such verbal rejection of DI fathers is an exceptional phenomenon among DI children and should, in the rare case where it does not remain a fear but becomes reality, be calmly interrogated as a provocation and/or an adolescents' way of addressing other, non-donation related problems in the family (e.g. Montuschi 2006a, 23–24). Thorn in Germany does not as comprehensively discuss this fear in her advice book, mainly touching upon it in connection with disclosure to adult donor-conceived persons (Thorn 2008b, 97).

British interview partner Tim Hampton said he felt confident that, should a verbal rejection of him as the father happen, he could look his children "honestly in the eye and tell them how much I love them and tell them I am sorry that this is the way it started and that I am sorry if that upsets them, but that it's just the way it is". He added: "And then it will go wherever it does". Both Hamptons told me laughingly that Sarah Hampton's mother apparently kept saying to them they must pre-emptively start telling their children to never ever say to Tim that he was "not the father". This made him comment, again with a laugh: "If you tell them not to do that, guess what is going to be the first bloody thing they do?"

Particularly the German families I engaged with voiced that if DI children say to their fathers "you are not my Daddy", it might be a sign of parental mistakes in kinship knowledge-management, "a symptom that something just went fundamentally wrong in the upbringing [Erziehung]" (Uli Linde-Feldman). German father Marc Schneider, who had read the DC Network publication discussing the fears around being verbally rejected as a father, said that even though he had been afraid of the scenario in the past, he now thought it would not "get to me anymore, because I now know how I would deal with it. I mean, the relationship is there and won't just disappear". Yet Schneider also expressed a conviction that a heightened interest in the donor might point to "the family not functioning quite right, there just not being a father figure, then there is more of a need to look for a father". My heterosexual German interviewees more often made such normative comments on child-rearing and knowledge-management than the other research partners. Typically, the conviction was expressed that choosing the right strategies for knowledge-management would make it less likely for the child to develop an interest in the donor, as already entailed in Marc Schneider's comment. Philip Steger, as another example of such tendency, said in our first interview:

> Philip Steger: "I think if you know from early on, that it [DI] is normal and one is raised, let's say, 'properly' that it is hopefully not a problem for the child. [...] I guess if a child has a decent upbringing, and a good home, then I hope that it will simply not become so important that it would get any problems."

German mother Silke Müller said she hoped that if she "simply let" her son "grow up knowing the whole thing was part of his history, meeting the donor would simply become insignificant for him". And Dörte Tönsch similarly stressed that openness about the donation and the right approach to the child's upbringing "would maybe lead to this wish [of seeking out the donor] never to develop". Berit Feldman remarked more generally that she would find it "brilliant, to be honest with you, if our children would just say, 'we don't care about the donor', that would be great".

My British interviewees remained more neutral on the potential interest of their children in the donation or the donor arising in the future. British mother Sarah Hampton even expressed a positive attitude to the possibility that their children would seek out the donor when turning eighteen:

> Sarah Hampton: "I would actually quite like one of my children to want to meet him. That might open up the chance that I got to as well and I would actually

like to see who he is and thank him… […] I know I have to be very careful not to push them [her children] that way."

Her husband expressed more ambivalent feelings about this scenario. He said that he found it difficult to imagine, but that his feelings might change in the future.

Recapitulation and Further Thoughts

My familial interview partners had typically either chosen active or passive disclosure as their overall knowledge-management strategy (as further analyzed in 7.3), which they predominantly developed in personal contact to interest groups. They welcomed the specific (lay-)expert advice and opportunity for personal exchanges available through the groups and the associated "psy-sciences". All parents morally condemned non-disclosure.

A common fear addressed through DI fathers was that the child would one day verbally reject them as fathers. Particularly my German research partners took a slightly paradoxical stance on knowledge-management, suggesting that disclosure could be seen as a means to prevent children from developing an interest in donor contact or the donation. In such reflections German parents meant to make a similar point to that expressed by Tim Hampton above: a taboo, particularly for children, can gain social significance exactly through its taboo status. Nevertheless, the implicit or explicit appraisal that if a child would want to explore his donor conception in detail in the future, this could be read as a sign of a failure of parental knowledge-management, potentially putting heightened pressure on child-rearing practices.

Freeman et al. (2009, 506) summarize several studies that have found regulatory uncertainty and lack of information on the donor to influence parental knowledge-management towards choosing non-disclosure. I would tentatively suggest that the paradoxical stance on knowledge-management as put forward by some German interviewees, might also be related to the ambiguous German regulatory situation. After all, telling one's children about gamete donation in an unclear legal situation such as in Germany makes the parents' points on the morality of their decision in itself paradoxical: not telling being seen as deceitful and hence dangerous to the family, but disclosure having the potential of producing numerous (legal) uncertainties for the child. Knowledge-management as apparent in my data hence became a balancing act between what was found to be morally and/or intuitively right—disclosure—and doing this in a way that would not make the children curious about their donor conception. For my British interview partners the legal situation seemed to produce less ambivalences regarding disclosure: they were more confident, some even curious about potential contact between child and donor and less likely to say that something had gone "wrong" if the child would start exploring the implications of its donor conception further.

7. Familial Knowledge-Management: Everyday Practices and Emerging Relations

This chapter focuses on everyday practices of kinship knowledge-management in the families I engaged with. It shows tangible practices, which are part of establishing oneself as a family-by-donation, rather than the broader opinions, histories, and strategies analyzed in previous chapters. The first section (7.1) concentrates on how parents built up an image of the gamete donor through clinical information during the matching phase. The section analyzes how this information became an image figuring in explicit and in more intuitive practices of knowledge-management. Inspired by Konrad's (1998, 2005a) concept of *nameless relations*, which she uses to describe diffuse forms of relatedness from the perspective of egg donors, I call the diffuse forms of relatedness apparent in how parents interact with the clinical donor information *administered relations*. I describe how families typically selected donors based on criteria of similarity and amiability. Both criteria were commonly addressed as of ambivalent hereditary character. Through the practices of interacting with donor information (characterized by the ubiquitous absence of photographs, a simultaneous clinical formatting of this information and a re-materialization of the donor in the imaginary), not only images of the donor emerged—parents became known in new ways as well.

The following section (7.2) focuses on vocabulary choices: which kin terminology the parents were using and how they constituted kinship through specific naming practices. Given the novelty of kinship-by-donation as an increasingly openly acknowledged family form, there is a lack of established kinship terminology. In this underdetermination parents were intervening with new naming practices. This *naming and terminology work* was typically both narratively re-constructed and performed within the interview situations itself. It entailed a relational positioning of the different people involved in the children's conception. It also commonly entailed advocating the kin-terms chosen (for example to always call the donor "donor" and not "biological father") to friends, acquaintances and the children's caretakers and teachers. Naming and terminology work, I shall argue, connects and dis-connects not only kin-persons in the present, but also establishes a connection to family members in the past. Those parents not conforming to the assumed "reproductive norm" (i.e. single mothers, visibly post-menopausal women, homosexual couples) seemed to engage in more inclusive terminology work than the heterosexual families.

The third section (7.3) showcases concrete practices of parental disclosure and analyses how the identified active (i.e. actively telling) and passive (i.e. reacting to questions) disclosers were telling their children about their donor-conception. Disclosing gamete donation, I argue on the basis of my fieldwork-materials, is a relational process resting upon the enrolment of objects, such as children's books, photographs, and collected materials, and is not only pertaining to individual families but also to their whole social world. The children's books about gamete donation used by the parents relieved them of having to constantly engage in "pioneering" knowledge-management through inventing individual disclosure-narratives. The disclosure strategy of *making known all along* (see chapter 6) was operationalized through numerous readings of the books to the children. Parents, particularly the active disclosers, worried their children's detailed knowledge of biological reproduction derived from the books might produce negative reactions from other parents. Mothers and fathers tried to prevent such imagined conflicts through further practices of knowledge-management involving their whole social circle.

The last section (7.4) analyzes subversive practices of knowledge-management. Often parents are trying to get in touch with other parents who have used the same donor, or, as they get older, the children themselves seek contact to each other. Some even try to get in touch with their officially anonymous donor. I discuss the grass-roots initiatives and the technologies and infrastructures involved in these subversive search endeavors. They typically make use of the internet and DNA analysis. These searches initiated by concerned parents or offspring tend to be independent of or undermine the official knowledge-management by clinics and past or present national regulation. I argue that such subversive practices lead to the emergence of different relations than the *administered relations* analyzed in 7.1: here we see the emergence of *wayward relations*, which are characterized by their unprecedentedness and related lack in established social roles. *Wayward relations*, as I will show, reaffirm notions of kinship as genetically grounded, but they go beyond simple notions of *geneticization*. Instead, they are not colonizing, as often argued within the *geneticization paradigm*, but complementary relations in the face of other, often failed relationships.

7.1 Getting to Know the Donor: The Constitution of Administered Relations

The parents-by-donation with whom I worked came to know their donors through the clinical information involved in choosing or being allocated a gamete donor (as analyzed in 5.2 from a clinical perspective) and integrated this knowledge into their own practices of knowledge-management. My argument in this section commences through firstly discussing the parental experiences with being matched to a donor. Then I turn to discussing the parent's criteria for donor-selection, the relationality involved in this, and what role choice played. I then make an excursus into analyzing the role of photographs in kinship knowledge-management. The section closes with an exploration into how the donor was imagined as a person and a brief recapitulation of the overall argument.

As part of constituting kinship-by-donation in clinics, parents are matched to donors—though on closer examination, as shown in 5.1, what or who is matched is debatable. It is not real-life persons being coupled here, but rather articulations of specific physical, social, and familial characteristics translated into clinical classification schemes and documentation practices and then matched according to local criteria. How did my parent research partners experience this process? They were treated in different fertility centers, with different matching procedures in place. The Schneiders from Western-Germany, who had ordered sperm from Denmark to their German clinic via the internet, were the only couple who had chosen a donor all by themselves through the clinical information to be found on the website of the Danish sperm bank. The other interviewees had to make sense out of the clinical donor information for the first time when they themselves were going through the registration phase at their clinic. Subsequently, during the matching phase (see 5.2), these parents-to-be were confronted with either their doctor's choice of a donor or a list of available donors.

The Hamptons humorously recalled their debates around choosing a donor from their clinic in Largecity:

Maren Klotz: "So how did that work, choosing or getting a donor?"
Tim Hampton: "Well, the choosing…"
Sarah Hampton: "-we had to fill in a sheet of what Tim looks like and…"
Tim Hampton: "-it was all…"
Sarah Hampton: "-quite bizarre! We had an argument about whether you (to Tim) were of small or medium build, didn't we? We had to get the nurse into the room… (general laughing)."
Tim Hampton: "Completely medium! I am not small! (laughs) Sarah was saying you are, you are! I was saying I am not!"
Tim Hampton (in more serious tone): "So you fill in that and then the hair color, eye color."
Sarah Hampton: "Hair color, eye color."
Tim Hampton: "Build, Complexion…"
Sarah Hampton: "And then preferences on educational background…"

On the basis of the articulation and recording of physical characteristics of Tim Hampton and the couple's wishes on the donor's education levels, the clinic provided the couple with a choice of two donors. The couple first chose the one whose education they particularly liked, but who was taller than Tim. After not getting pregnant after three rounds of insemination, Sarah Hampton started to feel increasingly "uncomfortable" about presumably having to "explain to children who were six-foot six when we are nowhere near that" and the couple decided to switch donors. The second donor matched all the physical characteristics recorded of Tim Hampton, but did not even have a university entrance qualification, while Tim has had postgraduate education.

British mother Holly Greenwood also recounted the process of choosing from a sperm donor list during our first interview:

Holly Greenwood: "We had the possibility of looking at three donor profiles and then we chose one. We got this very general information on eye color, hair color, education, body type, hobbies, so very general information."
Maren Klotz: "And was there something that was particularly important to you both?"
Holly Greenwood: "Well, I mean we did want somebody who kind of looks like my husband. There was one donor with brown eyes and no one in our family has brown eyes and he was totally against that. It was supposed to be someone with light eyes. So, similar physical characteristics were important to us, and education. We did want someone with a university degree."

While for Holly Greenwood the close physical resemblance between her husband and the donor was key in choosing a donor, the German Brazilian couple Tönsch declined a match along this rationale (also see section 8.1 on resemblance below). With Miguel Tönsch being a black haired South-American with a dark complexion their doctor had suggested a match with a sperm donor resembling these features. The donors registered at the clinic with the closest physical resemblance were Bulgarian and Croatian. Tönsch felt uneasy with the idea of this possibly prompting a child to "seek out roots with regard to these other countries" and this just making the donor insemination process "even more complicated [implying that being a German Brazilian family-by-donation was enough to deal with in itself]". Instead he assertively proclaimed how he wanted to get his son acquainted with Brazil through his "mother tongue" and possibly extensive visits to the country: "That's what I provide as a father!" He also repeatedly stated that he found the idea of a match based on physical resemblance absurd:

Miguel Tönsch: "The doctor said 'Maybe you should choose a donor who looks a little bit more like you'. And I found that to be nonsense. That's its own form of deception, he does not have to look like me. He is not my biological child, why do I have to look for someone who is just as dark-haired or whatever?"

His partner Dörte told me about eventually choosing their donor, who indeed had blue eyes and blond hair:

Dörte Tönsch: "He was doing community service work [instead of joining the German military] and probably needed money and had these nice hobbies: he liked sports and playing the violin. We felt comfortable with him doing civil service. Interestingly, there were several police men on the donor list and we agreed that, even though it is kind of nice that the law is standing its ground there as well (laughs), we did not really want a police man as a donor."

Rather than implying that being a police man was hereditary (as further discussed below), the Tönschs invoked their own political convictions in what donor they imagined to be likable as a person when presented with the need for making a choice.

The German Schneiders turned out to have been particularly crafty in their sperm donor selection. Unhappy with the limited information on donors available through their German fertility clinic, the couple instead chose to order sperm from the internationally operating Danish sperm bank Scan-Sperm. The doctors at their German clinic had told them that more information could be found in the donor profiles of the Danish sperm bank and they could just have the sperm sent to the German clinic.

Marc Schneider: "We really did not find that you got enough information in Germany. [...] For us, for Nadine, the question that we asked ourselves was: 'Can I love this child, if the donor possibly is an asshole?' Excuse my language!"
Maren Klotz (laughingly): "Not a problem".
Marc Schneider: "Essentially it is... Do I like this guy?"
Nadine Schneider: "Would I like him if I would meet him?"
Marc Schneider: "And who knows what the child would be like. And that's why our doctor recommended to us to use Scan-Sperm, because they have more information."

Although the information was more comprehensive in Scan-Sperm's German donor catalogue it still did not convey that certain *feel* for the donor's character, which the Schneiders were looking for. However, what they did like was the way in which Scan-Sperm's US website provided information. Eventually the Schneiders realized that the German and the US website of the Danish clinic most likely referred to the same donors:

Marc Schneider: "Scan-Sperm operates on the American market as well and there you can download much more comprehensive donor profiles. They do not have photographs, but a seven to nine pages paper in which..."
Nadine Schneider: "-questions can be answered in an open non-standardized way."
Marc Schneider: "Exactly, the donor can answer and the answer is left unchanged. They do not change or schematize it. They give all sorts of additional information. Genetic diseases in the family, at what age the granddads and grandmothers died. What is his favorite animal?"

During this conversation I was more and more baffled about the mass of information they could obtain this way. They kept adding more information they gathered through the donor database for U.S. based customers. The donor profiles revealed languages spoken, travel and food interests, eating habits, important life events, etc.

Nadine Schneider: "I had the feeling that I actually got a small impression of him [the potential donor], whether I would like him, through his answers."
Marc Schneider: "It is often not so important what they say, but how they say it…"
Nadine Schneider: "-how they phrase it."

Hence, what the Schneiders particularly liked about the US donor list was that, in their interpretation, the clinical formatting of it was actually kept to a minimum, making discernible the donor's personality. The couple started to closely examine donor profiles and they put a filter in place to make sure they would only find donors who matched Marc Schneider's height, ethnicity and eye color. They decided in favor of a medical student, whose donor profile they liked, although he did not match Marc Schneider's hair color. However, he did match Marc's hair structure, which Nadine Schneider described to me in detail in its specific "thickness". Wanting to avoid the much higher cost of ordering sperm directly from Scan-Sperm USA, the couple instead set out to make their own wayward match between the German and the American donor list:

Marc Schneider: "In the German list the donors have numbers, in the American one they have pseudonyms. We needed to find a match using the basic parameters such as height, hair color, eye color, profession, and that fit, it was not hard. […] We are sure that's him, it has to be him."

When Marc Schneider walked me through all the details of their story he was obviously enjoying showing me how clever they were to find their donor on both lists. With a glint in his eyes and a laugh afterwards he added: "I ordered via fax, paid by credit card and everything basically went as if ordering from Amazon."

Looked at more analytically, within all the parental descriptions of choosing a donor from a list or telling clinicians what they were looking for in a donor, two typical selection criteria emerged. These specific aspects of knowledge-management were firstly, the criterion of *similar-*

ity (which was in one case exchanged for *complementarity*) and, secondly, *amiability*. Similarity implies both physical resemblance according to the criteria set out in the clinic's files and similar educational backgrounds.[1] In the case of German single mother Maria Lieb similarity as selection criterion was exchanged for complementarity. Lieb, who had travelled to the USA for the donation given the difficult access to DI in Germany for single women, decided to choose a donor for his height to complement her rather small stature. Not being able to decipher American non-metric measurements, she chose a donor who was *extremely* tall and overweight. The later realization of this she called one of the "slapstick moments" of becoming a mother-by-donation.

The selection criterion of amiability I perceived in the Tönschs' discussion of not wanting a policeman as a donor and in Marc Schneider's frank assertion that the donor should not be an "asshole". Both similarity and amiability are simultaneously criteria within knowledge-management, which incorporate the concept of heredity *and* the concept of entering into a specific social relation—into what I call an *administered relation*—with the donor, as further discussed below. This ambivalence is particularly important to underline, because it could seem that similarity was only about heredity and amiability about the specific social relation. However, when Marc Schneider talked about amiability he also remarked (as already quoted above) "who knows what the child would be like [if he would choose an unpleasant donor]", seemingly implying he did relate child and donor in a hereditary continuity concerning amiability. Nevertheless, I simultaneously interpret his and his wife's discussion as also pointing to an emotional barrier against being *administratively related* to someone who neither Nadine nor he would like—just like the Tönschs intuitively preferred a conscientious objector to a policeman as a donor.

Laura Mamo (2005), in her study of sperm donor selection through US-American lesbian couples, has described an "extended form of kinship" she calls "affinity ties" (2005, 258), which is quite similar to *administered relations*. Mamo argues that couples construct such ties through the donor

1 All German and British clinicians I interacted with underlined that parents were typically not looking for a donor with *higher* educational achievements, but for a donor with *similar* education.

selection process. *Affinity ties* creatively incorporate physical and cultural aspects and thus go beyond a simple *geneticization*:

"Instead of users' understanding of genetics as determining futures, they negotiate and imagine ways cultural, social, and physical traits might interplay in potential children. At times, this results in maximizing competitive traits (i.e. increased height, decreased depression), but at other times it is a way to build and imagine shared connections. In all, practices of sperm selection, users themselves, and sperm bank services mutually constitute a technoscientific practice of kinship, which I have called affinity-ties." (Mamo 2005, 258)

Central to Mamo's well made argument is the concept of lesbian couples imagining a social connection to future children and an imagined increase in parental legitimacy taking place through the couple's donor-choice. Such creation of affinity ties is certainly similarly discernible in the selection processes based on similarity and amiability as introduced above. Yet my research partners did not only consider the donor's amiability in reference to imagined future children, as Mamo (2005) argues, but his or her amiability as a person continued to play a role for the parents long after conception. In other words, the donor's persona seemed to play a role beyond hereditary considerations and was continuously "re-materialized" on the basis of the clinical information within the parents' imaginations. That is why, inspired by Konrad's (1998, 2005a) concept of *nameless relations*, I have started to call donors a clinically *administered relation* to my familial research partners. *Nameless relations* are not first and foremost an emerging technoscientific practice of kinship in interaction with fertility clinics, such as Mamo's *affinity ties*, they also capture more long-standing imagined forms of diffuse relatedness, described from the perspective of anonymous egg donors. For my research partners, forging *administered relations* was not an explicit strategy, but rather a more implicit and intuitive practice of knowledge-management emerging out of the parental interaction with clinical information.

More aspects of what it means to enter into an *administered relation* through gamete donation as typical for my fieldwork material are well captured in the words of German mother Melanie Steger. Answering to an open question about what kind of issues surrounding being a family-by-donation the Stegers would like to discuss next, she said:

Melanie Steger: "I think it is more of a problem for women [than for the men] in DI families that the child comes from a strange man, because you wish the child would be from the partner you are living with. […] I had to call the sperm bank laboratory because of some questions I had once and they have women working there. And they said things like: 'Oh, yours is a really nice donor!' And I thought, oh, they are quite laid back (laughing). You know, when all of this is so strange to you and you think, well, that this whole method of conception is not 'normal', in quotation marks… But for them it was all normal and all relaxed. […] They said he is nice and quite fun and that I shouldn't worry…"

First she stresses the desire to have a child "together" (see section 4.2). She seems to have taken comfort from the notion that the "strange man" was "nice" and "fun", but does not address this as being of hereditary relevance. She rather brings it up in the context of discussing how she lost her "yuck" feelings about donor insemination. This again captures how amiability of the donor has been important to my interviewees beyond genetic considerations.

Moreover, the passage also captures what I see as further implied in the concept of *administered relation* (and will explore more in the sections below). I do not only mean to describe the donor as an *administered relation* to the parents, but rather argue that for my interviewees the knowledge practice of engaging with donor information held a relational character. Entering into an *administered relation* with the donor mediated through the limited clinical donor information also meant entering into relation with other people who were translating this information, such as the female laboratory personnel. And it also meant re-thinking oneself and one's partner in relation to this information. The Hampton's for example jokingly recalled, as quoted above, their negotiation of how Tim's body related to their clinic's articulations of the donor's body ("small or medium?"). Or, as also quoted above, German mother Nadine Schneider started to pay close attention to her husband's structure of hair, and single mother Maria Lieb thought about her own petiteness. The parents had to position themselves in clinically *administered relation* to the donor: as holders of a particular education, of particular bodies, and of particular ethnicities (also see 5.2 and 8.1). To discuss one more example of this process of changing one's own image through the prism of clinical donor information, Maria Lieb came to know herself as "Caucasian" for the first time when choosing a donor at the sperm bank in the United States. With "race" terminologies in Germany today not being as ubiquitous as in the USA, Maria Lieb had to learn to recognize that the term Caucasian in the sperm bank denoted donors "who look like me in some ways":

Maria Lieb: "So they had this list, of the, the type, if someone is rather, what's it called… Caucasian or something like that they call it, if someone is blonde and blue eyed, or if someone is rather… rather African or rather Asian."

It is discernible that she was unaccustomed to using American "race" categories and is trying to avoid using the term "race" by calling it "type" instead. She also appears to try and undermine the notion that "race" could be a clear-cut category by repeatedly using the term "rather".

Moreover it was not only recognizing oneself in a new light, specifically within new categories, but also having to weigh up these categories in relation to the donor, which was typical. This was particularly amplified when parents had the choice among available donors with different "features". (This was also the point where parental knowledge-management became physically incorporated into the bodies of the children born through the procedure, as analyzed in section 5.2). The Hamptons, for example, had to weigh up height in its relation to education (which was more important to them?), as discussed above. In other words, they had to weigh different aspects of similarity (or amiability), which they, possibly, never had to put in any relation before. German mother Berit Feldman recalled how friends from their DI interest group found these "balancing acts" irritating:

Berit Feldman: "Well, they said it was horrendous. They had five, sort of, men —and then they had to choose: Do we want someone who resembles us more or someone who goes rock climbing, like us. Oh god!"

Her statement that there were five "*sort of*, men" available aptly captures how within the clinical trajectory of knowing kinship-by-donation, patients/clients only became familiar with the donors as clinical articulations, not as living and breathing men (see 5.1 and 5.2). Berit Feldman perceived the assessment of these articulations as absurd. References to the absurdity of *choosing* a donor were in fact highly common among my research partners.

Aside from such often humorous references, my parental research partners were divided on whether they perceived choice within the donor selection process as positive or negative. The availability of as much donor information as possible and being able to choose a donor on the basis of this information was typically either addressed as a possible source of agency (for example in the way the Schneiders talk about their donor selection process above) or it was addressed as quite the opposite: as a possible source of jealousy and/or as ethically dubious. While German mother Silke Müller for instance wished that she would have had more choice on the sperm donor, her partner Marcel jokingly disagreed:

Marcel Müller: "To be frank, after all the shit that I had to go through, now getting a catalogue for my girlfriend to pick the best looking guy with the best smile—well, well, that would have been just what I needed…"[2]

The Stegers, who underwent DI because of a genetic disease, also critically discussed the theme of choice and said they liked that the genetically tested sperm donor was chosen for them through their clinic:

Philip Steger: "Choice to me in that context is negatively connoted… It is somehow negative. People who do it there [he is referring to the possibility of choosing from more detailed donor lists in the USA] are coming from the same situation to start with, but then, DI starts having the character of shopping."
Melanie Steger: "Yeah, yeah!"
Philip Steger: "And with us it never at any point, in any situation had the character of online-shopping or something like that. […] It was always really decent."

As apparent in the passage above, the Stegers invoked the theme of online shopping to denote treatment practices, which were dubious in their view, while the Schneiders (as cited above) actually used the same image to illustrate the perceived easiness of the treatment. Choice, while noticeably multiplying the relations drawn between different categories and persons, hence clearly had a contested status in my field recordings.

Brief Digression on Photos as Tools of Kinship Knowledge-Management

While discussing donor information, parents frequently addressed the lack of donor photographs. German single mother Maria Lieb, for example, commented:

2 These remarks were said in a situation of joking and mutual teasing; quoted out of context the passage might come across as more confrontational than in the longer interview context.

Maria Lieb: "Well, it was not like one would imagine with photos, but [you had to choose] only on the basis of certain characteristics. That is obviously an absurd situation."

Such parental references indicate that some research partners would have perceived photographs as the more intuitive basis on which to build *administered relations.*

In my field diary I often recorded the striking role the presence of photographs of children or extended family played when meeting my familial interview partners. Below is such a passage, where I discuss meeting the father and sperm donor in the German Arnulf rainbow family for the first time. As further explained in section 7.2 the father, Jacob Barry, is American—therefore I used an English sounding pseudonym:

Field diary Maren Klotz: As I was sitting down in the café, Jacob put a bunch of photos of [his son] Jonas on the table with the friendly but assertive statement: "So you can get an impression who we are actually talking about here!" I was actually taken by surprise. Not having ordered anything to drink yet, my notepad still sitting in my bag, I felt like I had not quite switched into an alert "fieldwork modus". So we started looking at the pictures together. I immediately found myself pointing out how Jonas resembles Lena [his mother], while at the same time thinking that I shouldn't have brought up the whole resemblance theme by myself. Funny—maybe also worth exploring analytically—how photographs seem to really "prompt" certain practices. I looked at each of the pictures Jacob had put on the table, Jacob followed my gaze to pick up which one I was focusing on and told me about every single picture how old Jonas was when it was taken. I found myself making appreciative "oh, see how cute he is!" comments."

The passage above refers to a particularly pronounced usage of photographs during an interview situation, but photos regularly were interactive parts of fieldwork situations, for instance as orientation for me when first being invited into people's houses or when research partners announced to me the birth of a new child via mail or e-mail. Commonly, during interviews or more informal interactions, research partners would occasionally get up to fetch a photograph of their family or children or lead me to such pictures being displayed on the walls of their houses.

Striking was also the account of British donor-conceived adult Bonnie Smith about how photographs had been involved in underlining her feelings of doubt concerning her father's biological parenthood. A few years before discovering her donor conception in her mid-twenties, Smith had found a box of old family pictures in the attic when housesitting for her parents. They were historical photographs of the paternal family. When her parents returned from their holiday and Bonnie Smith quite excitedly told them about her discovery her father "really flipped out." In a turmoil that was incomprehensible to her at the time, "he was stomping around the house muttering 'it's not your family, it's not your family!'"

Bonnie Smith: "That was when I grew suspicious. I said to my mum what on earth is he on about? […] And I'm interested in the family history and I loved getting all these photographs out and looking at them. […]"
Maren Klotz: "And what's your interpretation why he got so mad?"
Bonnie Smith: "It's weird isn't it? I think he just didn't know, couldn't cope with it, really."

When Bonnie got pregnant only one or two years later she deliberately asked the doctor at one of the check-ups for her blood group and compared it to her father's blood group, which she was well-aware of due to a medical condition he had. This confirmed that her father was not biologically related to her.

My argument about the prominent figuring of photographs in my fieldwork recordings is that photographs are relational kinship objects, allowing connections to be traced and made to persons and events in the recent and distant past and between bodies. Photographs figure as material components of communicative practices within which kinship is acknowledged. Both Bonnie Smith and I were at a loss what exactly upset her father when she discovered his family photographs (guilt about non-disclosure, rejection of Bonnie, acknowledgment of highly biologized kinship notions?). Nevertheless, he clearly seems to have been situationally unable to let her claim kinship via the photographs.

Photographs and photo-albums are thus part of the, in Smith's case contested, material infrastructures of kinship. They tenaciously prompt scripted behaviors in every day life, where resemblance, age or appearances are acknowledged. They are hence part of quite physically oriented acts of communication, as further explored in section 8.1 on resemblance-talk. Arguably, it was this embodied aspect of photographs as tools of knowledge-management that made it problematic for Bonnie Smith's father that she, physically apparently quite dissimilar to him, had discovered the family photographs. Because photographs are commonly part of *do-*

ing kinship, my parental interviewees repeatedly pointed to the absence of donor-photographs as a notable exception and hence unique identifier of *administered relations*. For the parents, *administered relations* were only built on the basis of clinical data (but see how photographs figured in the medical trajectory in section 5.2).

"Re-Materializing" the Donor into a Person

As became clear in narrative reconstructions through my interview partners and through my follow-up interviews with them, not only during the donor selection, but just as much over the years of being a family-by-donation, the parents used the limited donor information for further subtle practices of knowledge-management. What was typical was that the clinical information was used as a stepping-stone into the imaginary, where the donor was "re-materialized" into a person. As mentioned above, this turned out to be one of the typical characteristics of the *administered relation* between parents and donor.

Before analyzing the typical pattern, I want to describe an instance in which one family I engaged with used the clinical donor information to avoid imagining the donor as a person, shielding themselves *against* re-materializing him into an individual. The Feldmans had very little clinical information about their donor and had been clients in the fertility clinic described in chapter 6, which recommended non-disclosure and suggested potential non-compliance (up to burning records) with making available donor information. One clinical detail the Feldmans knew was their donor's clinical reference number: 173. The parents used this number to prevent the donor from becoming an imaginary person. In the past they had maintained a less distanced relationship to the sperm donor. They had for instance secretively thanked him in the birth announcement of their first-born: "We are grateful to all of those who contributed to him arriving", a message which only those of their friends and family who knew about the donation could decipher.

During the development of a familial every day life normality and the arrival of their second-born, however, they started to distance themselves from these earlier acknowledgements of the donor as a person. They also started to subtly distance themselves from the interest group discourse they had encountered where the donor was usually addressed as a gift giver (see 6.1). Instead, their knowledge-management tactic became to know him as a number:

Berit Feldman: "In the beginning I thought… I found it helpful what we learned in the group workshops [of Petra Thorn]: this gratitude with regard to the donor. Not this 'arghhh, we never want to meet him' but more like, super, he gave us a gift so we could become a family. But now I also realize… Well, I think it is something else, if our children in 16 years say they want to meet him, that's okay then. But I believe now, where we are only discovering ourselves as a family and with the whole legal situation in Germany being so unclear, and so few families… that's when I think it is actually really good that he is really far away. That's a number, that's not a person, that's quite nice."
Maren Klotz: "Are you talking about a real number?"
Berit Feldman: "Number 173 (laughing). That's what the doctor said: 'So, you have number 173 again'. And then he said: 'Okay, let's get this thing in' (laughs)."

This quote shows that it was partially the uncertain legal circumstances in Germany, which led the Feldmans to try to abstain from re-materializing the donor into a concrete person (also see section 6.2 for brief discussion of potential links between regulatory regimes and parental knowledge-management). It is also discernible how Berit Feldman is drawing on the distanced clinical language of her doctor to abstain from this re-materialization. How the donor has become a number for the Feldmans over the last years was not only narrated in the interview, but also performatively enacted in the situation. While Berit Feldman for example first described a person she was thankful to, she then switched to a neutral address ("that's a number" = "das ist eine Nummer" in German)—and ended with referring to the donor—or his sperm as "number 173" and "a thing". Uli Linde-Feldman reflected on this knowledge-management tactic:

Uli Linde-Feldman: "Well, I said, I only want to know the number, nothing else. Sometimes I think it would be tempting to see a photograph or something—but at the same time that's giving me the creeps. Because then it would be… At the moment *it* is really a number and that is good to live with. I think if it would be personified, I could imagine it would get complicated."

Uli Linde-Feldman also performatively enacted the donor as a number by using the neuter "it" ("*es*"). The quote shows Uli reflexively working through different options for knowledge-management and addressing his ambivalent feelings on potentially accessing more donor information, such as a photograph of the donor. He ends the passage with an affirmation that he and his wife preferred not to know the donor as a person and hence also did not want more information.

The other families I interviewed, in contrast, all imagined the donor as a concrete person. These imaginings were, however, just as much rooted in clinical information as the Feldmans' knowledge-management tactic was. In other words, parents did not just invent creative stories unrelated to the clinical information. While the Feldmans chose to refer to the clinical reference number to not make the donor a person, the other families—as already pointed out above—typically used minute details of the clinical information as a stepping stone to imagine the donor as an amicable person.

German father Philip Steger, for instance, took the fact that their sperm donor had to have an additional genetic test (for the disorder the Stegers were both genetic carriers of) as a starting point to imagine him as a particularly amicable person.

Philip Steger: "The donor, he has to be pretty decent, because they must have asked him: 'Here, you have to come in, give a blood sample that will be tested'. […] And that's where I thought: well, this will not be someone who simply does it, evidently also that, but *only* does it for monetary reasons. Instead, the donor must have thought about what he does there and if he says: 'Okay, I'll do it' then I thought that is a rather positive sign. […] I mean, it could have been quite a nuisance for him. If he had been a carrier, for instance, he would have been kicked out of the sperm bank."

British mother Shoko Nakamura, to recount another typical example of this process of imagining the donor, analyzed at length the different pieces of egg donor information which she had on "just an A4-sheet" and what she made of them. She explained she would like the donor if she would meet her personally. Her hobbies of "playing mandolin and rock climbing" Nakamura interpreted as pointing towards her being "nice, active, sort of positive to life". She also interpreted her Taiwanese-American donor's religion—Christianity—as pointing towards a possible altruistic person:

Shoko Nakamura: "She is a Christian, her family is Christian. So that might be connected to giving the egg. I mean, there is money, definitely, but there must be some, how do you say? -Altruistic thing…"

Hence, it was typical that parents used such minute pieces of information and imagined the donor as a likable person.

Commonly, and as already mentioned in several quoted passages, the parents imagined the donor as not solely driven by financial interests. German mother Dörte Tönsch explained that she liked overhearing how her clinic talked to men calling as potential donors on the phone. She had the feeling that the clinic personnel explained the complex steps to eventually be accepted as a donor so well that in her view it discouraged "nutcases who just want to make 100 Euros fast". Moreover, such familial narratives also showed that the families often did not clearly make a distinction between donation as an economic transaction and donation as a gift.[3] In other words, one did not taint the other. What parents typically did seem to feel uncomfortable with was the idea that the *only* motivation for the donation was money.

To review, parents came to know the gamete donor during the matching phase, and this knowledge later came to figure in explicit, and in more intuitive and minute practices of knowledge-management. Donor selection was typically based on perceptions of similarity and amiability of the donor. Both criteria were commonly ambivalently addressed as potentially having a hereditary component. Beyond such considerations the parents seemed to intuitively feel that they were entering into a social relationship with the donor, where his or her amiability was of importance not because of heredity, but because one did not want to be connected in what I have called an *administered relation* to an unlikable person. Within the associated typical knowledge practices of interacting with donor information (characterized by the ubiquitous absence of photographs, a simultaneous clinical formatting of this information and a re-materialization of the

3 Gift giving is, of course, a classical anthropological research topic (most famously according to Mauss 1990) and has also been explored in view of gamete donation (e.g. Konrad 2005a) or organ donation (e.g. Fox and Swazey 1992; Titmuss 1997). Key to the anthropological analysis is that, in contrast to a commercial notion of objects, where ownership is fully transferred between two parties, the gift is always bound up with the identity of the gift giver: that is where its power lies and where it obliges the recipient to reciprocate.

donor in the imaginary) not only images of the donor emerged—but parents became known in new ways as well. The concept of an *administered relation* connecting parents and donors hence implied a relational process.

To return to Konrad's (1998, 2005a) notion of *nameless relations*, which has inspired my idea of *administered relations*: the analytical work her concept does is to capture diffuse and distributed kinship ties emerging during anonymous egg donation. She argues from the perspective of British egg donors, who do not have access to information about the egg recipients. In other words, while receiving parents, such as my research partners, are comprehensively exposed to the clinical trajectory of information, donors are not. The donation process for them is defined through this complete absence of information. Konrad characterizes her concept as such:

> "...donors are partaking collectively in an exchange order of non-genealogical relatedness. This is both symbolized by, and embodied materially as, the discursive substance of anonymity." (Konrad 1998, 655)

While Konrad's work thus concentrates on anonymity not hindering diffuse forms of relatedness from the perspective of donors, the families I have worked with found themselves in a less diffuse relatedness to the gamete providers. The sperm and eggs donors were nameless to the families I have worked with in the literal sense, but the fragments of clinically formatted knowledge about the donor constituted *administered relations* squarely figuring between the imaginary spaces engendered through anonymity as described by Konrad and the constitution of particular forms of personhood and relatedness through clinical trajectories of knowledge.

7.2 Of Donors and Daddies, Fathers, (Co-)Mothers, Moms, and Mommies: Naming and Terminology Work

One central and explicitly negotiated component of kinship knowledge-management in all the families-by-donation I engaged with was what I have come to call *naming and terminology work*. I interpreted these comprehensive naming practices as knowledge-management tactics to place the donor in a specific relationship to the family and to emphasize specific past and present kin connections over others. Naming and terminology work was typically simultaneously narratively reconstructed and performed within the interview situation itself. It was never prompted through my questions, but rather only emerged as a relevant theme during analytic coding. This section commences by first discussing my research partners' naming practices with regard to descriptive kinship terminology, for instance how the parents referred to the donor. It then turns to discussing a second typical component of naming and terminology work: choice of individual pre- and surnames in the families-by-donation which highlighted connections to specific family members.

A typical example of the simultaneous reflection on and performance of naming and terminology work occurred when the German Steger family talked to me about which kin terminology to use in everyday life:

Philip Steger: "Well, we were thinking, what should we say, where are the differences? We are not completely sure yet, but we always want to say: I am the daddy [Papa] and…"
Melanie Steger: "-and the other is the…"
Philip Steger: "-and the other is the donor [Spender]…"
Melanie Steger: "-genitor [Erzeuger]."
Philip Steger: "That term [he is referring to 'genitor'], there I am not really sure yet, or… I don't know on which term we will agree…"
Melanie Steger: "-agree on…"
Philip Steger: "-agree on, because I don't think it's a bad idea to always use the same term. So I am the daddy and the donor just helped. […]"
Melanie Steger: "I also think, daddy has a completely different meaning, because the donor has not done any work in raising, or comforting or whatever… That's why I think, daddy is simply a completely different term. Of course, one always says: He is not my father (Vater). But a father is actually the one who raises the child…"

Hence, the Stegers were practicing their naming and terminology work in the interview with me. They agreed on Philip unequivocally being the Daddy of their daughter and mentioned both genitor and donor as possible terms for the donor—with seemingly a performative settlement of the issue through Philip, declaring that he was "the daddy" and the other "the donor". His wife Melanie also suggested the term father, which she identified to be more biologically fixed in its common usage than the term daddy, but acknowledged that she herself saw it rooted in care practices, rather than in biological reproduction.

A similar situation arose with the Feldmans, where again the narrative reconstruction of a past practice and the practice itself folded into one. What is specific to this situation is that the Feldmans drew me into the negotiation explicitly. Their conversation also brings up the theme of anthropological knowledge of kin terminologies:

Uli Linde-Feldman: "It is actually the case that the term father has been, in a sense, monopolistically occupied by me. It describes only me. […] There is no biological father [leiblicher Vater]."
Uli explains that the only possibility he could see the term father potentially being used through someone else would be if his wife Berit would leave him for a new partner who would also become involved in raising the children. Berit jokes around that she is not planning on a divorce at the moment. Then Berit says that the term father is an "ethnological term, laden with emotions" by this, as I understand her, denoting that the term implies a social role.
Maren Klotz: "I think ethnographers were also the first to point out that there can be a difference between genitor [Erzeuger] and pater. There are societies where…"
Berit Feldman: "-although, genitor is not what he is… he is not a genitor!"
Uli Linde-Feldman: "Well, he is actually a genitor… Or, isn't the doctor the genitor? [The German term "Erzeuger" has a similar connotation to 'maker' or 'creator']"
Berit Feldman: "No, genitor implies… Well, that he has performed an act and the like…"
Uli Linde-Feldman: "He has also performed an act…"
Maren Klotz (to Berit): "Hmmm, you're right… There is something active to the term…"
Uli Linde-Feldman: "But I think I could settle on 'genitor'."
Berit Feldman: "Really? No, I don't think 'genitor' is good."

The Feldmans eloquently unpacked how the donor, not having been present at the moment of conception, should therefore not be allocated an active role as they saw it implied through the term genitor. By also opposing the term "biological father" [leiblicher Vater], they further explicitly stressed the particularity of their family situation by linguistically separating it from, say, a patchwork family situation where the term "biological father" might be more appropriate.

The naming and terminology work of my research partners (and me) can be interpreted as a knowledge-management tactic to constitute the family in specific ways: because openly acknowledged clinical donor conception is an unprecedented way of building a family, traditional kin terminologies are not commonly found to fit, or they carry with them the implication of a specific relationship or roles found to be inappropriate by the parents. Hence, naming and terminology work is a relational knowledge practice which not only allocates the donor a "place" in relation to the family, but also positions the parent(s) and children in specific relation to each other, as I shall further show below. Lacking established vocabulary, the parents commonly explicitly debated the meaning of kinship terms, as apparent in the quotes above. These explicit reflections of kin terms and reflexive naming practices are one aspect of what I will further describe as the experientially acquired *reflexive kinship expertise* of parents-by-donation (see chapter 8).

For the heterosexual two-parental families-by-sperm-donation in my sample, naming and terminology work was typically an *exclusionary* practice—as for instance apparent in Uli's remark that he "monopolistically" occupied the term father. This was not the case for the single women and rainbow families I engaged with. It was also not the case for families-by-ova-donation, potentially because they were more assured of their kinship connection through giving birth. Single mother-by-choice Maria Lieb for instance did not concentrate on a separation of the terms father and donor, but of the terms daddy and father.

> Maria Lieb: "I somehow tried to differentiate relatively early between daddy [Papa] and father [Vater]. So that in a sense it becomes clear that she [her daughter] simply does not have a daddy in the usual sense of the word. That we are the family and the father simply helped me that I could have a child."

Thus, in the absence of a partner taking on the fathering role, excluding the term father seemingly became unnecessary for her. Instead, she only rejected the notion of closeness and familiarity incorporated in the term daddy, while acknowledging that the donor was indeed a father.

The Arnulf rainbow-family also juggled with finding the "right" kinship terminology, but having chosen to become a family-by-donation with known donor Jacob Barry who also acted as the father, their work concentrated on finding *inclusive* terminology, rather than an exclusive one. Birth-mother Lena was referred to as "mommy [Mami]" her partner Svenja was the "mom [Mama]" and Jacob was the "daddy [Papa]", for example. The Arnulfs had chosen this specific terminology, because Svenja's children from a previous heterosexual marriage called her "mom" as well, therefore it made sense to make Lena the "mommy" of the now two children born within their lesbian partnership, so that Svenja remained "mom" to everyone.

While in an earlier interview Lena Arnulf remarked that her partner Svenja's children from her previous heterosexual marriage simply referred to her with her first name, this was different four years later. Now, with their little donor-conceived brother Jonas addressing his mothers as "mom" and "mommy", Svenja's children had also taken on this practice. This is for example shown in clipping 7.1., depicting a drawing by Svenja's older daughter (then 1eleven years old). She is referring to Lena as "mommy" both in the drawing itself, and when later pointing out to me who is who in the picture.

With all families I spoke to, no matter how exclusive or inclusive their naming and terminology work was, this knowledge-management practice not only entailed a relational positioning of the different persons involved in the children's conception, it also commonly entailed advocating the terms chosen (as already apparent in one of Uli Linde-Feldman's quotes above) to friends, other family members, acquaintances and mostly nursery and school staff. The Arnulfs, for example, told me that in addition to the affective terminology of "mommy" and "mom", they felt like they also needed to "supply" the older children with a formal kinship term describing the lesbian partner's role in the family. As a formal kinship term they chose "co-mother [Co-Mutter]", which the two older twins started to use confidently in school. In Svenja Arnulf's interpretation this relieved her children from further explaining (since they had no clear understanding of sexualities yet)[4] that her lesbian partner Lena was "not an aunt, nor a friend…" Instead it enabled the children to refer to their own relationship

4 One anecdote told by Svenja and Lena Arnulf made me laugh: The twins, around the age of about ten then, had heard the term gay [schwul] applied to men for the first time, apparently during school yard banter. In an ensuing discussion with their mothers on what it meant, they declared that this was all very interesting, but that they did not know any "gays". (The Arnulfs have a social circle, which Svenja calls "homonormative", because the majority of their male and female friends and colleagues are homosexual). When told that Jacob, their siblings' Daddy and donor, was gay they called out "Noooooo?!", not disapprovingly, but in surprise and disbelieve.

Clipping 7.1: Drawing of the Arnulf rainbow-family made by Svenja Arnulf's daughter from a previous heterosexual marriage

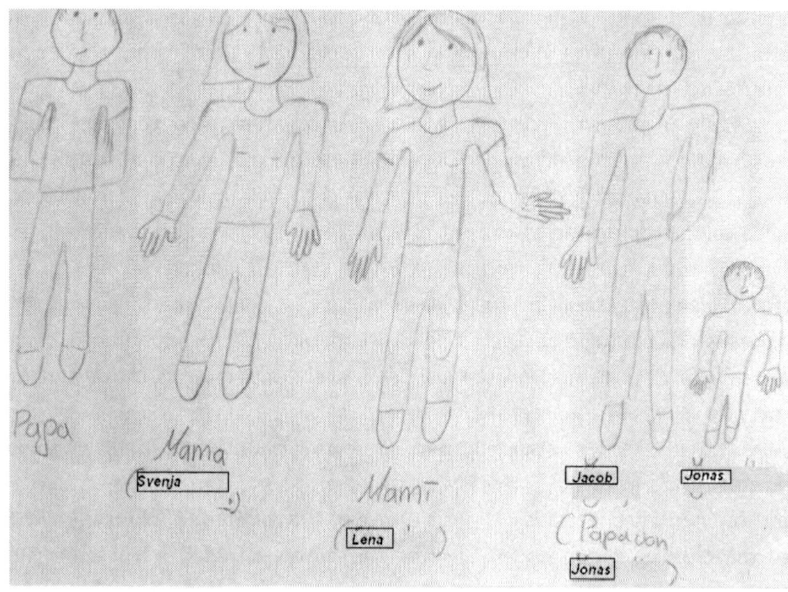

The drawing (from left to right) shows her "daddy", her "mom" Svenja, her "mommy" Lena, her little donor conceived brother Jonas, and his donor and father Jacob, whom she labels as "daddy of Jonas". She and her brother are depicted outside of the clipping on the left side. The drawing was made in an interview situation where I asked the Arnulfs to draw pictures of their family and talk to me about them.

with Lena, which they happily did from an age of about eight or nine onwards. In their DI conceived son's nursery school, Lena and Svenja Arnulf had also asked the personnel to use their affective kinship terminology:

Lena Arnulf: "Our experiences with the nursery school are only positive, which is really nice, I have to say. For instance, [I am impressed] that they [the teachers] learned who is the mom and who is the mommy, so they don't confuse the child, because he is still so little. […] The nursery school teachers, I think, they were happy that we told them right away, they really took it to heart. The children (at the nursery school) now ask 'are you mom or mommy?' Or they say (to Jonas): You have two *moms* and he replies 'I don't have two moms', because he does not have two *moms.*"

All of the other parents who were already talking about the donation to their children, had also instructed their day care center or school which kinship terminology to use, to make sure that the personnel did not refer to the donor as "your other father or the like" [Uli Feldmann].

Naming and terminology work thus involved the attempt at managing naming practices for a whole social domain, not just within the nuclear family. The Schneiders, for instance, discussed such a practice in the dialogue quoted below, which is also a typical—both reconstructive and performative—example of the exclusivity of naming practices as discussed above:

Nadine Schneider: "…we do not refer to the donor as father (Vater) or the like. I mean he does not have a role in the family, in that sense."
Marc Schneider: "Well, he does, he's the donor."
Nadine Schneider: "Yes, he is the donor, but not some other role."
(simultaneously with Nadine above) Marc Schneider: "That is a role."
Nadine Schneider: "With people who don't know much about it, who have never looked into the whole thing, the term father is often quickly applied and that is actually not what he is…"
Marc Schneider: "Just as much as we don't want the term genetic father [genetischer Vater] to be used. We have said this to the babysitter as well. That is the donor, not the father. These little things, we've also told the nursery school."
Nadine Schneider: "There is nothing with 'real father' [richtiger Vater] or 'biological' ['leiblicher'] or anything. The term father is not used [concerning the donor]."

The Schneiders above debate about the specific relationships that are implicitly "built-into" different kin terms and, as typical for the heterosexual families-by-sperm-donation interviewed, settle on the idea that Marc Schneider has an exclusive right to the idiom "father". Further, the passage shows how their terminological knowledge-management extends into their whole social circle, as typical for all families I engaged with.

Clearly, naming and terminology work is to be seen as an attempt to constitute kinship in specific relational ways through linguistic interventions. The crucial point to this practice is that it involves the recognition and often also privileging of certain relationships over others. This practice is one striking example of how parents are trying to manage the constitutive effects of kinship knowledge that Carsten (2007) has called for to be empirically studied (see 2.2). Given the novelty of kinship-by-donation as an openly acknowledged family form and thus the resulting lack in established kinship terminology and associated roles, an underdetermination arises into which parents are trying to intervene through their naming and terminology work. Exclusive and inclusive terms are situationally debated by the parents as reflexive kinship experts and then tactically applied to "make" donors, mothers, fathers, daddies, moms, and mommies.

Naming and Terminology Work for Pre- and Surnames

The German and British parents I engaged with did not only actively manage kinship terminology, but also commonly engaged in practices of knowledge-management with regard to individual pre- and surnames. For instance, several of the heterosexual families-by-sperm-donation established through these individual naming practices a specific connection between the children and the fathers' kin network. The Müller family had chosen their donor conceived child's first name from an old pedigree roll name-referencing Marcel Müller's paternal family line. Through this naming practice, mediated by the old document roll shown to me as a treasured kinship object during the interview situation, a connection was established to Marcel's cherished ancestry. The Feldmans, to take another example, were trying during my fieldwork to change their family name to "Linde". This was again an attempt, unsuccessful, as it turned out, to foreground a particular relation through the choice of the surname. Feldman was Berit's family name. When they married, Uli Linde-Feldman took on a double-barreled name and they decided that Feldman would be their family name.[5] However, this meant that although Uli was named Linde-Feldman, his children were automatically only named Feldman. By German law, a child's once chosen family name cannot be changed by the parents, for protection from varying parental relationships continuously resulting in an alteration of the child's name.

5 This official naming practice was put in place in 1992 after German officials started to worry about last-names becoming longer and longer when the first triple or quadruple family names started showing up with the children of the generation first allowed to take on double-barreled surnames starting to get married. Thus, double-barreled family names cannot be passed on to children.

Berit Feldman: "When we got married, 14 years ago, I said that I wanted to keep my name. And Uli said: 'Aw! But I want to have the same name as our children, I'll take on a double-name.' And with it was decided that our family name is my last name. [...] And when I got pregnant, we thought it would be kind of nice if our children had Uli's last name. We always said, the genetics from me, the name from Uli. And then I went to three offices and asked... I obviously had to tell them the whole story as well, so they don't think, hey, she's nuts. And then they said 'not possible'".

In the Feldman case, it seemed to be less the connection to a family line, as with the Müllers, but an additional recognition of Uli as a person at the heart of this naming work. The statement that he contributed the name and Berit "the genetics" also symbolically re-instated the duality implied in joint procreation and excluded the donor. After the conception of their second donor conceived child the Feldmans however progressively lost interest in further pushing forward such a name change. This was due to the complex legal action this would have entailed, but also because they said that they now just felt "normal" and other things, such as "getting the kids to bed" (Uli) were taking up their energy.

Individual naming practices in the Arnulf rainbow family, as a last example, differed in their inclusivity and in which specific relationships they foregrounded. Jacob Barry, donor and father of the two children of Svenja and Lena Arnulf, repeatedly told me the story of how his first child Jonas got his name.

Jacob Barry: "Did Svenja and Lena tell you this? Eleven days before Jonas was born, my father died. Then we were still discussing possible names and I suggested, we could maybe name him Jonas, after my father. [Barry's father is American, and the name Jonas exists in English and German]. And they went ahead and did it! But—they did not tell me anything. On the day of his birth, when I saw Jonas for the first time, I was at this hospital room window with Svenja [the co-mother], a nurse, and a doctor. [He was not in the labor ward during Jonas' birth, but waited in the hospital]. That's where I saw Jonas for the first time! And the nurse asked: 'And what's his name?' And Svenja said 'Jonas', and I could have almost cried. They did not tell me anything before, not anything."

The relational symbolism in how Jacob Barry recounted this situation could not be more pronounced. Co-mother Svenja, who he would be in rivalry with had the Arnulfs have chosen a dual and exclusive family model instead of an inclusive one, brought him the news that the child was named after his father—thereby emphasizing the connection to Jacob and Jacob's family, while at the same time also exerting a parental authority. She was the one who named and who then brought the news of this naming practice. It was notable that this example of naming work does *not* emphasize a connection between the parents in the absence of joint procreation, as was typically the case with the heterosexual families. In other words, it was not co-mother Svenja who was recognized through this practice, her role was self-evident it seems. Instead it was Jacob Barry, the donor, to whom a connection was underlined. Whereas the other examples above emphasize exclusive parenthood in the absence of a so-called genetic link, the foregrounding of Jacob Barry's family through the Arnulfs' individual naming and terminology work emphasizes inclusive parenthood in the absence of a conjugal relationship between Jacob and birth-mother Lena.

Based on my fieldwork materials, naming and terminology work on both the level of kinship terminology and the individual level of practices involving pre- and surnames seems to be a central and explicitly negotiated tactic of kinship knowledge-management for families-by-donation. (I will further analyze it as also being a reactive tactic to anticipated confrontations in section 8.3). In its reflexive employment, typically involving longer discussions in the interviews, it differed from the more intuitive knowledge-management discussed in section 7.1. However, it was also entangled with these more intuitive practices, because it involved allocating a specific role to the donor figure. It thereby contributes to the specific relational constitution of families in the face of a terminological underdetermination of kinship-by-donation, due to the novelty of openly acknowledged donor conception. As a practice it connects and dis-connects not only kin-persons in the present, but also establishes a connection to family members of the past.

This knowledge-management practice, to come back to Konrad, differed from the "multi-directional flows of relatedness" (1998, 660) leading to a "generalized diffuse relatedness" (1998, 661) she describes from the perspective of anonymous donors. The parents, in contrast, often used naming practices explicitly as a way of managing what Konrad calls flows of relatedness. For example, by including the donor through talking about him or her, but commonly excluding him or her from the core family unit through not allowing the donor to be known as "father" or "mother". The parents were also underlining their difference from so-called patchwork families through this naming practice, because terms such as "biological father" marked the existence of previous sexual relationships in patchwork families. Those parents not conforming to what I will discuss as the "reproductive norm" in section 8.4 (i.e. single mothers, visibly post-menopausal women, homosexual couples) seemed to engage in more inclusive terminology work than the heterosexual families, particularly the bi-parental families-by-sperm-donation. This was probably the case because the sperm donor could most clearly be perceived as a rival to the male's role as a father (and lover) in families conforming to the assumed heterosexual norm, while other families found themselves "outside" of the norm already, due to their sexualities or chosen method of reproduction.

7.3 Telling the Child

As analyzed in chapter 6, the parents of my sample had typically developed an overall active or passive approach to disclosure. This section analyses their practices of telling the children in more detail. I analyze how the approach of *making known all along* (chapter 6) was operationalized in practices of reading the books on gamete donation to infants. I shall argue that such available children's books relieved parents of a "pioneer" status when telling their children about their donor conception. I also found that parental disclosure was embedded in wider practices of trying to adopt kinship knowledge-management for the whole social domain of the family. This section commences through firstly giving a short overview of the disclosure practices of my interviewees. I then turn to a detailed analysis of how disclosure was handled with the help of the books and close with the discussion of extending knowledge-management to outside of the nuclear family.

During the time of my fieldwork not all of the passive disclosers had actually started to talk about the donation with their children, because the children simply had not asked questions about reproduction yet. The German-Brazilian Tönschs were waiting for the moment, when their son Alvaro would start asking questions. Their other child, Helene, was still a toddler. At the end of my fieldwork the Stegers had three children and none of them were asking questions yet. British single mother Shoko Nakamura's son Ochi or the Dünke's surrogacy conceived daughter were also not yet asking about reproduction.

The Müllers older "naturally" conceived son Moritz had been told about his little brother's DI conception when he was around seven and started to ask questions about reproduction. His little brother was also still too small to ask questions. The older children of Svenja Arnulf from her previous heterosexual marriage had been told about their younger siblings' DI conception, because they asked about their co-mother Lena's pregnancy. The younger Arnulf children themselves, six and three at the end of my fieldwork, had not talked about the details of DI conception or sexualities with their parents yet.

All the other families had told their children. The Kings' donor-conceived children were already young adults and had been told long ago when they were in kindergarten and asked "where the babies come from". The Feldmans, the Schneiders, the Greenwoods, and the Hamptons were all already talking about DI with their children, although the children were still very young (under six at the end of my fieldwork)—following an approach of active disclosure. The Taylors had also followed an approach of active disclosure with their ova-donation-conceived son and their younger "naturally" conceived daughter. Both Taylor children were already teenagers during my fieldwork. Single mother Maria Lieb had also actively started telling her daughter from a young age onwards.

As already mentioned in chapter 6, children's books were not only a central part of the emergent interest group canon of knowledge-management, but also figured centrally as "tools" for disclosure among the families I interviewed. Exemplary for the passive discloser's usage of the books was how German mother Silke Müller recounted her usage of Petra Thorn's German children's book on donor conception in heterosexual families:

Silke Müller: "It was interesting with Moritz [her son, about seven then; only his younger brother is DI-conceived], I mean, when is the right time to tell? I could practice with Moritz, in a sense. So I was being quite good and read all these books on 'when is the right moment to tell' and so on. But then, erm, how are you going to really do that? You know, when is it really the best moment? You actually do get a bit jittery…"
Marcel Müller: "Of course."

Silke Müller: "The whole thing: how shall I really phrase it? How will he take it, what will the reaction be like? And then it was, it was so easy, really no problem at all. It simply all fell into place, because my son at some point asked: 'Mom, where do babies actually come from?'—or something along those lines. And I just thought: Marvelous—let's get the book! [laughs]. And I went: 'Normally it works like this, but with me it worked liked this'. And he just went, 'okay, but now I want to play some more Star Wars'. Children just take these things so easy and it is no problem whatsoever to them. They take in the information and they do talk about it every once in a while, but not necessarily in that exact moment. One really should not be afraid of that moment. And I think for me, it is good we can practice. We can grow with it so it also won't be a problem when Jan (her younger donor-conceived son) is older."

Silke Müller waited for questions regarding reproduction to arise before she chose to talk about the donor conception to her older son—but then used the "DI education" book to explain. In my fieldwork data I found a pattern that children mostly started to ask questions about reproduction, pregnancies, or sexuality when their mother was pregnant with a sibling. In the Arnulf rainbow-family, such questions were particularly complicated to answer, because the Arnulfs simultaneously needed to explain DI, sexual orientation and family forms. This is for instance discernible in the interview passage below where Svenja Arnulf and her partner Lena talk about how Svenja's children Mareike and Karl from a previous heterosexual marriage started to inquire about the "facts of life". At the time referred to during this interview the two children were about eight years old.

Svenja Arnulf (to her partner Lena): "Well, when you were pregnant [with DI-conceived first-born Jonas] Mareike [Svenja's daughter] really started to ask a lot of questions…"
Lena Arnulf: "How a child grows in your tummy and so on… Although, what they actually know about sexuality with regard to us…? They [Mareike and Karl] did actually say: 'Oh, we thought you had sex with Jacob [donor and father of Jonas].' And I went: 'Oh no, we went to the doctor!' They actually briefly had the question if I would move in with Jacob, or Jacob with us, because he is the father. Actually, at first they thought that their own father [Svenja's ex-husband] would be the father, because that seemed logical. You know how children are… 'No, Jacob will be the father.' 'Will he move in with us?' '-Naw…' That was that, and then: 'Oh, not even sex? Well…' [implying they lost interest then]."

The Arnulf twins worried that their co-mother's pregnancy would change their own situation. They wondered what kind of relationships, to stay within the kinship studies terminology, were actually arising from this particular act of reproduction. Being children of a divorced couple themselves, and probably having come across stories about parental break-ups among their peers, they were asking themselves if their co-mother's pregnancy was somehow in conflict with her relationship to their mother. Realizing the inclusivity (rather than the exclusivity they might have already encountered as a norm) of their family and that everything would stay the same at home, they seemingly lost interest.

While the Arnulfs' family situation was quite distinct from that of most of my research partners, what was actually typical for the overall sample in both the interview passages above was the difficulty of combining the disclosure about the donor gamete conception with more general sex education (for some of the misunderstandings this produced among the children also see section 8.6). Silke Müller told her son Moritz how it worked "normally" and then how it worked with regard to his younger brother. The Arnulf twins were faced with trying to understand how her co-mother got pregnant, while at the same time trying to understand how it worked for people other than their two mothers—and then learning to keep this apart. Such disclosure situations thus marked a first learning process for the child that families come in different shapes and sizes, but that some of these shapes are more widespread and/or considered the norm.

The active disclosers were not only invoking the children's books in their attempts to tell their children about their donor conception in situations where the children asked specific questions, but were already reading the books to their children before they could even talk. How Holly Greenwood talked about her usage of the book "My Story" (see section 6.1) was typical for this approach:

Holly Greenwood: "I got the book from the DC Network website. They had several publications, for lesbian couples, single women, eggs donation, sperm donation. Would you like to see the book?"
Maren Klotz: "Yes, please". [longer pause while we get the book and some food from the kitchen and play with Holly's then one and a half years old daughter]. "And when did you start reading it to her?"
Holly: "Hmmm, I don't know, when she was eight months maybe? It's clear she doesn't understand it, but it is simply for us, so that we practice telling her."

Maren Klotz: "What do you find especially helpful about the book?"
Holly Greenwood: "Maybe saying things like 'sperm' or 'insemination' in front of my child [laughs]."

For Holly Greenwood it was the element of "practicing" through reading the children's book, which she marked as particularly important in the interview. Using the book as a parental training-tool to "practice" disclosure was also discernible as a theme in the passages quoted further above.

Reading the books on gamete donation to very young children was the operationalization, so to speak, of the kinship knowledge-management strategy to make the donor conception known *all along*, as analyzed in chapter 6. German father Marc Schneider's account below was typical for the active disclosers concerning this operationalization.

Marc Schneider: "I have read the book by Ken Daniels and I bought just about every children's book about this topic [DI conception]. I have quite a nice library about the whole subject now. [...] And I decided then to tell my son very early, because that's supposed to establish phrasings in the brain, which later on will make sure that he says 'I have known this all along'. I think he was a year old, when I started telling him and at some point we started to also use Petra Thorn's children's book."
Maren Klotz: "I know that book..."
Marc Schneider: "-and he likes to look at it every once in a while, and from time to time I read to him or you [to wife Nadine] also sometimes talk to him, it depends... Not at the moment..."
Nadine Schneider: "-rarely so at the moment...
Marc Schneider: "-not something like..."
Nadine Schneider: "-we don't have to look at the book every single week."
Marc Schneider: "No, not at all. It is simply, if it comes to mind sometimes, because he also enjoys it. He knows that he... 'Should I tell you your story again?' and he finds that quite interesting then."

In the beginning of the quote above, Marc Schneider repeated parts of the DC Network canon on knowledge-management verbatim as laid out in their brochure on early disclosure. While the interview passage is typical for my sample concerning the children's book usage through the active disclosers, it is also exceptional in conveying Marc Schneider's particular interest and knowledgeability of the international canon of knowledge-management. When it came to children's books and popular science or self-help books about DI from all over the world, Marc Schneider had become an expert and was when I met him in fact thinking about translating some of the internationally available children's books into German. With this he was a particularly pronounced example of parents turning themselves into what I will more comprehensively introduce as *reflexive kinship expertise* in section 8.1.

Active and passive disclosers alike made recurring remarks how reading the books was "practice" or "training" for the parents to feel comfortable with their disclosure decision. Many of the actively disclosing parents underlined how their children at the first reading were not able to understand the words yet and the reading therefore took place *only* for them, the parents. The following quote from my first interview with the Hamptons captures this quite well:

> Sarah Hampton: "We've started reading the My Story book very, very early. More for us, to get used to using the words. Because… -it's quite difficult to use… Because to talk about eggs and sperm and reading that to a young child is a difficult thing."
> Tim Hampton: "Oh yeah, the first few times we did it was…."
> Sarah Hampton: "Yeah. So we started thinking, should we use different words? And, in the end, we just read the book and we are comfortable reading it now and using those words."

As shown here, parents following the approach of early active disclosure typically needed to overcome a reluctance to talk about biological substances with their children. Since the children's books (as analyzed in chapter 6) all conveyed knowledge about biological reproduction (however leaving out heredity and sexuality), parents needed to "practice" getting used to reading to their children about sperm or eggs. Parents commonly stressed how it was hard to "find a child-appropriate language to explain" (Philip Steger), to make the donor conception become "a tellable story, in simple words" (Dörte Tönsch). The books were typically addressed as a solution or answer to this struggle, relieving the parents of having to invent such a "tellable story" themselves.

In my fieldwork materials, it appeared that as a tactic of knowledge-management the usage of the children's books was quite different from the naming and terminology work analyzed in 7.2. While kinship terminologies were extensively reflexively interrogated through the parents, the narratives the books conveyed were not. They were rather accepted as tools for knowledge-management validated through their embeddedness in the interest group canon and as containing established ways-of-knowing kinship-by-donation. The frequent use of the books had the effect that young children apparently sounded very much alike when they talked about gamete donation (as analyzed in 8.6)—because the children were often repeating the book text. The books were hence part of a process of normalizing kinship-by-donation and canonizing knowledge-management (also see Knecht et al. 2011). Through this the parents were relieved from individualistically acting as *kinship pioneers* during disclosure, loosely drawing on Rayna Rapp (1999).[6] They did *not* have to engage in unprecedented knowledge tactics like those parents starting to disclose assisted conception or starting rainbow families, say, 25 years ago did.

The children's books should however *not* be seen as solely an end-product of parental networking endeavors and associated processes of a canonization of knowledge-management. Instead, they have figured in the center, sometimes even as starting point, of these practices of networking and canonization. The British DC Network, as an example and as traced in section 6.1, actually came into being around the activity of putting out the very first "DI education" book in the 1980s—and succeeded with this in the early 1990s. Furthermore, the children's books not only stood at the center of interest group formation and at the center of individual parental knowledge-management containing preformatted narratives for disclosure, they also played a role as material objects for knowledge-management. The books could be materially handled—thereby, at least in the parents' understanding—also signaling interest or disinterest in the subject of donor conception by the children, irrespective of their abilities of actively verbally exploring issues. It was for instance a typical practice among the parents of my sample, active and passive disclosers alike, to leave the book in the child's room—and thereby bestow the child with

6 Rapp has famously used the term *moral pioneers* for the hitherto unprecedented moral-philosophical deliberations women have to engage in to make sense of the availability and of the results of prenatal screening. I would argue, hence the reference to Rapp through speaking of *kinship pioneers* that the users of reproductive technologies are also often confronted with seemingly unprecedented decisions in how to *do kinship* with the newly available techniques. However, I do not want to imply that such families necessarily face comparable moral dilemmas.

agency regarding knowledge-management. The Hamptons, for example, made the following remark:

Tim Hampton: "We read it to him for a while, we regularly read it to him for a while."
Sarah Hampton: "But now it is just in the bookcase."
Tim Hampton: "And now if he wants that rather than another one of his books, he has that."

The quote below by German mother Nadine Schneider is another example of the typical role the books played as material toys:

Nadine Schneider: "The book is with him, in his room on the bookshelf, so he can always pick it up. And, I mean children, they play all the time, they move everything out of the shelves and out of the cupboards… His favorite game at the moment is the going-on-a-trip-game and there he takes everything from the shelves and puts it onto his trolley and then carts it to wherever. And of course other children then also handle the book and that's okay."

The books thus shifted disclosure from being a potentially embarrassing one-off talk about the facts of life, as it is a much deplored cliché for parental knowledge practices irrespective of kinship-by-donation, to being more light-hearted and playful. Bestowing the books with the status of toys under the children's control furthermore was typically seen as part of a gradual process of disclosure within which the children and their playfellows were actively participating.

Some of the parents also mentioned to me that they had explicitly kept parts of the paper-work associated with the donation for their children to look at and handle. This was similar to the common practice among parents to keep some of the objects associated with their children's birth, such as the bracelets used for identification in neonatal care units. Parents thereby compiled informal kinship-archives including information on the donor and the treatment—in Germany commonly against the treating physician's advice to destroy such materials (see 6.1). These informal archives were not described as being part of everyday life, but of rarer situations of talking about donor conception with the older children of my research partners. Maria Lieb, for instance, told me how looking at the little box in which she kept the donor information was one of the situations in which she explicitly discussed the donor conception with her daughter.

As already explored in 7.2, parents commonly extended practices of knowledge-management to outside of the family. A typical worry of my interviewees was that through early disclosure their children might have problems when talking to others about what they had learned from the books on donor conception. Uli Linde-Feldman for instance mentioned that he wanted to ensure teachers would not intervene:

Uli Linde-Feldman: "Our children are in pre-school and in a nursery school and we told everyone there from the beginning. We just said, if the child says something, we need to tell the nurses. We don't want her going: 'No kid, you got something wrong there', that's actually important."

German father Marc Schneider, as another typical example, stressed that he wanted to avoid potential confusion of his son's ways-of-knowing kinship-by-donation through informing everyone in their social circle about the donor conception.

Marc Schneider: "Quite a lot of neighbors know about it, all of our friends know, the teachers at the kindergarten know, because… Because we are telling our son, we obviously want to avoid that someone might react awkwardly if he says something. 'What kind of nonsense are you talking?' or why does a three year old know how babies are made… Well, other parents might take offence with that. That's why we are explaining it to those people he sees a lot. And then we are also trying to establish the necessary basic knowledge about the whole thing so that that actually works out well."

The accounts of situations where the young children were talking about their donor conception outside of the family (analyzed in 8.6) notably did not convey negative reactions from others, only an occasional parental uneasiness. Whether this means parental knowledge management was highly successful in normalizing donor conception for their whole social domain, or negative experiences did not find their comfortable place within the interviews I conducted, has to be left open. What I want to stress, however, is that for my research partners, telling their children about gamete donation entailed many more related knowledge practices than "just" telling their children about gamete donation. In other words, disclosure involved wider practices of knowledge-management than merely informing the children. My research partners were commonly trying to ensure that not only their children but also their whole social domain knew about the donor conception and hoped that that would shield their family from potential confrontations. This sometimes even extended to choices of nurseries, schools, or places to live. The Schneiders, for instance, had almost decided against sending their son to a Catholic kindergarten, but were then convinced otherwise during a consultation with the nursery teacher who had turned out to be involuntarily childless herself and highly supportive of their decision to use DI.

To summarize for this section on parental disclosure, the children's books relieved the parents I interviewed from having to engage in "pioneering" knowledge-management all the time. The ways-of-knowing achieved through the usage of the books however needed to be constantly defended against anticipated frictions arising from a lack of knowledge on kinship-by-donation by others. Particularly active disclosure (i.e. those parents who told very young children about gamete donation instead of waiting for questions on reproduction to arise) was perceived to be in need of explanation to the wider social circle. Parents worried their children's detailed knowledge of (parts of) biological reproduction as conveyed in the children's books might produce negative reactions from other parents. All in all, disclosing gamete donation turned out to be a relational process both in resting upon the enrolment of objects, such as the children's books and collected materials, and in its tendency to actually become not a knowledge-management process confined within individual families, but pertaining to a whole social domain.

7.4 Subversive Knowledge-Management and Wayward Relations

I have previously analyzed how my research partners came to know the donor as what I called an *administered relation* (7.1): the fragmentary image of a person compiled out of the accessible clinical trajectory of knowing kinship-by-donation (5.2) and the families' imagination. This section, in contrast, focuses on subversive search endeavors followed by parents or children-by-donation to find officially anonymous donors or so-called donor-siblings.[7] These subversive practices of knowledge-

7 Donor-siblings (a term often used by persons concerned) are half-siblings conceived through the gametes of the same donor. Conventionally, half-siblingship however

management typically make use of the internet and also often rely on DNA analysis. Commonly, these practices have a grass-roots character. The searches tend to be independent of, or even undermine the official knowledge-management of clinics and past or present national regulation. Because of their independence from the clinical trajectory of knowing kinship-by-donation, I have come to call the forms of kinship emerging from such searches *wayward relations*. Acquiring kinship knowledge through these searches helps persons concerned to assert agency over the past. This past is often perceived to be characterized by a lack of knowledge over kinship, particularly for donor-conceived adults. Persons concerned also assert agency within the creative search endeavors themselves, making crafty use of knowledge on genetics, genetic testing and IT technologies. I will show how donor conceived adults have started to network and set-up their own unofficial registries largely unnoticed by the wider public and policymakers.

Wayward relations reaffirm notions of kinship as genetically grounded, but go beyond simple notions of *geneticization*. Instead, they are viewed to be complementary (not colonizing) relations in the face of other, often failed relationships. They also show a tendency to connect for connection's sake, termed the "imperative to connect" by Knecht (2009b) and Edwards (2009a). Ultimately, the subversive knowledge-management practices discussed below show a socio-material uncontainability of kinship knowledge at odds with anonymous donation regimes and ultimately challenging clinical and state monopolies on managing kinship information (Klotz 2012). *Wayward relations* are thereby to be viewed as part of an ambiguous development towards a diminishing domain of privacy.

This section commences by briefly presenting examples of subversive practices of knowledge-management and *wayward relations* in my fieldwork data. I then discuss the presumably not widely known initiatives, infrastructures, and technologies such practices make use of. I describe four examples of subversive searches and the establishment of *wayward relations*

implies a previous sexual and often also romantic relationship between the parents. Donor-siblings are only genetically related through the chance allocation of a specific donor through the clinic. To use the term "siblings" in this context is thus ambivalent. Nevertheless, given the unprecedentedness of such relations and associated lack of an established vocabulary, I have decided to stay with this emic expression. I however do not want to suggest that genetic kinship is socially meaningful *per se*.

in more detail, focusing on single-mother-by-choice Lieb, the German Schneiders, and the two British donor-conceived women I interviewed. I conclude with an interpretive discussion of the described practices and phenomena, focusing on the "imperative to connect", the nature of *wayward relations*, and the infrastructures implicated.

Examples of Subversive Knowledge-Management and its Infrastructures

German single-mother-by-choice Maria Lieb, who used a US sperm bank to conceive, turned to a US-based internet contact registry called Donor Sibling Registry[8] to find out more about her donor and to locate donor-siblings. The German Schneiders, who had used the Danish sperm bank Scan-Sperm, were contemplating the possibility of prospectively locating their sperm donor through the supposedly "unidentifying" information he had supplied and also thought about registering with the Donor Sibling Registry. British mother-by-egg-donation Shoko Nakamura was staying in contact with the North-American physician who had treated her, to potentially use him to find out more about her anonymous donor and/or potential donor-siblings of her son Ochi. The two British adult donor-conceived women I interviewed, Bonnie Smith and Lydia Rivers, and one of two donor-conceived children of research partner Susan King were registered with the British contact service UK Donorlink.[9] Bonnie Smith had thereby found a donor-brother and they were together searching for their anonymous donor. The German donor-conceived adults whose activities I was mainly following through their public website[10] had set up an unofficial registry for German donor-conceived children and potentially interested donors through the US-based genetic genealogy service FamilyTreeDNA.[11] And, as briefly touched upon in chapter 5, after becoming aware of British parents trying to subversively network via clinical donor IDs to locate donor-siblings, the British HFEA had set up a donor-sibling registry itself. This official HFEA sibling registry was, however, only open to donor-conceived adults, not to the parents.

8 www.donorsiblingregistry.com
9 www.ukdonorlink.org.uk
10 www.spenderkinder.de
11 www.familytreedna.com

Such practices of subversive knowledge-management to establish *wayward relations* rely on specific initiatives, infrastructures, and technologies. The Donor Sibling Registry (DSR) was founded through a North American mother-by-donation in 2000 (see its logo in clipping 7.2).

Clipping 7.2: Donor Sibling Registry Logo (Source: website www.donorsiblingregistry.com)

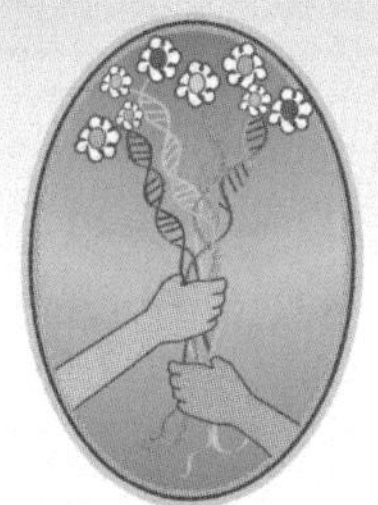
THE
DONOR SIBLING REGISTRY
EDUCATING, CONNECTING AND
SUPPORTING DONOR FAMILIES

The DSR logo depicts flowers with stems made out of DNA strands.

The DSR has developed from a website that enables networking between donors, parents, and donor-siblings into a large interest group. It releases publications, collaborates with academic research, and presses for further self-regulation in the market-driven US reproductive medical sector. At the heart of its service, however, lies its website, which was originally set up to facilitate familial networking via the unique donor codes[12] used in the USA and now also allows networking around other available information, such as the names of treatment centers and doctors involved. It does not connect people along DNA tests, but rather enables members to assign themselves to already discussed information. Members can also set up a new thread themselves. The website further enables searches and anonymous and non-anonymous contact options. Membership (which is

12 US fertility centers assign unique numbers to each donor (e.g. Freeman et al., 2009, 506). This is not common practice in Europe.

fee-based) in the registry is growing fast, reporting over 36,000 members in early 2012, in late 2007 it had been only 10,000 (Freeman et al. 2009, 506). Freeman et al. have been among the very first researchers to analyze the registry's activities (but also see recent publications by Hertz and Mattes, 2011, who do not singularly focus on the DSR but generally on donor-sibling tracing through various registries by single-mothers-by-choice exclusively; and Jadva et al., 2010).

Almost 10,000 so-called matches between donor-siblings or families and donors have been facilitated through the service, as reported on its website in 2012. The DSR promotes the idea that it is socially enriching and satisfies a natural curiosity for donors, parents, and particularly donor-siblings to get in touch online or even form closer relationships. It also promotes the idea that it might be useful for medical reasons to do so, as for instance promoted through the mission statement depicted in clipping 7.3.

As reported by Freedman et al. (2009, 507–508), parental desires to search for donor-siblings out of "curiosity" and, less frequently, to help a child have a "secure sense of identity" were given as the main reasons to join the DSR. Single mothers and lesbian couples were most active in searching and together comprised two thirds of the registry's membership. The last third was comprised of donor-conceived persons,[13] heterosexual parents, and donors. The DSR caters to all forms of donor conception, but centers on sperm donation (as do the few studies on the DSR's activities), which reflects the much higher number of donor-siblings potentially conceived through sperm donation. Although heavily US-based and in English, the DSR has also opened to clients of internationally operating sperm banks and fertility clinics all around the world. Because it tries to put in touch so-called donor-siblings, it has the capacity to circumvent clinical restrictions on identifying donor data. Once one donor-conceived child turns 18 years old and can access the data on their donor, this information can be shared with the other, potentially much younger children. (Such potential for sharing information was also reported by Hertz and Mattes (2011,

13 Families might also be using one log-in together. From the reports on the DSR website it seems like there is more direct donor-sibling-contact and searching going on than the membership of mostly parents would suggest. Older children seemed to follow-up on parental searches or conduct them together with their parents.

Clipping 7.3: DSR Mission Statement (Source: www.donorsiblingregistry.c om)

The DSR Provides:

- Donor-conceived people the opportunity to locate critical medical and health information from their biological donors
- Donors the chance to anonymously or openly share family, ancestral and genetic details with their offspring
- A place for mutually desired communication to begin for donors and their donor-conceived offspring
- A site for donor-conceived half-siblings to connect and extend their family ties
- A comprehensive, secure, and positive environment of information, studies, support, and resources for parents and their children
- Advocacy for the rights of donor-conceived people and education about the issues, and challenges of their community
- The opportunity to connect even without having a donor ID or number

1141) as one reason for parental networking). I presume that this subversive capacity of donor-sibling registries has also been one of the reasons for the British HFEA to set up its own official registry, whereby it can control that only offspring over 18 years of age can access the network. Since there are no unique codes available in Germany and in the UK, using the DSR involves far more "detective work", e.g. the location of potential other identifiers (such as the donor IDs some British parents collected) and subsequent DNA tests.

The British registry UK Donorlink (UKDL) has through its large press coverage (e.g. Dreaper 2006; Frean 2004; Lambert 2009; Morrison, 2006) sometimes appeared like a British version of the much used DSR. UKDL however is, in comparison, minute in membership and employs different technologies for matching than the DSR. UKDL recently reported to have less than 200 fully registered members and facilitated less than 30 matches

(UKDL 2012, 12). UKDL was set up by activists and counselors originally involved in post-adoption self-help work with a UK Department of Health grant (currently under review) to enable British donor-conceived persons, conceived before gamete donation became comprehensively regulated in 1991, and former donors to get in touch. It operates with DNA tests and a databank. Members are informed if another member is likely to be a donor-sibling or the donor, based on the tests. A fee is charged for the DNA test; otherwise the service is free. UKDL commissions an external laboratory to perform the tests. The laboratory is not available directly to registry members to explain or discuss test results; all communication is handled by UKDL.

One of the British donor-conceived adults whom I interviewed, Lydia Rivers, reported that she had problems using UKDL's service and they had told her this was due to staffing problems. She for instance learned that her DNA samples had not been sent out to the laboratory for analysis almost four months after they were taken. She had also been told that a maternal DNA swab was additionally necessary (more about the testing options below), which led to conflicts with her mother who initially refused to take the test, because she was reluctant about her daughter joining UKDL. The likelihood of a mother favorably agreeing to take a DNA test in order for her adult child to find the donor seems distant, because adults joining UKDL had after all often found out about being donor-conceived by accident, not because their parents had chosen to disclose. This testing practice might thus be one reason for the small numbers in membership. That the taking of DNA swabs needed to be officially witnessed might have provided for a further threshold. The registry additionally had negative press coverage during the time of fieldwork, because of a "false match" (see clipping 7.4).

What had happened? The "matching" of donor-siblings via DNA analyses always operates with probabilities. This is firstly due to the arbitrary reduction of the chromosome set during the development of gametes, making it theoretically possible that half-siblings share hardly any characteristic DNA sequences. And secondly it is due to the laboratories needing to incorporate population-genetics, because correlations in DNA sequences can either point to the likelihood of being closely genetically related, or to two individuals coming from a highly insulated, i.e. "in-bred" popula-

Clipping 7.4: Daily Mail headline (Source: Pryer, 2010)

Despair oft the DNA ‚sisters': In a terrible mistake that casts new doubt on DNA profiling, it turns out they weren't related at all

tion. Thus, what happened at UKDL was not a straightforward mistake as suggested through the headline in clipping 7.4, such as swapping samples, but an incautious interpretation and communication of the testing results. Paternity or maternity testing is less complex than half-siblingship testing. Furthermore, the genetic sequences analyzed for testing paternity or half-siblingship mostly differ. Paternity tests currently commonly operate with analyzing so called STRs (single tandem repeats), while degrees of relatedness are easier to establish through testing for similarities in so called SNPs (single nucleotide polymorphisms), which are also analyzed for genetic ancestry research (see Hauskeller, 2006 for the discussion of different available DNA testing technologies from a genomically informed philosophical point of view).

UKDL at the time of my fieldwork operated with the testing method used for paternity testing, which explains why they were encouraging new members such as Lydia Rivers to also send in a parental DNA swab, because this would make potential half-sibling matches through the STR analysis more reliable. Additional parental swabs are not needed for SNP analysis testing for siblingship. In internet forums facilitating exchanges between donor-conceived persons, which I monitored for my research, UKDL was criticized for using tests perceived as outdated (see one example of such a criticism in clipping 7.5).

The clipping discusses the usability of so-called ancestry research sites for subversive knowledge-management (also utilized by the small German

Clipping 7.5: Discussion among donor-conceived persons worldwide on genetic genealogy and the testing technology used by UKDL (Source: www.australiandonorconceptionforum.org.)

> To all that have undertaken some genetic genealogy, whether they be offspring or donors. A donor conceived person has set-up a project group on FamilyTreeDNA for donor conception.
> I have included a message from her below:
> The goal of the project is to identify half-siblings (mom not needed!!) among adult offspring, as well as for former donors to locate their donor children. It's also going to look at the possibility that some clinics/doctor's were using donors who themselves were related (brothers or father/son). Also in clinics like Harley Street which donors often provided for many/all of the doctors, perhaps over many many years – so age and doctor is not an accurate determiner of possible relatedness.
> Also, a note on UKDL: Unlike UKDL which uses CODIS markers, and like [redacted] and I found recently, these markers are not accurate enough to determine half-siblingship, and why there's been so much shadiness with UKDL.....these tests look at hundreds of thousands of SNPs across the genome. So the accuracy of the test is impeccable, especially in determining immediate relatives.

donor offspring community active on the internet). Over the last twelve or so years commercial services based on genomic testing technologies for research on ancient and recent ancestral and ethnic "origins" started to appear mainly online. The tests have been critically discussed concerning their rather arbitrary linking of individuals to highly specific places or groups of people. If one employs a different genealogical gaze, ancestry evidently grows exponentially. More crucially for these tests, DNA transmission (and analysis) is in itself arbitrary and reductive, as mentioned above.[14] However the tests have also been described to be reflexively interrogated through their users rather than simply being accepted for their essentialist message. Hauskeller (2006) for instance describes them as a means to claim and strategically employ identity in a post-colonial scientific world. Companies such as FamilyTreeDNA (see clipping 7.6),

14 Gametes only contain half of a person's chromosomes and the process of meiosis leading to such reduction of DNA sequences is arbitrary. Furthermore, DNA analysis employed in ancestry research often makes use of tracing only female or male ancestral lines. This is the case because of the more or less unchanged matrilineal transmission of mitochondrial DNA and, similarly, the patrilineal transmission of the Y-chromosome.

GeneTree[15] or AncestryByDNA[16] now have been joined by even more controversial companies such as 23andme[17], which concentrate not only on genetic ancestry research but also on the calculation of risk susceptibilities and are mainly marketing their services through the internet.

Clipping 7.6: Part of FamilyTreeDNA Webpage (Source: www.familytreedna.com)

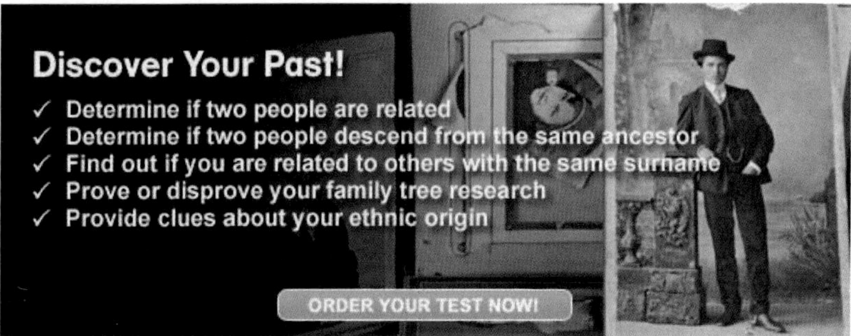

One feature that the internet-based genetic genealogy services offer, in addition to the tests employed to find donor-siblings of both genders, is Y-chromosome testing and the linking of specific DNA sequences to specific last-names. (The background to this roughly summarized is that due to the patrilineal heredity of both last names—as a historical practice—and Y-chromosomes, there are many correlations between family names and specific base sequences on the so-called male chromosome. One could say this is a classic case of socio-material co-production). There has been one reported case where the employment of such a service through a donor-conceived teenager has led to the discovery of his supposedly anonymous sperm donor in the US (Motluk 2005), which has, however, not led to broader policy discussion on donor anonymity in the UK or Germany.

Crucial for the appropriation of commercial genetic genealogy services into subversive practices of kinship knowledge-management has been the growing internet-led networking and associated "self-expertization" of

15 www.genetree.com
16 www.ancestrybydna.com
17 www.23andme.com

donor-conceived individuals.[18] The commercial testing sites themselves were initially set up to profit from the much larger community of hobby genealogists.[19] However, donor-conceived adults, without access to donor-information and highly critical of this practice, started to use such services for their own wayward searches. They did so largely unnoticed in the press or social science research. Clipping 7.7 for example depicts part of a discussion among donor-conceived individuals about using Y-Chromosome testing.

Clipping 7.7: Discussion in Web-Forum on using Y-Chromosome testing (Source: www.australiandonorconceptionforum.org)

> I joined up with the name project that was associated with that name. Within that project, people are grouped according to DNA results. Two of the people in my group [redacted] had also tested these other 9 markers as it was part of a batch done with another company. I was able to get mine as additional tests with FamilyTreeDNA. With FTDNA there are a whole bunch of other markers you can test for under the advanced orders.
> The results matched, further strengthening the link.

A typical example for such networking and expertization practices is young US-American blogger Lindsay Greenawalt, who holds academic degrees in biology and IT, and has devoted much of her blog (see clipping 7.8) explaining to other donor offspring the pros, cons, details and probability

18 For websites networking donor-conceived individuals independent of parental interest group formation e.g. see www.spenderkinder.de (operating from Germany) and the English language sites http:// tangledwebsorg.wordpress.com; www.idoalliance.org; www.canadiandonoroffspring.ca; www.searchingformyspermdonorfather.org. Also see http:// australiandonorconceptionforum.org for extensive discussions among donor conceived persons from all over the world of genetic genealogy research and websites.

19 For ethnographic analyses of hobby ancestry research for instance see Edwards (2009a), Nash (2002), and Timm (2010).

calculation basis of different genetic testing technologies. (She is also the person referred to in the forum-post depicted in clipping 7.5).

Clipping 7.8: Greenawalt's Blog (Source: www.cryokidconfessions.blogspot.com)

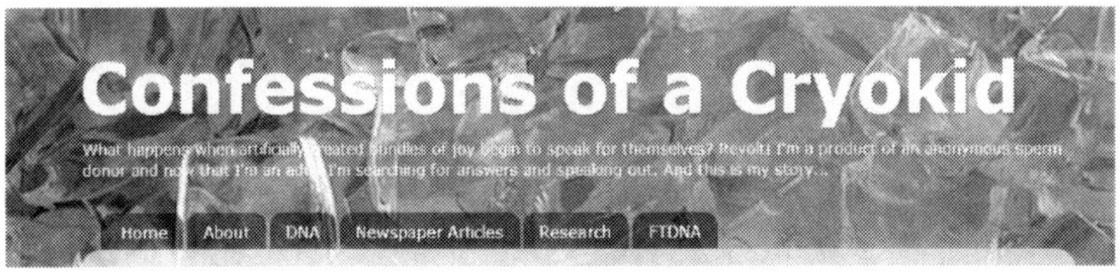

Greenawalt has networked with similarly concerned individuals over the last couple of years in an attempt to create her own website and database for sibling- and donor-searches. However, in 2011 she announced that she was collaborating with FamilyTreeDNA to facilitate the "first and only worldwide DNA project for donor-conceived adults and former/current donors through FamilyTree DNA" (part of the announcement in her blog depicted in clipping 7.9).

The testing technology employed in this endeavor is a combination of Y-chromosome testing for males and autosomal testing via SNP analysis, to enable surname correlations and donor-sibling tracing. A twist is added to the new project: the searches include the larger group of hobby genealogists registered with FamilyTreeDNA. A sperm donor could, for instance, be using the site for his hobby ancestry searches and now be found through the searches of the donor offspring. Furthermore, it would not even have to be the donor himself—a close relative would also be flagged as a match (see discussion of such a case in clipping 7.10).

Despite this US-focus of FamilyTreeDNA, it has also become home to the wayward German donor-offspring and donor registry in December 2011. The approximately twenty German speaking adult donor-conceived individuals publicly appearing on their website www.spenderkinder.de now suggest taking the FamilyTreeDNA test to all German-speaking donor offspring or donors interested, as mentioned above. On the website they announce that "given that some clinics have destroyed the donor data, we had no choice but to search for the donor or half-siblings ourselves", be-

Clipping 7.9: Blog announcement of new donor sibling registry hosted by FamilyTreeDNA (Source: www.cryokidconfessions.blogspot.com)

WEDNESDAY, JULY 13, 2011

Official Release: Donor Conceived DNA Project!!

I am excited to announce the creation of the *first and only* worldwide DNA project for donor-conceived adults and former/current donors through Family Tree DNA.

Project website: Donor Conceived DNA Project

The main goals of the project will be as follows:

1. A central location for donor-conceived individuals to locate half-siblings
2. A central location for former and current donors to locate their biological children

Other goals of the project are to provide awareness to donor-conceived adults, former/current donors, and parents of donor-conceived children to the benefits and successes of using DNA tests to identify not only half-siblings but to give direction to the identity of the biological parent, and to analyze the DNA of donor-conceived adults in an anthropological light.

low this the price (199–289 US dollars) and the procedure for ordering the test kit online are explained (see clipping 7.11).

The infrastructures on which subversive practices of knowledge-management rely are hence largely determined by the capacities for transnational networking caused by the internet in conjunction with advancing genetic testing technologies. The implicated "expertization" of donor-conceived persons is, however, different from the growing influence of interest groups on scientific knowledge production as discussed in section 6.1 We do not see the combination of experiential knowledge with scientific knowledge gaining currency *within* policymaking and scientific research, as commonly discussed for interest groups activism. Nor do we see the introduction of psy-knowledge as a new strand of scientific knowledge becoming effectual in the field, such as identified above as specific for the fertility sector. Rather, complex infrastructures and knowledge are utilized practically unnoticed to make *wayward rela-*

Clipping 7.10: Forum discussion on donor searches (Source: www.australiandonorconceptionforum.org)

> One of my friends in the states had it done recently and was able to work out who her donor is from it. She had a "suspected" name to start with but was able to locate this person through the family tree of her closest match, a second cousin. Thereby confirming the identity. At this stage it is "easier" for those in the states (as that is where most of the people who have taken the test reside), but at least it is a positive sign that the FamilyFinder test can be used to work out who your donor is.
> Time for me to start saving.

tions. While some of the described registry initiatives were used and/or advertised predominantly through parents (for instance the DSR), others were predominantly used and advertised through the donor-conceived (for instance UKDL, and the FamilyTreeDNA registry).

Case Discussions of Wayward Relations

A more detailed analysis of subversive knowledge-management being used to build *wayward relations* is necessary here before the phenomena can be more fully interpreted. German DSR user and single-mother-by-choice Maria Lieb offers an excellent example:

Maria Lieb: "I have found out that Lotta has about 30 half siblings. I hope the father would still like to meet her now that there are so many others. […] But at least she is among the two or three oldest, so there is a good chance. […] I am also wondering whether he really is who he claims he is. I mean I googled this project at the university, which he claimed to be working at, and that actually exists. But I am not really sure everything he reported to the sperm bank is true. How could they check that? I mean I also found out that he is donating at different banks, and that is against the official policy of these sperm banks. That also explains why there are so many half-siblings…"

Clipping 7.11: Web-announcement of the opening of the unofficial German donor (offspring) registry (Source: www.spenderkinder.de)

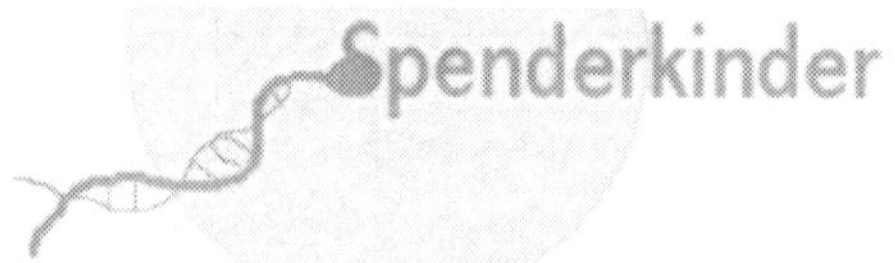

Unsere Suchdatenbank: Family Finder

Da einige Kliniken die Daten der Spender vernichtet haben, bleibt uns nichts anderes übrig, als selbst nach dem Spender oder Halbgeschwistern zu suchen.

Wir benutzen seit Dezember 2011 den Family Finder Test der amerikanischen Firma Family Tree DNA (FTDNA), um Halbgeschwister und Spender zu finden. Wer also herausfinden möchte, ob er oder sie mit uns verwandt ist, sollte am besten diesen Test machen!

Family Finder kostet 289 $ und muss direkt bei FTDNA bestellt werden, es gibt aber regelmäßig Sonderaktionen, bei denen der Test nur 199 $ kostet. Wir empfehlen und nutzen den Test, aber haben keinerlei Verbindung zu oder Einfluss auf FTDNA. Die meisten in der FTDNA-Datenbank enthaltenen Personen sind keine Spenderkinder, sondern Menschen, die an ihrer genetischen Abstammung im weiteren Sinn interessiert sind und entfernte Verwandte suchen.

Wie funktioniert der Test?

Der Family Finder Test muss im Internet Shop von FTDNA bestellt und per Kreditkarte bezahlt werden. Ca. 2 Wochen später erhält man das Testkit mit zwei Sticks, mit denen man einen Abstrich der Mundschleimhaut nehmen kann. Außerdem muss man ein Release Form unterzeichnen, dass FTDNA die Email-Adresse an mögliche Verwandte weitergeben darf. Proben und Release Form schickt man zurück zu FTDNA und erhält ca. 6 Wochen später eine Nachricht, wenn die Daten in die Datenbank aufgenommen wurden.

In der Datenbank von FTDNA sind momentan 10.000 Genprofile enthalten, die mit allen neuen Testergebnissen auf eine mögliche Verwandschaft abgeglichen wird. Bei einem Treffer sieht man den von dem möglichen Verwandten angegebenen Namen und kann ihn per Email anschreiben.

It turned out that the donor's own subversive donations at several banks had been discovered through some of the parents Lieb was now in touch with via the DSR. One father had by chance realized that the information provided by the donor under two different numbers was very similar. During my fieldwork, Lieb's contact with the other families was only loose: a few e-mails had been exchanged over a longer period of time. Lieb nevertheless mentioned that she would be quite interested in travelling to the USA at some point to have her daughter meet her donor-siblings. There was also an emerging reciprocity in information exchange among the parents: Lieb, for example, mentioned she was thinking about scanning and sending her original donor information sheet in return for those of other parents. A subject of worry among the connected parents was that five of the 30 donor-siblings had turned out to have a severe developmental disorder (see section 8.2 on medical history for more comprehensive discussion).

In the absence of any clear social roles defined for donor-siblingship between the 30 children, Lieb herself reflexively interrogated what kind of relationships were emerging:

Maria Lieb: "I don't know, do donor-conceived half-siblings and their mothers and fathers have anything in common, are they connected?"
Maren Klotz: "That would be one of my questions as well, what is it that's actually happening between people there?"
Maria Lieb: "I actually found it quite moving. Even though we only exchanged e-mails, but when they wrote e-mails of how their children were like, to think of the potential parallels… also to exchange photographs…"
Maren Klotz: "Incredible."
Maria Lieb: "Yes, but it was also shocking that there were so many half-siblings and the thing with the disease…"

With her curiosity about information on the donor and other siblings and positive appraisal of potential contact, Lieb seems to be quite a typical DSR member. The little research available on the new phenomenon of building *wayward relations* reports that while one third of all registrants on the DSR are single-mothers-by-choice through sperm donation, they form the strongest group both in looking for donor-siblings (which is far more common in general) and in looking for the donor (Freeman et al. 2009, 507). Curiosity is reported as the main reason for searching among registry members in Freeman's questionnaire study of almost 800 registry members. Potential real life contact between donor-siblings and to the donor was evaluated positively, both as a possibility and in retrospect after contact had been established.

What was different in Maria Lieb's case was the large number of donor-siblings she was able to locate, in contrast to the typical estimated to be between three and five donor-siblings, according to Hertz and Mattes (2011, 1137) or Freeman et al. (2009, 511). Both groups of authors report that the kind of social contact established varied considerably, from what Hertz and Mattes have termed a "genetic backup system" (2011, 1137) (where networking seems to foreground the exchange of knowledge deemed medically relevant), through (most common) loose web-based associations of parents where photographs of the children and other information were exchanged, to less frequent real-life contact, which mostly centered on only a few of the other families found who were deemed simpatico and easy to reach geographically.[20]

Hertz and Mattes conclude from combining their analysis of dominant themes in qualitative survey responses and the quantitatively assessed importance attached to the exchange of photographs that "…a kinship system built on the randomness of donor-shared siblings still means that blood carries significant meaning and genetics cannot be completely ignored. As the quotes indicate, physical resemblance and shared traits acted to further motivate one to pursue contact" (2011, 1152). The medium by which resemblance was explored through their respondents was photographs, provoking "raw emotion", feelings of connectedness to the other families and "moments of awe" (2011, 1139), which were quite similar to what Maria Lieb told me. While I find Hertz and Mattes' opening sentence above ambivalent (why, for instance, speak of the traditional kinship metaphor of "blood" in this context?), their findings on the centrality of photographs in the making of *wayward relations* resonates with my analysis of photographs as central kinship-objects (see previous section 7.1 and following section 8.6 on resemblance).

In another example of subversive knowledge-management, German DI family Schneider mainly discussed the potential *future* possibility of establishing *wayward relations*. Because they had conceived with the internationally operating sperm bank Scan-Sperm and had located their donor —in a subversive search endeavor—in both its German language and its US-American donor list (7.1), they had the option of registering with the DSR to look for donor-siblings. Father Marc Schneider was aware of the website's existence and expressed some interest in potentially us-

20 In their study covering several registries and particularly focusing on single-mothers-by-choice Hertz and Mattes (2011, 1139) for instance found that only 21.3 percent of the 289 families in their study who had actually located other donor-sibling-families had met those in person, while 74.9 percent had exchanged e-mails, 63.9 percent had exchanged photos of the children, and 20.7 percent had talked to each other on the phone. Freeman et al. also point out that real-life contact with donor-siblings and the—considerably less frequent—contact with donors was far more often pursued through single-mothers and lesbian couples than through heterosexual couples (2009, 510). The thereby ensuing relationships were framed as figuring somewhere between kin and friendship (2009, 512).

ing it in the future. He said that he had checked the DSR unsuccessfully a few years earlier trying to find information on their donor. After that, he had not explored the option further. His wife Nadine Schneider said to me that she found the thought of donor-sibling networking "a little strange, because actually one is not really related if one thinks about it". Both she and her husband agreed during the interview that they would probably settle on letting their son decide whether he wanted to establish *wayward relations* in the future. This attitude was typical for most of my parental research partners. Moreover, the Schneiders told me of a DI family they were friends with who had used the DSR, similar to the practices described through Hertz and Mattes (2011), and exchanged photographs. The other family had apparently found striking resemblances between the children, because they all seemed to "take after the donor" (Nadine). Still, the Schneiders found the idea of "having to meet just because of that" (Marc) "simply all a little abstruse" (Nadine)—dismissing the idea that physical resemblance could lead to building *wayward relations* (as discussed above concerning Maria Lieb's experiences).

Concerning the donor, the Schneiders expressed ideas about potential for future subversive searches without the use of the DSR. Lawmakers in Denmark, the home of their sperm bank Scan-Sperm, have not required that sperm donors be identifiable. Using Scan-Sperm at the time for the Schneiders thus meant that the procedure was fully anonymous, as much as it would have been *de facto* anonymous under German regulations back then as well. The clinic had in fact informed them that they had destroyed all identifying records on the donor, though Marc Schneider doubted that this was the case: "They say they have destroyed his 'real' data because he is not in the active donor stock anymore, but we doubt that they've really done that". Not long after the Schneiders used Scan-Sperm, new German regulations introducing a fragile non-anonymity (GewebeG, 2007) left the Schneiders in an ambiguous position. They had chosen Scan-Sperm for their comprehensive donor-information (see 7.1), to then realize that this meant they had cut-off their son from ever legally seeking the donor in real-life. Marc Schneider said that they had stored the donor's profile electronically and as a paper file, so their son could later look at it (also see the brief discussion on kinship-archives in section 7.3). Marc Schneider added that he doubted the security of the donor's anonymity, should their son ever be earnestly interested in tracking him down:

Marc Schneider: "So I think, to trace someone nowadays would not be so hard; there was some information in the profile, for instance… he [the donor] put down what he studies and when he will finish. So, what I am saying is (laughs), I think we actually have enough information to potentially find him."
Maren Klotz (joking tone): "Denmark is not so big after all."
Nadine Schneider (laughing): "Not at all, exactly. And how many universities do they have where you can study medicine?"
Marc Schneider: "It will come down to a fairly small group of people, should our son ever go after him."

To two British donor-conceived adults whom I have interviewed, donor-sibling contact and potential contact to the donor were both highly important. Bonnie Smith, the woman who had stumbled onto her father's family photographs in 7.1, had found a donor-brother via the DNA analysis administered through UKDL. She was eager to point out that the "match" with her donor-brother was a "good" one:

Bonnie Smith: "Donorlink, they say you're so many times more likely to be related than not, and it can be that you're a hundred times more likely to be related than not, or something like that… In our case they said we're nine million times more likely to be related than not."

Smith is an only child, she was twenty-six at the time of the interview and happily raising her then one and a half year old son in a partnership. The relationship to both her parents was described as close, although she was angry about having to find out about the donor-conception herself. Bonnie said that despite the discovery of her DI conception "My dad will always be my dad."

After receiving the call from UKDL about the sibling match and the question whether she still wanted her contact details to be released, she first started exchanging e-mails with her donor-brother. In fact, feeling shy about how this encounter would unfold, she had asked UKDL to only forward her e-mail address to him and declined to speak to him on the phone (as he would have liked from the start) for a couple of months:

Bonnie Smith: "It was just because speaking on the phone to someone you don't know very well is quite difficult. Actually, I think I would have been less nervous about a face-to-face meeting. We waited a bit [but wrote back and forth]. And then we got drunk and then phoned (laughs)."

The two had known each other for about 18 months when I interviewed Bonnie. They were on the phone with each other frequently, about once a week as Bonnie told me, and were also eagerly writing messages online. However, they had only met in person once in the previous year. Bonnie explained that, although only living a few hours apart by train, meeting up more often just seemed too difficult, with them both having very little money to spend, but also with both being quite reclusive. Nevertheless Bonnie referred to her donor-sibling with strong affection, calling him her "brother" throughout our interview and repeatedly referring to conversations the two had had about donor conception or what her brother's likely opinion on some of the issues we discussed would be.

When I asked how meeting face-to-face with him had been, she reflected:

Bonnie Smith: "Obviously, I was a bit nervous. He looks like me, which is very surreal… And, as the day went I kind of recognized some of my facial expressions in him. And that was very weird. It was a unique situation, obviously. You know, you're there thinking: Oh, I want this to go well, I hope he likes me… But then also feeling weird, feeling like we're going to be sort of connected now forever anyway. That's the thing: he is always worrying 'you're gonna get fed up with me' […]. I'm always going: 'No, I'm not gonna get fed up with you. You know, we're connected, that connection is never going to go anywhere!' I kept saying to him: 'Unless you're about to confess that you're a serial killer, we're pretty good!'"

Bonnie clearly referred to her donor sibling as close kin, recognizing resemblance and connectedness. However, their relationship was also new and "weird" and hardly based on face-to-face contact or any interaction with the other's family and friends.

At the time of my fieldwork the donor-siblings were scheming about further subversive searches, making use of other online networking services than UKDL. Finding donor-siblings or potentially the donor himself was not important to them due to medical considerations (see the more detailed discussion 8.2 on medical history). Smith rather described that for her it was important to find out how the donor "was like as a person"—and that her brother was more interested in other donor-siblings than the donor. However, she did not dwell much on what the reasons for their searches were, presenting them as self-evident. Smith talked about their plans for further searches and how this might involve acquiring their donor's clinic ID, his "nickname", from old patient records:

Bonnie Smith: "Somebody that I met online who was conceived there [a particular clinic] approached them and got quite a lot of information from them, including his donor's nickname. What this person is going to do is post this online. Chances are, you're going to find somebody who will go, ooh, my donor is known as that as well. [...] Basically it's chasing these hints up. There might not be any records though. And they're not obligated to give them to us; it's a bit rubbish. But I think only when we've exhausted every possible avenue... Only then will we let it go. Because you've got to do everything you can, to try and find out what you can. That's how we both feel. That we won't rest until we've done everything and then at the end if we've still got nothing, at least we tried."

The second British donor-conceived adult I interviewed was thirty-year-old Lydia Rivers, who had also registered with UKDL. I was among the first persons to be told about her donor-conception and during our interview she often appeared to be very upset, sometimes crying. The interview with her was very complex in the way she was conveying her story and at the same time reflecting upon it: moving back and forth between different positions to take on what had happened to her. At age 27 she had found out from her mother about her donor-conception when her younger brother had joined the Army and was preparing to be sent abroad. In a mixture of raw emotion about his life being in danger and a worry concerning DNA analysis in the potential event of his death, their mother had told the two siblings about their donor-conception. The mother was unsupportive of Rivers' searches for half-siblings, as mentioned above, expressing a lack of understanding why her daughter was pursuing them. Apparently, apart from the siblings, not only all maternal and paternal relatives—including cousins—but also all other close friends and neighbors had known about them being donor-conceived, but never told them. Rivers described this as extremely hurtful and presented her family history as marked by a break-down of relationships: a fierce parental divorce, a strained relationship with her mother and her brother, a renouncement of any relationship to her father long before she learned about her donor-conception, and a somewhat unstable relationship with her partner and father of her two children.

At the time of my fieldwork Rivers had not heard back from UKDL on a potential match. When I asked her what her hopes were should UKDL inform her about a donor-sibling she told me:

Lydia Rivers: "I would hope that I would be matched to someone who wanted the same thing, which would be… -to be siblings. It would be strange, because you are adults and you have not grown up together and you really have not a lot in common other than the fact that you are half-brother or -sister. I would want to have a sibling bond with them. Spend a holiday or anything like that (laughs). To actually spend time getting to know them. They would probably have children of their own as well, which would mean my children would have cousins. And I would want to, once I got [to] know that person, introduce them to my children as their aunt, or as their uncle. Not just as a friend of mine… -because that's what they would be."

A potential scenario, which scared Lydia as she made clear in the interview, was that a prospective donor-sibling would have other ideas about how their relationship could look. She told me that another UKDL member she had spoken to was very distraught, because her donor-sibling wanted no face-to-face contact, just the swap of a few photographs to compare possible resemblance. Lydia appeared to be troubled by the possibility of this happening to her as well. She had also spoken to a former donor at a UKDL meeting in London, who expressed uncertainty about actually wanting to meet with potential offspring. This she found "shocking" and generally incomprehensible why anyone would join UKDL without being certain about wanting to establish closer relationships to anyone located via the register.

Concerning her donor, Lydia believed it was extremely unlikely she would ever find him through the contact registry, comparing it to playing the "lottery". She was quite self-reflexive in describing how "the idea [of the donor] I have in my head is a really romantic conception of fatherhood, because I want him to be everything that I haven't got". She also expressed that she wondered if he really was a medical doctor, like they had told her mother at the clinic. Lydia was the first of her family to obtain a university degree and described to me how she, with her intellectual abilities, had always stood out in the family—making her wonder if the donor-conception might be the reason for this. After sharing these reflections she, however, followed by saying that she did not straightforwardly believe in intelligence being hereditary. Maybe only some aspects were, she concluded in our interview. Lydia expressed a worry about UKDL potentially closing because of lack of funding and was anxiously waiting to hear back from them.

Interpretive Discussion

Having examined the infrastructures and networking endeavors that make subversive practices possible and after exploring examples of subversive knowledge-management in my fieldwork materials, especially the experiences of Maria Lieb, the Schneiders, Bonnie Smith and Lydia Rivers, I call the thereby arising or envisioned relationships *wayward relations*. Unprecedented and lacking associated established social roles, these relations are wayward in their often officially unintended character and circumvention of past or present national regulation. *Wayward relations*, just like *administered relations* in 7.1, again hold a relational character: they are a way-of-knowing and thereby connecting to others and to oneself. Parents explored their own interests and role, asking questions of what connected donor-siblings and if such a connection would be meaningful for them as parents. More importantly, adult donor-conceived persons made themselves into experts in genetic testing technologies, got to know themselves as holders of specific genetic sequences (I even came across donor-conceived individuals exchanging their haplotypes and -groups via internet forums), and discovered themselves in the face of their donor-siblings.

In the different cases, literature, and infrastructures discussed, three seemingly typical aspects of *wayward relations* play out in differing constellations and balances. First is what has been called the "imperative to connect" (e.g. Edwards, 2009a; Knecht, 2009), an emergent cultural pattern where making connections becomes a moral good in itself. Second is the complementary and often latent character of *wayward relations*. By this I mean that actors are turning towards the newly sought genetic connections to complement other relationships, which were for instance experienced as unreliable. And thirdly, we see the tendency towards a "diminishing domain of privacy, anonymity and ability to remain silent (unknown)" (Edwards, when discussing the wider implications of the research activities she witnessed in ancestry research, 2009a, 9).

Knecht (2009b) and Edwards (2009a)—and also see Strathern (2005, 11)—conceptualize the imperative to connect as a wider cultural pattern at work also within contemporary kinship phenomena. Edwards for example ethnographically describes the growing interest in "family treeing", i.e. ancestry research, in the north of England, which "marries, amongst other things, the technological and the mystical, empirical research and imagination, kinship and class, thus connecting facets of human being that are often, in analysis, kept apart" (2009, 18). Drawing on Green et al.'s (2005) research[21] on information technologies and place-making and extending it to kinship studies, Edwards interprets her informants' detective work to unearth past genealogical connections and their strong reliance on IT infrastructures as part of a wider social imperative to connect: where *making connections* becomes a joy and celebration of the serendipitous moment.

Knecht (2009b) arrives at similar conclusions when observing activities of "transfamilial networking" between adoptees, donor-siblings, interest groups, experts and genealogists within communities of families-by-donation or adoption. She sees the imperative to connect implicated within the theme of fragmentation experienced by families where conception and parental roles have been distributed in non-traditional ways; it is a mode of *re-embedding* relationships and roles in newly defined family realms. Edwards suspects that the contemporary currency of the imperative to connect is both "inflected by a post-industrial landscape and recent experiences of social and economic upheaval" and "exercising some of the emotional capacities that would otherwise be exercised by organized religion" (2009a, 17). Both Knecht's and Edwards' assertions show the imperative to connect not only as a newly emerging pastime and celebration of connections, but just as much as a form of counter-movement to late-modern experiences of fragmentation.

21 Green et al. have originally analyzed various projects of so-called Europeanization via the information-technological "connecting-up" of institutions, where making connections started to appear as a moral, social, and economic goal in itself and could be seen as at odds with other notions of place-making. They for instance describe that "tensions were often expressed between an imperative to connect that required the objects connected to be made compatible with one another by placing them on an abstracted technical scale (i.e. through removing the contexts that made them incompatible) and the responsibility to ensure that the interconnections resulted in the production of particular kinds of places—an integrated Europe, a socially responsible city, a competitive region" (2005, 810).

Within donor-conceived Bonnie Smith's assertions of how she wanted to "try everything" to find the donor and her presentation of the rationales for establishing *wayward relations* as seemingly self-evident, the notion of the imperative to connect seemed to resonate. It similarly seemed to resonate in the searches motivated by "curiosity" as done by Maria Lieb and the Schneiders, and discussed in the literature as the main reason for the enormous success of the Donor Sibling Registry. However, especially in the ways the two donor-conceived women talked about their subversive practices of knowledge-management and real-life and imagined *wayward relations*, the motivations of both connection and curiosity were joined by conflicts over information-sharing, relationships perceived to be unsatisfactory, and by a sense of lost agency. In the two cases the notion of the imperative to connect as a counter-movement to fragmentation, not as celebration, seems to be implicated, along with Carsten's (2000, 2007) notion of reclaiming agency over one's past by acquiring kinship knowledge, as discussed in section 2.2. In her work on adoptee reunions with so-called birth kin Carsten argues that one would starkly simplify these activities if conceptualized as first and foremost a sign of *geneticization*. Instead, these searches for kin should be understood as pointing to the contemporary "importance of establishing continuities […] between past, present, and future" (Carsten 2000, 689). In my fieldwork materials, genomic sequences (not blood as proclaimed by Hertz and Mattes above) are part of establishing such continuities. I would argue that the actors thereby assert agency not only over their past, but also in the actively and creatively performed searches themselves—through their crafty mastership of genetic knowledge and information technologies and generally through becoming active performers of searches rather than just passive subjects of official regimes of knowledge-management.

For donor-conceived adult Rivers, for example, who found herself surrounded by failed relationships, there was comfort that DNA (analysis) offered a new register of tracing relationships: procreative ones in the past and newly to be established siblingship in the future. Contacting UKDL (and looking at websites set up by other donor-conceived adults) she described as a first step in coming to terms with the late revelation of her donor conception. She expressed a hope and desire that maybe those new relationships would be more durable, even though she acknowledged that they would not "just" come into being through discovery, but would then also need a temporal and personal investment. However, what would actually happen once a connection via DNA was established still proved to be uncertain, as she worriedly pointed out by referring to all those UKDL members who apparently were leaning more towards using the register to establish "latent ties" (Hertz and Mattes 2011, 1141), as apparently common for *wayward relations* if one follows Hertz and Mattes. In this context Carsten reminds us of the always fragile complementarity of *wayward relations*, because the coming together of one's biological kin unaccompanied by the "flow of time that is central to the experience of kinship (…) can only partially reconnect the past with the present and the future" (2000, 700).

Wayward relations are hence an example of using the "constitutivity" of genetically substantiated kinship-knowledge in a complementary fashion, not a colonization of relationships through genetics. In her insightful review of the scholarly discussions surrounding the idea of *geneticization* as, essentially, a determinist threat to social life as first introduced by Abby Lippman (1992), Mamo argues:

> "geneticization fails to recognize the dense networks of agency and constraint on both sides of the lay/practitioner divide which constitute newly emerging arenas of medical, technoscientific practices of genetic knowledges. Feminist scholars enter here with the assertion that patients (users) respond to developments in genetics and other new health technologies and knowledge in ways that (can) challenge the strong deterministic thesis implied by a notion of geneticisation." (Mamo 2005, 239)

The *wayward relations* that my research partners were working on seem to re-affirm the traditional notion that genetics can establish relationships, but within their complementarity, creativity, asserted agency, and unprecedented implication of technologies they add what Edwards (when analyzing recent ancestry research) has called an "early 21st century complexion" to the old project of validating Western kinship (knowledge) by looking to biology (2009a, 5).

Part of the proclaimed 21st century complexion of *wayward relations* was evidently afforded through their strong implication with information technologies and DNA analyses. These phenomena make it increasingly difficult for a corporation or regulatory regime, to contain knowledge on biological reproduction, making anonymity harder or nearly impossible to maintain in the realm of gamete donation. The internet and its defining capacity to network huge numbers of people, with large amounts of data, and bridging vast physical distances provides the crucial infrastructure and is therefore not an underlying "structure" or "channel" for *wayward relations*, but co-constitutive of subversive practices of knowledge-management. For some of those *wayward relations* which were not or hardly based on face-to-face contact or only a future "back-up", for instance, it was the specific capacity of online relationships not only to enable contact over physical distances but, more importantly, to remain latent and then be re-activated after longer periods of time without this being viewed as socially inappropriate.

It was striking how self-evidently the participants in my fieldwork, including myself, yielded to search-engine logics. Finding the donor's "nickname" would already give one enough information for posting and googling and a few million male Danes could be light-heartedly envisaged being scanned in the search for one specific donor. Furthermore, the availability of commercial genetic genealogy services on the internet and the growing associated databases (FamilyTreeDNA currently stores test results of almost half a million individuals) are displacing state monopolies on kinship information contained in official records and registries, as discernible in the German example. Ultimately, these developments show what I have called the *informational* uncontainability of kinship(-knowledge) (Klotz 2012).[22] This development holds unexplored implications for the national regulation of donor-anonymity and questions of data protection, and seems to be the seldom-considered socio-material undercurrent to worldwide diminishing regimes of donor-anonymity. As Edwards points out above, the astonishing potency of subversive searches for kinship knowledge, be it for kinship-by-donation or adoption or general ancestry research, have a slightly uncanny side, not because such practices colonizingly *geneticise*, but because they (might) colonizingly connect.

22 I am not arguing that kinship or kinship-by-donation *in general*—whatever this might be—has evolved from something contained to something uncontainable within the Industrial West. Rather, I am specifically referring to kinship knowledge, in this case in the shape of DNA "information", and its official regulation.

8. Familial Knowledge-Management: Confrontations and Tactics

Gamete donation is not what makes our family. Usually towards the end of our long interview sessions my interview partners felt it important to stress this point. Family life to them was predominantly about daily care practices, not about being a family-by-donation, as it could appear in an interview situation. British father Tim Hampton's statement below was typical in underlining how everyday chores and worries figured in the forefront of family life, and not the details of assisted conception, which I kept asking about:

Tim Hampton: "Most of the time I am waking up thinking I didn't get much sleep last night. Hell, how am I gonna get through the day without making a big mistake at work and, and be able to end work so I could come home and read the kids their bedtime stories. That's what I am spending most of the time thinking about (laughing). It's certainly not: Oh it worries me, the donor sperm (laughing)."

These narratives about bedtime stories, childhood diseases and—a recurring theme—lack of sleep, I took as a prompt to switch to a specific part of my interview manual. I acknowledged and summarized the descriptions of how DI did *not* matter that much, to then ask about outside prompts, which made them think of being a family-by-donation again. In this chapter I not only discuss and analyze these various confrontations, but also which typical knowledge tactics the families developed in response. (The term confrontation I use only in the sense of prompting thoughts of the donation, not as connoting a negative experience). Thus, in contrast to the more long-term and strategic practices analyzed in other sections, this chapter foregrounds tactics of kinship knowledge-management developed by the family as reactions to everyday life confrontations invoked by others: friends, neighbors, or the pediatrician. It is thus also an attempt to again reconstruct past situations from a cautiously realist perspective.

I shall start the chapter with comprehensively discussing the most common everyday confrontation by far to do with being a family-by-donation: talk about physical resemblance (section 8.1). I explore how families chose two different tactics in response to such confrontations, "play along", i.e. non-disclosing resemblance-talk, or disclosure. I note how resemblance for my interviewees was predominantly positively recognized through others even in the absence of genetic relatedness. In contrast to other research within kinship studies, where resemblance-talk was experienced as an extremely negative confrontation (Becker et al. 2005), my interviewees approached the subject creatively and reflexively and did not report negative situations: they tactically played along with it instead and began to interrogate it as a cultural script, rather than a question of straightforward perception and cognition. I argue that resemblance-talk figures as a ritualized practice to welcome a new family member. It focuses on physical bodies and rests within the confines of hereditary thinking, finding its limits through "race", while simultaneously undermining it through its flexibility.

The following subchapters contain briefer discussions. Medical history (discussed in 8.2) is identified as the second most common confrontation. I note here that for most of my interviewees the absence of parts of a medical history for themselves or, more often, their donor-conceived children, was not discussed as inherently problematic. Neither a tendency towards genetic self-management (e.g. Novas and Rose 2000) nor extreme unsettledness about not being able to answer medical history questions (e.g. Finkler 2001) was discernible.

Some of my interviewees also reported additional confrontations, which are taken up as more limited case-discussions. Section 8.3 focuses on confrontations through exclusive or geneticized kinship terminologies, such as references to the donor as "the *real* father". Section 8.4 discusses confrontations with which those families not conforming to the "reproductive norm" (i.e. homosexual families, single mother families, or families where the mother was visibly post-menopausal) were confronted. Section 8.5 focuses on the conflation between infertility and impotence and the assumption that biological reproduction is the ultimate fulfillment of heterosexual relationships. The last section (8.6) analyzes what happens when the child starts talking about the donation and thereby intervenes in parental knowledge-management.

A theme introduced in the first section and followed through all successive subchapters is how through dealing with the confrontations my parental interviewees make themselves into what I call *reflexive kinship experts*. The confrontations lead parents to explicitly debate otherwise taken for granted aspects of kinship, such as resemblance between parents and children because of heredity, or that everyday culture is infused with references to joint reproduction. Parents instead began to point to the often flexible and ritualized dimensions of such assumptions. They developed their own theories of where these flexible and ritualized dimensions stemmed from, mostly stressing the "stubbornness" of mundane everyday life practices.

8.1 Resemblance-Talk: "The old folks would always say 'Just like Daddy', no matter how the child looks like"

Every family I engaged with during my research acknowledged that it was what Becker et al. have called resemblance-talk—"comments and queries about a child's physical resemblance to parents and other family members" (2005, 1301)—which presented the most pervasive confrontation with the donation. British mother Sarah Hampton, for instance, told me that it was resemblance "more than anything" which situationally brought DI to the forefront again for their family. Or German father Uli Linde-Feldman summarized: "A really central theme is the whole resemblance story, the 'he-looks-so-much-like-you'—story". In this chapter I firstly sketch out aspects of the discussions of resemblance-talk in the anthropological literature. I then turn to discussing how resemblance-recognition is part of relational processes of individuation, to then turn to a longer analysis of the flexibility of resemblance-talk as experienced through my research partners. Subsequently the parental tactics of knowledge-management in reaction to resemblance-talk are analyzed. I close with a brief analysis of the *limits* of resemblance.

Becker et al. have described resemblance-talk as highly problematic for families-by-donation. According to the authors it underlines the families' deviant status in the face of a norm of biological relatedness and heightens concerns about potential problems arising from an open acknowledgment of the donor treatment. They argue:

> "discourse on resemblance reinforces the assumed natural order of things and supports a hierarchy of legitimacy, in which a clear physical resemblance to family members confers greater legitimacy, while the legitimacy of those who lack a resemblance to the family is questioned, subjecting them to stigma." (Becker et al. 2005, 1301)

Interestingly, while my study also points to the centrality of resemblance-talk, echoing Becker et al.'s description of its experience as absolutely central for families-by-donation, my interview partners expressed far less critique about or concern with it. (In fact, the Feldmans were the only family that described resemblance-talk as making them feel uncomfortable, as further discussed below). Becker et al. stress how, for their interview-partners, it "exacerbated ongoing concerns about how best to control the information that a donor had been used, e.g. uncertainty about their disclosure decision (or lack of one)" and for some it prompted "a recurrent sense of loss as resemblance-talk reminded them of their infertility and the missing genetic link to their children and other family members" (Becker et al. 2005, 1302–1303). Aside from their larger sample size and the US-American focus of Becker et al., there are similarities between the research: for instance, participation in the American study was also predominantly self-selective, parents-by-donation were interviewed recurrently and questions on resemblance not prompted, but only followed up if raised by interviewees. However, while my research partners also underlined that resemblance-talk was indeed the most common confrontation to do with being a family-by-donation and therefore required reactive tactics of knowledge-management—this experience was typically *not* addressed as problematic. It was rather registered with interest and reflexively interpreted.

German father Philip Steger, for instance, raised his conviction with me that resemblance-talk was just a convention, not really tied up with the recognition of physical shapes:

Philip Steger: "Well, the old folks in the village in Allenfels, they'll go 'Oh, just like Daddy', no matter what. That's normal. It does not play any role how the child looks like. They would always say that."

Mother Dörte Tönsch—with her children not physically matched to Brazilian father Miguel—communicated her astonishment at a situation where she took resemblance-talk as a prompt to tell about the donation, only to find it had been forgotten a week later:

Dörte Tönsch: "Yes, of course sometimes people ask questions… The other day at the pediatrician, the assistant goes: 'But your husband is a classical South-American, with black hair and dark eyes?' And I said: 'Yes, but I already told you last week, when you asked me the same thing: the child has been conceived through donor sperm'. And she goes: 'Oh yeah, right, I forgot.' I mean, that's astonishing, you would think when you tell folks something like that, they would probably remember, because it probably does not happen so often. But I guess it is actually not that uncommon anymore, in society. That people actually treat it fairly normal, but the questions "Wouldn't the child have to look Brazilian now", those will also remain. On the other hand, my boss, when he saw Alvaro for the first time, he said he had a Brazilian nose [all laugh]."

Anthropologists Marre and Bestard, discussing transnational adoption, have argued that "resemblance expresses continuity between individuals and is a good starting point for reflecting on how the constitution of a person through kinship is not limited to isolated individuals, but refers to people that relate to one another" (2009, 64). In this vein, I interpret resemblance-talk as it presents itself in my fieldwork materials not as an unambiguous confrontation with a norm of biological relatedness where there is an "underlying message" to be deciphered that "a genetic connection is vital" (Becker et al. 2005, 1308). Nor do I interpret it as the straightforward cognitive recognition of similar physiological shapes. I will rather treat it as touching upon the characteristic kinship tension of corporeal continuity as described and discussed in Chapter 4 and as a situational practice through which to relate to new persons—children—in specific ways. Resemblance-talk is to be seen as an interplay between the recognition of different physiologies and a pervasive cultural script for the interactive "placing [of] the new [child's] body into the group of the family body and constructing the new individual body as a family member" (Marre and Bestard 2009, 65).[1] What seems central to me is that through the experience of reflecting far more on what resemblance-talk might actually "mean" compared to families where resemblance could always unquestioningly be attributed to connected biologies, families-by-donation have become what I call *reflexive kinship experts*, who recognize both the highly complex variants of *corporeal continuity* (see Chapter 4) and the scriptedness of resemblance-talk.

Resemblance as Relation and Individuation

Marre and Bestard (2009, 66) have commented that, paradoxically, resemblance-talk is both about the relational placement in a literal and metaphorical family body and about individuation. Interviewee Philip Steger touched upon this tension when he reflected about resemblance from a broader perspective:

Philip Steger: "I really don't care. The child is like it is, and who it looks like is essentially of no concern. That has never been important to me and I also noticed in the past how I… I did not hate it, but always found it totally silly, when someone said to me: 'Ah, here's little Helmut!' Well, that's because my father is called Helmut. That's when I said: I am Philip and not Helmut (laughs)."

Thus, the scene recounts how Philip Steger symbolically becomes the individual Philip in relation to his father Helmut. Steger himself denounces the relationality potentially arising from resemblance (thereby symbolically negating a connection to the donor) and stresses individuality instead: the child is like it is.

However, other parents struggled with recognizing individuality in the absence of a clear impression of the donor's physiognomy. The Feldmans and Maria Lieb, for instance, experienced the assumed resemblance between their children and the donor as an *additional* confrontation (additional to the resemblance-talk employed by others) through their *own* perceptions.

Berit Feldman: "When Moritz started to slowly develop his facial features, that was sometimes… That you sometimes had the feeling, and I've heard that from

1 Also see Bestard (2009, 19) as cited in chapter 2.3.

other DI parents as well: who is looking at me there? There is a third unknown person looking at me through him."

And Maria Lieb reflected on occasionally wondering about the sperm donor's appearance when looking at her daughter:

Maria Lieb: Sometimes, when I don't really know… -You see, sometimes children's faces change considerably. Then I've had that, that I thought, I wonder how he looks like. Sometimes I find she looks more like my family, but then some things are really unfamiliar…"

Both mothers recognized the physical changes their children were going through and experienced this as a—literally—strange process, because the physiological changes were not placed in a relational network of "known bodies". As discernible in many more instances of my fieldwork materials, individuality of the children was sometimes not easy to ascribe through the parents, because, as made visible through the analysis of resemblance-talk, it is conventionally recognized within a relational matrix that is partly "hidden" during gamete donation. In other words, I am arguing that Western individuality becomes recognized and enacted in a matrix of relationships. These relationships are partly recognized as a connection between bodies that are supposed to resemble each other. Since a connection to the donor was assumed, but the parents did not know what he or she actually looked like, this occasionally produced effects of the uncanny. This is pointedly captured in Berit Feldman's statement above that someone else was looking at her through her son.

Flexible Resemblance-Talk

Families recounted how typically situations of resemblance-talk took the form of a positive recognition through others, rather than a negative calling into question of resemblance. Uli Linde-Feldman, for example, told me how his colleague commented that he really "could not deny this child" when first seeing a photograph of his son. Through mentioning that resemblance-talk made them think of the donation, the parents acknowledged that they connected likeness to heredity. The continued experience of *positive* resemblance-talk, however, led them to actually reflexively de-construct this connection, as I will further discuss below. Tim Hampton fondly recalled his first experience with similarity recognition:

Tim Hampton: "We were sitting in, in this restaurant by the sea and he was in his pram as these two older ladies were sitting on the next table and they said: 'Oh isn't he lovely!' One said: 'Oh gosh, doesn't he look like his dad?' And, erm, I mean really, I felt really pleased, actually. It was the first time anybody said that."

All my interview partners were full of similar stories of a flexible tracing of physical resemblance. On a personal level, I found the narrative reconstructions of such instances through the Tönschs most striking, because I had earlier perceived a noticeable non-resemblance between son Alvaro and his father Miguel when meeting them for the first time.

"After we had introduced ourselves, we all played a bit with the child. I immediately noticed that it obviously had not been 'matched' with Miguel's dark appearances: a blond and blue-eyed child. Their, most of all his, reasons for this lacking phenotypical matching are, so Miguel told me in the interview later, rooted in their personal politics: if one decides to go for sperm donation, one should not hide this through an 'as if' donor selection. I found this line of argument simpatico and sensible. However the mixture of Alvaro's explicitly Brazilian name and his, to me, explicitly 'non-Brazilian'[2] appearance also strangely touched me as establishing facts for Alvaro: he will always have to explain why that's the case, at least that's what came to my mind." (Fieldnotes Maren Klotz)

The Tönschs, in contrast to what the ethnographer noted in her diary, were always full of accounts how much Miguel and Alvaro—and subsequently also new baby sister Helene—looked alike to others. It was not only the "Brazilian nose" already quoted above, but also how Helene had "exactly the father's eyes", for instance, or how the "neighbor said, she looked Alvaro in the eyes once, and she knew this was our child. Even though his eyes are so blue..." (Dörte Tönsch).

2 I am aware that Brazilians come in all shapes and sizes. I am invoking this diary passage here for autoethnographic purposes to evoke my own immediate sense of resemblance and non-resemblance and the categories that then came to mind, regardless of their sensibility under more careful analysis.

Tactics of Knowledge-Management

Nevertheless, even though positive acknowledgements of resemblance prevailed, the families I spoke to all felt like they had to develop reactions to resemblance-talk: tactics of knowledge-management, of finding the right balance between non-disclosure and disclosure in order to ensure a comfortable running of daily life (for a more general discussion of this concerning assisted conception see Knecht et al. 2011). What seemed typical was that such tactics needed to be developed over time: while at first resemblance-talk was commonly used as a prompt to tell others about the donation or produced situations of uncertainty whether to do so or not, its continued flexible experience led parents more often to engage in what I started to call *"play along" resemblance-talk*: parents join the talk about physical characteristics without disclosing the donor treatment.

Sarah Hampton, for example, recounted how she slowly got used to resemblance-talk: how it was "really weird in the beginning", e.g. when people talked about the (in comparison to her blue and Tim's light brown eyes) strikingly dark eyes of her children. And how she grew "much more comfortable with that" and would use resemblance-talk as a prompt to disclose more seldom:

> Sarah Hampton: "People go: 'Oh haven't they got beautiful eyes' and, and I kind of got used to saying: Yes, aren't they lovely (laughs)."

Becker et al. have described for their study that parents developed "a variety of creative strategies for managing resemblance-talk [...] including plausibility arguments, passing, and strategic silence" (2005, 1307). On the level of the practices involved in what I called "play along" resemblance-talk, my research partners probably engaged in similar behavior as denoted by Becker et al. However, I chose to call the tactic of not disclosing the donation (as apparent in the quote above) "play along" resemblance-talk instead of passing, because I did not want to suggest that my research partners were trying to pass for anything when not disclosing the donation during resemblance-talk. Instead, the tactic of *playing along* could also be described as the reflexive recognition of resemblance-talk as a pervasive cultural script for performatively welcoming and placing a child within a family. Parents quite light-heartedly experimented with this cultural script. Melanie Steger for instance told me:

Melanie Steger: "A lot of people say, because our daughter has got these extremely blue eyes, they go: Wow, she has really blue eyes, from whom did she get those? And I always think: I know from whom (laughing). Then I always say: She's got those from me. Because I also have a slight blue touch to my eyes. Then I always say: She's got those from me."

Both Sarah Hampton's and Melanie Steger's laughter seems to underline a playful sense of satisfaction with their chosen tactic and a light-hearted joy of being able to sometimes knowingly withhold information on the donation—and thereby also regaining some control over the situation. The Tönschs told me that if they were not in the mood to talk about the donation "because people inevitably have further questions then and you don't want to chat about that with just anyone" (Dörte Tönsch) they simply made remarks that the kids seemed to be "taking after" Dörte and left it at that. They have also had the recurring experience that using resemblance-talk as a cue for disclosure did not lead to negative reactions:

Dörte Tönsch: "Its like you [to Miguel] said, it is not that people are taken aback. But they then think: 'Okay, fine, nowadays one probably should not expect that things are just like they always were in the past'. I mean, if I walk through Eschenkrug [a quarter of Großstadt with an extremely high birth rate among women well in their thirties] and see how many folks are pushing twin-prams, you also notice… I don't ask anymore, but if someone wants to tell me, that's fine…"

Resemblance-talk thus seemed to encourage flexible views on *what makes a family* on the side of the people the Tönschs told, instead of exacerbating concerns about heredity for the Tönschs as a family.

Deciding on the "Right" Tactic

In the on-the-spot decision making process whether to just engage in "play along" resemblance-talk or actually talk about the donation, whether the persons starting the resemblance-talk had much continuous contact with the children played the decisive role. Holly Greenwood, typical for such accounts in my fieldwork materials, explained that she was using resemblance-talk as a prompt to tell acquaintances about the donation when she felt like "they should know the truth", because of the amount of contact with her daughter:

Holly Greenwood: "For instance my neighbor from across the street, she has a daughter who is three weeks younger than my daughter. They will probably grow up together, so I used it [what she earlier called "resemblance-chat"] and told her, because I am also telling my daughter."
Maren Klotz: "And what did your neighbor say then?"
Holly Greenwood: "She thought it was interesting and asked a few questions [about donor anonymity], but actually I would not even care if people had a problem with the donation. I think it was the right decision and she is a much wanted, a loved child…"

The tactic of telling those who have much contact with the child or the children ties in with my discussion of the process of disclosure becoming a process of knowledge-management going far beyond the nuclear family (see chapter 7). Holly Greenwood's specific phrasing that people should know "the truth" also resonates with the casting of secrecy as a threat to personal relationships as analyzed in chapter 6.

The Feldmans were the only family outspokenly ambivalent about resemblance-talk. Uli Linde-Feldman described how for him, feelings of insecurity and a subjective pressure to tell prevailed when people commented on an apparent resemblance between him and his son:

Uli Linde-Feldman: "People always think: Ah, I bet that really makes you feel good. But the opposite is the case. Many folks think that's positive. That's where I say: no, it's really stupid, because it makes me feel really strange. It makes me feel like I have to tell anyone who does it."

The Feldmans did not seem to perceive resemblance with the same playfulness as most others of my interview partners. Uli Linde-Feldman was not, like Tim Hampton for instance, pleased about resemblance-talk involving him and his children. Instead he felt like he had just at the time of our first interview slowly come to terms with it. He mused that he, having studied psychology, maybe addressed and worked through issues making him feel uncomfortable more consciously than others. In the interest group he attended with his wife, where most others did not raise such issues, he asked himself: "Am I the psychologist, who says: hey, don't fool yourselves… Or am I somehow different?" Even though Linde-Feldman told me that most difficulties with the confrontation through resemblance-talk were behind him, he still sometimes looked at those children in the neighborhood who strongly resembled their parents with sadness. He said to me that one boy in particular looked like "his father in a miniature version" and that this made him reflect that "it is probably really nice, to see yourself walking around like that". In doing so, he expressed a desire for what I have come to call corporeal continuity. Although he also wondered about the nature of resemblance-talk (more below), he was less enthusiastic in stressing its flexibility. He attributed the pervasiveness of positive recognitions of similarities between him and his children more to "the doctors having done a good job", in the sense of actually *physically making* resemblance in the clinic.

The practice of clinical physical matching was not questioned through any other family than the German-Brazilian couple Tönsch. Most other participants viewed it as a knowledge-management tactic in itself, shielding them from an obvious "visibility" of the donation. Holly Greenwood, for instance, in retrospect, narrated the birth of her daughter like the positive confirmation of a knowledge-management tactic, taking its beginning with the matching process in the clinic. She explained to me that she and her husband chose a donor for his physical similarity to her spouse:

> Holly Greenwood: "And it worked out so well! Directly after giving birth, when the midwife saw Teresa she immediately said: 'She looks just like Daddy!' (…) When she was an infant, most people said that she looks like her father. One really does not notice at all, one would never think that she is not our biological daughter. The clinic really did a good job [with regard to the "matching"]."
> Maren Klotz: "And your husband? Was he pleased by this?"
> Holly Greenwood: "Yes of course! Yes, yes. Now people notice that she looks quite similar to me, but when she was really small, really the majority of people said that she looks like her father."

Consequently, I would like to add that reactions to confrontations through resemblance-talk for my research partners did not only consist of "play along" resemblance-talk or openness, but also of a tactic set at an earlier point in time: the physical matching between parent and donor according to various articulations of physical characteristics (see 5.2 and 7.1).

However, both the "non-matched" Tönschs' pervasive experience of positive resemblance-talk and most of my interview partners' seemingly growing conviction that resemblance-talk was mainly a convention also point to something analytically notable: matching might be part of the parental knowledge-management tactics surrounding the donation, but positive resemblance-talk in my view is not simply a sign that the doctors have done "a good job" as noted by Uli Linde-Feldman above. To elaborate: my fieldwork materials oscillate between stories on the complete flexibility of resemblance and, in contrast, how it is objectively there and can be clinically produced. Trying to strike a balance between more materialist and more constructivist thrusts of interpretation, I argue that the pervasiveness of positive resemblance-talk shows how Europeans talk relatedness—thereby doing kinship—along physical bodies. In doing so, they ritually connect bodies of families or families of bodies. These bodies do take on certain appearances through hereditary processes (and a lot of other things). However, they also—exactly through these very same hereditary processes (and a lot of other things)—are unique. The practice of noting resemblance as a recognition of likeness within this unique outcome of procreation is partly so flexible because we are *never*, in contrast to Linde-Feldman's description of the neighbor's child, miniature versions (which, taken literally, would mean clones) of our genitor or genetrix. Unique bodies, as the outcome of the materialities of duo-genetic reproduction, leave room for interpretation. Physical resemblances between persons are thus clearly not unambiguous and their recognition is part of practices and "cultural perceptions of identity recognition" (Marre and Bestard 2009, 66), as shown in the ethnographic work on their local or cultural variation. Malinowski's descriptions of the "denial" of physical resemblance between maternal kin through the Trobriand Islanders is the most famous ethnographic example of the flexibility of resemblance recognition.[3] This flexibility underlines how kinship is about corporeal continuities between persons, but—as also discussed for habitualized mannerisms and language in chapter 4.1—it is not always about straightforward biological reproduction.

3 The denial of physical resemblance between siblings, Malinowski, in his notorious mix of *othering* and empathetic ethnographic description, describes as at first seeming "savage indeed, so lop-sided, distorted and quaint it does appear" (1957, 173) to then go on and describe in great detail the beliefs and practices around legitimate and illegitimate resemblance recognition for the Trobriands, making them seem not so "lop-sided" after all.

The Limits of Resemblance

I have myself been declared on different occasions the spitting image of my mother, of my father (who has never been declared to resemble my mother), and as bearing no family resemblance whatsoever. Given the prevalence of resemblance-talk in the form of a positive recognition in my collected data, I asked myself what hints my fieldwork materials gave on the limits of this flexibility? What makes bodies *not* alike? There were a few but telling instances in my data indicating a potential answer. The questions asked of Dörte Tönsch, whether Miguel was indeed a "real Brazilian", provide a hint. Most tellingly I found a line in one interview with the Stegers. In this section of the interview, as quoted in parts above, Philip Steger talked about how resemblance-talk was just "normal" and in no direct relationship whatsoever to how a child "actually" looks. It is, he observed, something people do "no matter what". Melanie Steger, however, intercepted laughingly: "You're right, yes—as long as the child was not actually black". It seems likely to me that this is indeed where the inclusivity and flexibility of the European cultural script for *making relations* through resemblance-talk comes to a halt: at "race".

German father Marcel Müller—who is "white"—noted in the interview, when discussing donor choice and matching, that "after all we are paying him [the doctor] well for making the right decision" and followed this assertion with the qualification that the right decision would mean that no "Black" or "Chinese" would be chosen. (Also see Becker et al. 2005, 1303 for a passage where this scenario is voiced as a fear through informants). Moreover, DI conceived adult Bonnie Smith told me that she was planning to talk to her son about her donor conception, partly because of his unexplained "exotic" appearance.

Bonnie Smith: "I can't hide it. It's important, he needs to know. It's funny because my son has characteristics that we don't know where they come from: he's quite dark-skinned, not, you know, white, white-skinned, but quite olive."

Such passages should be read in contrast with other passages in which, as we have seen, resemblance was noted, noticed and narrated along unique and—most importantly in the case of children—also perpetually changing children's bodies. Tactics of knowledge-management often took on a light-hearted note, elusively shifting between conscious but playful "deception", non-hereditary notions of corporeal continuity, or reflexive acknowledgements of resemblance-talk as "nothing more" than a cultural script which one happily plays along with. Thinking about the limits of resemblance-talk, however, the entanglements of kinship with heredity and race come to the foreground. While I found the flexibility of resemblance striking, it was still far from infinitely variable: Melanie Steger was probably right about her husband's musings that the old folks in the village would *always* welcome a new child with resemblance-talk would find its limits if a "white" mother and father would visit them with a child conceived through a "black" donor or vice versa.

Resemblance-talk for the families of my research thus remained flexible as long as it rested within what one intuitively knew about racial markers and the theoretical boundaries of heredity probabilities, even though those were articulated as extremely wide in most instances. This resonates with Schneider's postulate that kinship knowledge is tied up with scientific knowledge on heredity in "the" West (see 2.2), while also showing that resemblance recognition is not a simple transference of biological knowledge into everyday life.

Moreover, this points to the wider entanglements of scientific knowledge and "race" as one classificatory category for human physical variability. It is a category with a violent past and present, which elevated status cannot be explained by its simple physical *out-there-ness* just as much as resemblance recognition cannot.[4] Both resemblance and race thus must be seen as complexly interwoven with "transnational and historical signification" and their "intersection with other perceptible attributes" linked to "historical social hierarchies" (Thompson 2009, 133).

The Making of Reflexive Kinship Expertise

As the last point to raise in this section I would like to discuss how, as already briefly touched upon above, the persistent experience of positive resemblance-talk has turned my research partners into what I call reflexive

4 Also see chapter 5.1 for the discussion of ethnicity during the matching process. For a more comprehensive discussion and informed postcolonial critique of race categories within reproductive medicine—as already mentioned in chapter 5—e.g. refer to Bergmann's (e.g. 2012a, 2012b) research or to Thompson (2009).

kinship experts. They did not need to read about Trobrianders praising resemblance between father and children, while laughing at the idea of a resemblance *between* those very same children (Malinowski 1957, 176) to start thinking about resemblance-talk as a variable cultural practice rather than a straightforward cognitive activity. It was repeatedly described as only a convention, surprisingly flexible, as a part of everyday life, as a compliment, as normal: a "standard component of everyday chit-chat" (Holly Greenwood). It has led my research partners to reflect on resemblance-talk as a cultural script quite extensively within their social circle.

Even Uli Linde-Feldman, who attributed positive resemblance-talk mainly to a doctor's skill in clinically making "a certain resemblance" so that "one later does not say this is a totally different child", told me about his conversations with friends interrogating resemblance:

> Uli Linde-Feldman: "I've started talking about it [his uneasiness with resemblance-talk] with other guys… They said to me: 'Listen, people doing it are not trying to get to you, they actually want to say something nice to you. And when they want to say something nice, most Germans don't come up with anything smarter than 'he really looks like you!' Maybe this is actually something ethnological [turning towards me]. One thinks one gives the Alpha male a good feedback by saying 'I can see that you fathered this child.' There are no rivals in the horde. I am only letting you know, one can see that this child is yours."

The passage above is a very explicit example of the interview as a relational knowledge practice in itself, stirred to considerable extent by the role I am allocated in the field: Linde-Feldman attributes specific "ethnological interests" to me, which he assumes to lay in the realm of evolutionary theoretical frameworks far beyond my social/cultural-anthropological lens. I assume that this view of what the ethnographer might be interested in stems from a particular image of ethnology prevailing within his own studies of psychology.[5] Into his musings he invokes recapitulations of discussions with friends, anticipations of my own interpretation, and possibly his own academically-stirred explanations. The passage also shows the reflexive making of kinship expertise: his own experiences have led

5 Consequently, I do not interpret his statement as a straightforward evolutionary interpretation of resemblance-talk, but more as a reflexive musing on his cautious recognition of resemblance-talk being potentially more than just an affirmation of a clinically made physical similarity.

him to acknowledge—in continuous conversation with his social circle —the prevalence and simultaneous scriptedness of resemblance-talk. He also invoked different registers of explanation, from people wanting to be nice, to the articulation of an evolutionary script confirming group status or successful procreation.

Holly Greenwood's following account was typical in how it shows that this expert status has also led my interviewees to closely observe how other concerned parents handled situations of resemblance-talk:

Holly Greenwood: "I also find it really interesting to hear how other parents deal with it, with this whole resemblance theme. For example this mother of twins [whom she previously talked about as a member of her interest group, with the twins conceived through eggs donation], every time the girl says something like 'Look Mommy, your hands look exactly like mine!' the mother takes this as an opportunity to communicate to her that this is not possible at all. I would never do that, I would say: 'Yes, very nice…' This does not imply that one says: 'Yes, we're biologically related now!' But if she [Holly's daughter] would say: 'Hey, I have the same eye color as you, Daddy', he would say: 'Yes, you're right, we both have blue eyes.'"Thus, Greenwood observed how another mother interpreted any references to resemblance to be directly linked to concepts of heredity—or at least always used them as prompts to tell her daughter about the donation. Greenwood found this inappropriate and, when recounting the incident for me, invoked examples of corporeal continuities not linked to heredity or "play-along"-resemblance-talk.

Concluding Discussion

I would like to stress that my research partners conceptualized resemblance-talk as the most persistent confrontation in their everyday lives with their decision to have the donor treatment. Most of them, however, did not experience this as an inherently negative confrontation with straightforwardly *biologized* notions of kinship, as put forward by Becker et al. who argue that through resemblance-talk "the notion of blood relatedness is expressed" (2005, 1301). In conversation with Marre and Bestard's research (2009) and my research partners' own interpretations and observations I interpreted resemblance-talk as the rather flexible performance of a cultural script for the relational placing of a child within a family. Accordingly, the tactics of knowledge-management adopted by my interviewees mostly consisted of light-hearted practices of "play-along" resemblance-talk or an openness, which was sometimes also politically motivated.

About the reasons for the differences between Becker et al.'s findings and mine I can only speculate. They could be related to openness about gamete donation having increased or also to differences between Europe and the USA. What I find most likely is that not so much our data, but our interpretative frameworks differed. The authors conceptualized resemblance and its recognition as causally linked to the cognitive recognition of discrete similarities and as being a rather straightforward pointer towards *biologized* notions of kinship, while I did not. Nevertheless, both physical bodies and probabilistic concepts of heredity also did play a role in how resemblance was known in my own research materials. For example, the significance of physical shapes and heredity was underlined through the accounts of how confrontations with resemblance change when children's bodies change. This points to both the contemporary aptness of Schneider's postulate on the rooting of kinship in scientific knowledge, but also to how it might be productive to empirically break down this postulate and discuss its more minute entanglements. For resemblance-talk it became clear that probabilistic concepts of heredity and race, encompassing notions of corporeal continuity, the familial practice of knowing bodies in relation to other bodies, the performance of a cultural script and the recognition and narration of unique and changing physical bodies all opened up different legacies and entanglements—rather than unequivocally pointing to the recognition of genetic kinship.

My research partners reflected on resemblance-talk, and through this turned themselves into reflexive kinship experts, who—just like me—interrogated resemblance-talk as a cultural script. They called upon scientific or politicized explanations for this script, but most prominently on understandings of everyday life holding "stubborn" standardized practices of interaction.

Their expertise provides an interesting empirical illustration of what the new kinship studies postulate: that reproductive technologies are actually part of a complex and intertwined destabilization of "nature" and "culture". There is an ongoing debate if and how one can empirically tackle the question of how "the substitution between nature and culture, or the increasing space occupied by technology in reproduction, affect the kin relations involved" (Carsten 2003, 174). Part of the question is how to do so without appearing to be "complacent about some celebrated 'implosion' of nature and culture" (see Franklin 2001, 319; for some more general remarks also see Mol 2002, 19–21). And to keep in mind that despite the stunning "advances in the area of assisted reproduction" which lead to "changes in kinship ideology" being "declared by some to be inevitable", others argue that central elements of "kinship ideology have remained unchanged" (Ragoné 2004, 342). Beneath large scale concepts of *nature*, *culture* or *ideology*, the kinship expertise of my informants shows how third party assisted conception leads actors to reflexively unpack inherent parts of *doing kinship*, such as resemblance-talk, which otherwise mostly remain implicit, and thereby resemblance-talk actually becomes a subverting practice. It pays heed to the entanglements of kinship with knowledge on heredity, but, through its pervasiveness, scriptedness and flexibility undermines any straightforwardly geneticized perceptions of kinship.

8.2 Medical History: "Not that we're aware of"

How advances in molecular biology might be leading to a redefinition of what it means to be in and of a family body has been diversely discussed within kinship studies (e.g. Featherstone 2006; Finkler 2000, 2001, 2005; Konrad 2005b) and the wider social scientific literature concerned with the so called new genetics (e.g. Bunton and Petersen 2001; Novas and Rose 2000; Rabinow 1996). Scholars have concentrated on how concepts of family, personhood, and, say, pastoral care might be transformed through a re-framing of the older understanding of diseases "running in families" within the probabilistic risk language of genetics. Kaya Finkler has focused on how the ubiquitous register of medical history in everyday interactions with physicians might lead to a medicalization/geneticization[6] of kinship

6 In her work Finkler herself mostly speaks of medicalization, rather than geneticization. Since she only empirically focuses on genetics/genomics in healthcare and the

and has described how it proved to be a painful confrontation for a group of adoptees she has followed in her research. She argues that the persistent experience of not being able to answer questions pertaining to one's so-called medical history was the main cause for this group of healthy individuals to try and find their birth parents. She cites one adult adoptee with the sentence "'When you go to the doctor and you do not have a medical history you are not a person'" and argues that most of her research partners "felt like 'aliens' because of the lack of a biological family medical history. Every time they went to a physician they were questioned about their family medical history, and they could not provide one" (Finkler 2001, 241). As a ubiquitous genre she sees medical history to be related to the geneticization of kinship:

> "Whereas family and kinship relations are fluid and can be tampered with to expand or truncate a significant same group, the genetic definition of family and kinship is grounded in biologically produced ties, especially when people enter the medical stream and are asked about their medical family history." (Finkler 2005, 1061)

Within my own fieldwork materials, medical-history-talk proved to be a less frequently described and discussed confrontation than resemblance-talk. It was also far more often prompted through my questions than the discussions surrounding resemblance. All in all, it nonetheless seemed to be the second most common confrontation addressed by my familial interviewees.

However, the sense of deprivation described by Finkler above was not discernible in my data, potentially because my interview partners were mostly parents and thus possibly less alert to such everyday confrontations than the donor-conceived or adoptees themselves. While one might have hypothesized that parents would worry for their children's lack of medical history, this rarely came up. Incidentally, one of the adult donor conceived women I interviewed explored medical-history, or the lack of it, with similar apparent despair as Finkler's interviewees. I am, therefore,

---

associated risk discourses, I mainly discuss her work within the focussed discussions on geneticisation (also see 9.2), to which she also relates her works. Commentators on Finkler's work have also underlined that the way she is using the concept "medicalization", she actually seems to be referring to "geneticization" (e.g. see the comments on one of Finkler's articles under Finkler (2001)).

going to briefly explore the issue of medical history with regard to being a potential confrontation to the grown-up children conceived through donor treatment that I spoke to, and only then elaborate further on my findings with regard to the parents I interviewed.

Lydia Rivers, the donor-conceived woman whose case was first discussed in chapter 7.4, had used the registry UK Donorlink to look for donor-siblings or her donor without success. She said to me:

> Lydia Rivers: "I joined Donorlink when I was pregnant with my daughter. Because it suddenly made me think about… where I was from. Not only in an emotional sense, also in a practical sense—what happens if I am getting some genetic disease? [A disease] that I don't even know. I cannot do anything about it, if that's the case, but… But there was no real screening back in the 70s. I could have any genetic disease. Because… at least when you know who your parents are, you know when things run in the family. You'll be prepared and when you don't…it is a bit of a Russian roulette, really, in terms of your health. And I am just worried about that, for my children…"

In order to convey her worries about not knowing anything about her father's medical history, Rivers chose language that was as similarly drastic as that used by Finkler's interviewees. However, I have previously discussed her case (chapter 7.4), as, first and foremost, that of a person trying to reclaim agency over her past, retrospectively marked by her experience of unequal sharing of information and a related betrayal of trust. Rivers spent most of the interview exploring the various ruptures of past relationships entangled with her mother's very late revelation of the donor conception to her and her brother. She did not explore the theme of medical history in more detail than above or in relation to any particular diseases that she was fearful of. When asked again what she would be interested in, should she really find her donor, she again did not mention medical history, but discussed her wish for a close relationship. Thus I actually did not interpret her statement above, although in despairing language, as a sign of an escalating "ideology of genetic inheritance promoted by the new genetics" (Finkler 2005, 1061). Instead I interpreted it as yet another way to address her sense of injustice, deprivation of knowledge and deprivation of agency. In other words, medical history, first and foremost, proved to be a confrontation because it reminded her of this deprivation. Rivers' idea of establishing new relationships—afforded by genetics—I interpreted as an attempt in Rivers' case to complement other, often failed relationships. This attempt did not appear to be a sign of the colonization of social relationships through genetics, as implied through the geneticization paradigm (e.g. Lippman 1992).

In contrast, the other donor-conceived adult, Bonnie Smith, who I was able to interview during my fieldwork, , did not express much interest in medical history. This was the case even though Bonnie had made the awkward experience of being placed briefly on a monitoring regime for a genetic disease she was actually *not* at risk of due to her donor-conception (see 6.1). Smith's parents' obvious lack of worry that she would be at risk contributed to her growing sense of suspicion that she was not genetically related to her father, and she was eventually told about her donor conception when confronting her mother with her father's "wrong" blood group. In the discussion quoted below I am prompting the theme of medical history through my questions:

Maren Klotz: "I was just wondering whether genetics is something that is important to you?"
Bonnie Smith: "I guess it's not something I have thought about a lot. But obviously I thought I'd genetically inherited my dad's disease gene. Erm..."
Maren Klotz: "There are many scientists who are arguing that now that we know the genetic code to this, this, and this, we still do not know what to do with it. So I did not mean to imply with my question that it necessarily is important..."
Bonnie Smith: "Maybe in the future at some point it will be more important. I think, for me at the moment it's more the relationship. It is not so much about my donor's medical history. Obviously it would be good to know his medical history. But it's more about who he is as a person. More than anything, yeah."

Hence, despite being prompted, Bonnie explained that medical history was only of marginal importance to her and the donor interested her mainly as a person.

Both the British and the German parents of my core sample did mention their children's medical history as the second most common everyday confrontation, but except for Maria Lieb (as discussed below), none of them expressed concern about such situations. Typical for this was how German mother Dörte Tönsch talked about doctor consultations below:

Maren Klotz: "And this theme of a confrontation with being a family-by-donation and biological relatedness, is that only apparent in those situations [containing resemblance-talk] we just talked about?"

Dörte Tönsch: "It also came up with physicians, because they might for instance ask 'are there allergies in the background?' Then one thinks… Then one says: 'not that we're aware of', because that is really the case. I mean, on my side I don't know about anything and with the donor we definitely don't know, so we are not aware. When this happened for the first time, I thought that they [the sperm bank] will have actually considered that the donors are preferably people who do not have something [a disease]. But even the pediatrician [whom Dörte told]… I don't even know if she found this so important that she noted it down or not."

Similar to the reactive tactics of knowledge-management concerning resemblance-talk ("play-along" non-disclosing resemblance-talk or disclosure), for medical-history-talk parents also engaged in on the spot decision making processes whether to lay open the donation or employ the tactic of "play along"-medical-history-talk, as apparent in the quote above. However, *when* to employ which tactic and *what* the confrontation might say about kinship was not as reflexively interrogated as it was for resemblance. It seemed that disclosure towards physicians was intuitively made when parents thought "it might be important" (Dörte Tönsch). With none of the children of my research partners being chronically or severely ill, this was commonly done only when discussing allergies and eyesight. In these cases, the parents assumed a hereditary component, but did not explore this further in the interview situations nor did they address the lack of a medical history itself or the confrontation with this lack as a problem.

Only the Schneiders told me how they found it slightly odd that their pediatrician did not seem to know how to react to their disclosure:

Marc Schneider: "I find it astonishing that even pediatricians… For instance this pediatrician we talked to when he [their son] needed his spectacles… Well, maybe this even was about something else. In any case, she asked whether there is a previous history of this with me. And I went: "No, doesn't make any difference either, because this is a sperm-donation-child [Spendersamenkind]". And she just stared at me and changed the subject very very quickly."

Here, then, Marc Schneider mentioned the doctor's potential awkwardness as a problem, not the donor-conception itself. The only instance in my fieldwork materials where medical history was mentioned by parents in a more problematic context was when Maria Lieb recounted the subversive investigations into her donor (see 7.4). However, it was not the lack of a medical history that was discussed as problematic, but what she found out: as mentioned above, five of her daughter's unforeseen thirty donor siblings were diagnosed with a developmental disorder on the Autism spectrum. The question of a hereditary component to this disorder is currently much debated in the media. With her daughter having long passed the age that the condition normally presents, Maria Lieb was only mildly worried that it would still appear. On the other hand, she told me:

> Maria Lieb: "My daughter is a very withdrawn child. And I can actually imagine that it is actually genetically determined [genetisch bedingt] that she is so very introvert. She can play alone for hours and does not miss people around her. Sometimes this makes me think. But I am glad to know that this might be related."

Lieb also speculated that the donor potentially had the developmental disorder himself and had become a sperm donor because the disease had kept him from pursuing real-life sexual relations. I wondered if for Lieb, who had lived very reclusively as a single-mother-by-choice for a few years (see 8.4 and 8.6), the notion of her daughter's reclusiveness being hereditary also provided comfort: the thought meant that her chosen lifestyle, which at the time of our interviews she had started to view more critically as overly withdrawn, had nothing to do with her daughter's behavior.

I would like to summarize for this section that, mostly due to its portrayal in Finkler's research (e.g. 2000, 2001), I expected medical-history-talk to be a pervasive and problematic confrontation with the donor conception for my research partners. However, although the second most common confrontation discernible in my data, it was typically not addressed as warranting reflexive interrogations and explicitly formulated tactics of knowledge-management as was apparent for resemblance-talk. Parents intuitively decided whether to engage in "play along" medical-history-talk or just disclose the donation, because they—without further unpacking this for me—assumed a hereditary component to the condition they consulted the doctor about.

Adult donor-conceived Lydia Rivers was the only person within my fieldwork materials who addressed the lack of a paternal medical history in similar desperation as described by Finkler. I interpreted this in the context of Rivers' family history: not first and foremost as a sign of the geneticization of kinship, but as the simultaneous mourning of the loss of agency over her past and an attempt to reinstate it by means of the register of medical history, among others. In the social scientific discussions surrounding geneticization (for a more extended discussion see 9.2) the most extreme ends of the debate either diagnose "notions of predestination and a sense of fatalism" (Finkler 2000, 7) prevailing among persons with *risky* medical histories and "fragmentation, internal conflicts and turmoil" (ibid., 5) among those without one altogether. Or they bring forward, arguing in almost diametric opposition, that one can discern a growing "genetic responsibility" entailing instances of active self-management, as analyzed through the late-Foucauldian perspective of Novas and Rose (2000, 458). For my own research partners, the corporeal continuity of diseases was unequivocally accepted, but medical history was scarcely discussed as problematic and or as potentially enabling.

8.3 Kinship Terminology: "Will they meet their real father?"

One further reported confrontation which was addressed explicitly by some—not many—of my interview partners, were situations where colleagues, friends, and other acquaintances would use kinship terminology viewed as offensive: for instance when the donor was described as "the *real* father". The knowledge-management tactic in how to deal with such confrontations I have comprehensively discussed as *naming and terminology work* in chapter 7.2. This section thus briefly links back to my earlier argument.

Confrontations through exclusive kinship terminology were commonly described through parents-by-adoption I interviewed for another research project.[7] The so-called birth parents of adoptees were referred to by others as "the real parents". The adoptive parents I interviewed recounted such confrontations as hurtful and widespread. They always countered them with angry rebukes that "of course we are the real parents!" For the families-by-donation engaged through this research, such confrontations seemed to be more scarce. They were first and foremost

7 The project was the aforementioned longitudinal study on kinship and different forms of assisted conception (Humboldt University Berlin, SFB 640/C4).

visible as anticipations in the great care the parents themselves took to constitute kinship in specific naming practices and to inform their entire social world about the terminologies preferred. As described in detail in 7.2, this typically included letting others know to not call the donor by any recognizably parental idiom, such as *genetic father*, *biological father* or *genitor*. This was done in more detail for sperm donors than for egg donors, to avoid any assumptions of a previous sexual relationship between mother and sperm donor.

As real life experience, confrontations with the "wrong" kin terms were scarcely recounted. Uli Linde-Feldman was among the few to do so:

> Uli Linde-Feldman: "It is funny, when you let people in on the whole story for the first time, how they get all insecure with their language and say things like: 'Oh well—and will they be able to meet their real father?' That's where I usually grin and say: 'I *am* the real father!'"

Thus, Linde-Feldman here reacted exactly like the adoptive parents I interviewed, with an immediate rebuke. Mostly, it however seemed like the anticipatory knowledge-management taking place through the parents actually foreclosed such confrontations. That such confrontations were more common for parents-by-adoption might also be related to an actual parental relationship—however short—having previously existed at least for birth-mothers, but potentially also for birth-fathers.

8.4 Not Conforming to the Reproductive Norm: "Is it true that Jonas has two moms?"

Those of my familial research partners who were homosexual, single, clearly post-menopausal, or, like the Stegers, known by their social circle as carriers of a genetic disorder, had to live with people inquiring how they were able to conceive. I summarized such typical confrontations as arising when interviewees did not conform to *the reproductive norm*, i.e. when reproduction itself already made visible to others that assisted conception was likely to be involved. None of my interviewees invoked examples of such confrontations when I directly asked about what everyday life situations brought the donation to mind again. I rather interpreted them as confrontations myself when analyzing and coding other discussions I had with my interviewees.

Lesbian couple Svenja and Lena Arnulf, for example, often told me about everyday life situations where they had to explain themselves to others. In the interview passage below they told my colleague Michi Knecht and myself about reactions from their son's kindergarten group:

[Lena Arnulf talks about the kindergarten their donor-conceived son Jonas attends and explains that she does not know how many parents know about their family situation.]
Lena Arnulf: "…but now the children have asked for the first time: 'Is it true that Jonas has two moms?'"
Michi Knecht: "Does Jacob [Jonas's father and donor] pick him up from kindergarten sometimes?"
Svenja Arnulf: "Not often."
Lena Arnulf: "But that is actually always the next question then, about a male parent. That is always… The other day the children asked me: 'Does Jonas have two moms?' 'Yes, he does.' 'Has the Daddy died already?' 'No, he also has a Daddy!' (laughs)."

The Arnulfs seldom conceptualized such confrontations as problematic in interviews, but recounted them with an interest in how others were reacting to their family form. Svenja Arnulf once described to me how she could switch between perceptions of normality:

Svenja Arnulf: "Mostly, we are living in a kind of 'homonormativity'. By this I mean that what we are living…—that's the stronger reality for me. Also, because we get together with so many similar families and I am always out and about in my own 'homoworld' [she works in a gay rights organization]. So that's my normality… Sometimes, when I see a heterosexual couple, then I think, 'oh right, this is the real world'. Even though I lived this myself once, it seems so far away."

Her description thus conveys pointedly how the Arnulfs did not constantly perceive themselves as different in a heteronormative world, but were only occasionally reminded of the particularity of their family form. Nevertheless, although they were rare, there were confrontations to Svenja's and Lena's family life which they experienced negatively. They both remembered how irritated they felt, for example, when Lena's parents sent a greeting card for their son's birth only to the birthmother Lena and to father and donor Jacob Barry. Or they could talk for hours about the difficulties of filling out official forms in a way which translated their three-parent reality into administrative ways-of-knowing.

Given that such confrontations were not only related to having used DI to conceive (which my heterosexual interview partners could flexibly invoke in many situations, as discussed above), but more generally related to their lesbian parenthood, engaging in any *as-if* knowledge-management tactics was not an option for the Arnulfs, who identified as gay rights activists. They expressed that they saw their family also as a political project, involved in a struggle for the acceptance of homosexual parenthood and a breaking-up of the heterosexual bi-parental reproductive norm. The Arnulfs conveyed this was one of the reasons to participate in my research.[8]

The other interviewees not conforming to the reproductive norm were more ambivalent about putting their reproductive decisions in a wider political context. Although not apolitical in general, single mother Maria Lieb for instance explicitly stated that she did not feel like "politicizing" her private life. She told me how she had consciously given up her lifestyle of the 1980s, which had been shaped by the feminist credo that "the private is political" and during which she had lived in lesbian relationships. Lieb sometimes chose to not further explain the donor conception of her daughter and to instead just "invent a one night stand". She went through phases when her daughter was still quite young where she isolated herself to avoid confrontations:

Maria Lieb: "I think sadly, because I did not feel comfortable with it [the DI conception], I isolated myself more than I would have done otherwise. I never wanted all those questions, which might come up if you're striking up friendships. So it was a step, which changed my life more than I would have thought. I did not isolate myself on the job, but with parents I met in playgroups or the like, I never wanted to get too involved. Because one of the next questions then always was 'and how does he look like?', 'and what does he do?', 'and why did you two split up?'—and those were all the things that I did not feel like talking about."

Hence, for Lieb the temporary inability to develop a reactive tactic of kinship knowledge-management led to isolation. However, she later over-

8 They even asked me to not anonymize them within this book, because they felt like they did not want to hide. I, however, chose to refuse their wish, not only because University regulations oblige me to anonymization, but also because the Arnulfs' children were too young to give consent to potential non-anonymization.

came this through her daughter's own openness and working with a counselor (see 8.6 below).

In case of post-menopausal mother-by-egg-donation Shoko Nakamura, I assumed that her visible age (55 at the conception of her son Ochi) might also lead to questions from people she met during her everyday routines. Nakamura, however, told me that even though she had decided in principle to tell anyone about the donation who would ask about her age and how she had been able to conceive, this never actually happened. She did not further interrogate why this was the case. I would assume that acquaintances obeyed the widespread convention to not ask a woman about her age.

Moreover, Nakamura's potential status as a single-mother-by-choice was not discernible to outsiders, for instance to her loose acquaintances from the South Korean Mother's Club she had become involved with after Ochi's birth: she lived with a male housemate who also sometimes cared for her son. Her donor, although not co-habiting, also acted as Ochi's father. In fact, although not in a romantic relationship during and after Ochi's conception, she did not identify with the label single-mother-by-choice within this unusual care arrangement. In general, Nakamura was not an interview partner to reflect much on outside labels for family forms and did not—in contrast to the ethnographer—perceive her situation as extraordinary. Neither did she reflexively interrogate her relationship to an assumed reproductive norm, like the Arnulfs did, for example.

Nakamura however referred to various confrontations her age had produced when interacting with public authorities. The most severe example of this, which she found to have been "an extremely strange experience", was that after she had registered Ochi with the South Korean embassy to get his passport, they later doubted she was his birth mother, because she was over fifty. She then had to "prepare extra documents, like a translated list of all my gynecological appointments during pregnancy and a letter of confirmation from the doctor who had delivered Ochi". The donation itself was never discussed during this process, but rather whether her age was not an indication of "illegal adoption or the like" (Nakamura). Thus, proof of pregnancy (as also enshrined in British law, which legitimizes motherhood via birth and not via genetics) warded off official confrontations prompted through her non-conformity to the reproductive norm.

I want to summarize for this section that those of my research partners who did not conform to the traditional heterosexual family were confronted with questions on reproduction—and had to develop situational tactics in responding to these questions—simply because they were not assumed to be able to reproduce without assistance: where did their children come from? Who was part of their family? And was all of that legitimate? The Steger family, as mentioned above, also had to deal with such confrontations. Their first daughter's death, from the genetic disorder that Philip and Melanie were previously unknown carriers of, had of course not gone unnoticed among colleagues and acquaintances. Thus, sometimes people they did not know very well still asked how their following children had been conceived. All of the families had developed their own situational tactics of reacting to such confrontational questions. The Stegers disclosed the donation if someone directly asked about their hereditary disease and just sadly thought about their first daughter when asked how many children they had and which one was the first-born. The Arnulfs' family life was bound up with the wider political struggle for lesbian rights and inclusive formats of family. They thoughtfully and often humorously reacted to all questions regarding their family with politically motivated openness. Maria Lieb instead sometimes chose to not disclose the donation. Shoko Nakamura seemed to be embedded in such unusual social relations that this actually stopped acquaintances from asking questions. It also seemed to stop her from feeling like she should close ranks with politically more intelligible family forms, for instance with women who clearly identified as single-mothers-by-choice. What was a shared experience for many families, however, was that how they knew their family sometimes proved to be hard to translate into administrative ways-of-knowing.

8.5 Biological Reproduction as a Confirmation of Heterosexual Love and Virility: "Well done, nice shot!"

The next to last form of confrontation I would like to draw attention to in this chapter consists of situations within which biological reproduction was addressed as a confirmation of heterosexual love and of virility. These confrontations did not lead to reactive tactics of knowledge-management, as I shall show below, but to reflections on normative perceptions of kinship and masculinity through my interviewees and their social circle. I will firstly discuss the theme of joint reproduction. Then I turn to discussing the conflation of male impotence and infertility, including a discussion of how my interview partners reflected on notions of masculinity.

Confrontations through the first theme mainly pertained to the heterosexual couples in my sample who had used sperm donation, although the Arnulfs also told me that the absence of joint biological reproduction had once been dismissively described to them by esoterically-inclined friends to make homosexual relationships inferior. Uli Linde-Feldman for instance recounted the following situation capturing such a confrontation pointedly:

Uli Linde-Feldman: "My cousin got married within this shamanic ritual. And during the ritual they kept saying these uninspired sentences, like 'the earth grounds you and the sky'… whatever, 'skies you'… And then they talked about children, because they have a child together: 'In your child, both your bodies and both your souls reproduce in one'. Later on family members said to me: 'What a load of crap! How do you feel, Uli, when they say stuff like 'your love was unified through procreation'?' They were actually quite angry."
Berit Feldman: "Really? That's how they reacted? How nice!"
Uli Linde-Feldman: "Yeah, yeah, they were quite irritated and said: 'How insensitive!' […] So my 'clan' deals really quite sensitively with the whole thing, they have actually started reflecting on such things a lot".

Thus, the Feldmans conveyed their experience of a situation where biological reproduction had been hailed as the ultimate confirmation of heterosexual love within an esoteric ritual. Other family members, aware of the donor-conception, had also experienced the ritual as a confrontation and later shared their impression with Uli Linde-Feldman. The situation hence shows how emergent kinship-expertise described above (8.1) not only leads those immediately affected to reflexively interrogate negotiations of kinship that are otherwise taken for granted. In addition, this emergent reflexive expertise was also shared experientially by those within close affective relationships with the parents and made them aware of the often implicit ideal of *shared corporeal continuity*, such as discussed in section 4.1.

A related confrontation mentioned by some of my male research partners was the conflation of impotence and infertility. Here, too, infertility/

fertility was interpreted as a sign for something else: not just the heterosexual relationship, but also as a sign for virility—or a lack thereof. I also want to discuss general reflections on masculinity through my interviewees in this context.

Mother-by-egg-donation Shoko Nakamura interrogated how male infertility was different from female infertility, and donor conception hence potentially experienced differently:

> Shoko Nakamura: "I suppose for men it might be different… […] After you have given birth, the egg, it is not really a big thing. But for men, I can imagine, whether that's my sperm or not, it is a different thing. Because it is always abstract, isn't it? The man is in a bit of a sad position, isn't he, in this reproduction process. A man is always watching, from outside of the fence, and women, women experience. They get pregnant and give birth. I'm really glad I experienced that, because otherwise I would have missed this big thing which you, we, are allowed to experience."

Thus, according to Nakamura, men would feel their masculinity was in question when using a gamete donor in a more significant way than women's femininity. She also speculated that they would more easily attribute significance to their (missing) physical contribution to the conception of a child. Infertile male interviewees did not explicitly compare egg and sperm donation, as Nakamura did, unprompted by me. And, in contrast to Nakamura's expectation, they also did not straightforwardly underline the importance of biological reproduction, although the loss of parts of a corporeal continuity was sometimes mourned.

British father Tim Hampton reflected on male infertility as such:

> Tim Hampton: "It would be a big deal for anybody, dealing with infertility. But there is a… I think there is a peculiarly, peculiarly male bit of shame associated with it. It is a deep male shame. Some would say it is natural—but I don't think it's that—but there is a deep male shame that comes with not being able to father children…"

Hampton said that when first dealing with his diagnosis, he "literally struggled to say 'I'm infertile'", but with the help of a counselor learned to mourn his fertility and openly acknowledge his shame and through that ultimately came to terms with it. He also described how the rough locker room jokes of his football teammates—"very men's men, macho men" (Hampton)—were among the mundane, everyday confrontations with his infertility and through this also with being the father of a family-by-donation, which he simply had to live with. Hampton described how he told them about his son's donor conception and his own infertility for the first time:

Tim Hampton: "At first I could not tell them, I just couldn't, and I was ashamed that I couldn't. I promised myself that I would tell them when we had the baby, so [starts chuckling]… When our son was a week old, they came round to meet him, all these big guys… And one after the other they walked in, saw the baby and then I, I told them. I said: 'I just got something to tell you' and they, they had presents with them, and they went, 'oh, right?' And of course they were then, and have been since, completely supportive."

Thus, Hampton felt supported through his teammates. Nonetheless, his openness meant that there would be jokes making use of the conflation of infertility and impotence and vice versa: "We call this 'taking the piss' in English and what that means is that you pick on people, but only close friends do it to each other" (Hampton). His reaction to his teammates' jokes was mostly to just play along. He confronted one "merciless" but "not nasty" teammate once and asked "if he actually knew what he was talking about" (Hampton).

My other male infertile interview partners did not address as openly if and how the diagnosis affected their own sense of masculinity. When asked directly they negated the question whether it played a role for them and implied they were "above that" (Miguel Tönsch), but sometimes commented on conflations of infertility with impotence or vice versa, fertility with potency. Uli Linde-Feldman for example laughingly recounted how some of the men he regularly practiced for a marathon with said about Berit's pregnancy: "'well done, good shot!'—really on this embarrassing sexualized cliché level…". Or Philip Steger told me that locker room humor was explored as a common confrontation among interest group members:

Philip Steger: "I've never met a guy there [an interest group for families-by-donation] who had any problems that he was not the genetic father. […] But there are these everyday situations, which everyone has to live with and which we talk about: after football, you've had three beers, and then, erm, under the shower someone says about your pregnant wife: Well done, well done—or something like that. Where it might be just a bit too much for you for a short moment or you feel like you are not entitled to say anything…"

The jokes implicitly conveyed that a man should be congratulated on his fertility as having done "well", which connoted not only fertility, but also meant being a potent lover. Given my interviewees' complaints about such conflations I found it ironic that some of the clinics were actually discursively perpetuating the link between fertility and virility in their sperm donor recruitment campaigns (see 5.2). Except for Tim Hampton, none of my male interviewees talked about taking the confrontation through "male jokes" as a prompt for discussing their status as fathers-by-donation. Both forms of confrontations—representations of biological reproduction as an integral fulfillment of a love relationship and locker room jokes ambiguously conflating being "good in bed" with fertility—were rather just observed and internally noted. But they were nevertheless interrogated in their normativity, also in conversation with the families' social circle, and in that sense were part of the families relationally and reflexively making themselves into kinship experts.

8.6 The Child Talks: "If we have eggs in the kitchen, we also need sperm for Daddy"

As analyzed in chapter 7.3, my research partners had started disclosing the donation to their children at an early age, often before the children could talk, with the help of specific children's books. These parental methods of disclosure entailed that as soon as the children could talk, the parents' roles as exclusive knowledge-managers vanished. I thus treated the children's own addressing of their donor-conception, as the last of my examples of parental confrontation to do with being a family-by-donation to be analyzed. In this section I explore the specific dynamics of disclosure this produced.

With the young children having neither fully grasped conventional concepts of heredity, sexuality nor what adults meant with "privacy", typically humorously recounted confrontations arose for the parents I worked with. The Schneiders account below captures this pointedly:

Marc to Nadine Schneider: "Didn't he once say to you after shopping 'shouldn't we buy sperm as well?'"

Nadine Schneider: "No, wait a minute, that had to do with the kitchen… [laughs] He has this toy kitchen, and he also has eggs in this kitchen. And one time he had this idea that 'if we have eggs in the kitchen, we also need sperm, for Daddy' [Maren Klotz starts laughing]. You don't expect that to happen. We were a bit baffled there [laughs]. And that's why we said, we have to tell other people, so they don't look at him funny if he says something like that."

Thus, an additional (to some of the aspects of resemblance-recognition as analyzed in 7.1) confrontation internal to the families proved to be the children's talk about the donation. Within the narrative reconstructions of such situations, their comical side was commonly stressed. It also was typical for both the German and the British children to retell the exact words featured in the children's books on gamete donation. The Feldmans, for example, recounted how their son started to refer to Thorn's children's book (Thorn and Rinaldi 2006) in everyday situations:

Berit Feldman: "I have read the book by Petra Thorn with him quite often and…"
Uli Linde-Feldman: "-and we were out on a walk and then he suddenly went: 'you went to see a doctor, and then you were very sad, and then you went to the doctor again, and then I came'—or something like that."
Berit Feldman: "And on Sunday, I was at my old workplace and I said to him: 'Look, this is where I used to work'. And then he said: 'Where was I when you worked there?' and then I said 'Well you had not been born yet' and then he went: 'Ah, that's when you were sad, and then you went to the doctor and got sperm" [we all laugh].
Uli Linde-Feldman: "And he doesn't have a clue what that means, but still…"
Berit: "And there were people walking next to us and I just went, huh… (laughs). I just thought, oookay…"

The quotes the Feldmans were attributing to their son are almost a word-for-word retelling of Thorn's book (see section 6.1 and clipping 6.10). The parents commonly conveyed feeling uncomfortable with their perception that their young children were talking about the donor conception without, from the parents' point of view, actually understanding what they were saying. This led to occasional worries that a dramatic "light bulb moment" (Sarah Hampton) of realization would follow at some point. These occasional worries were, however, rebutted, as parents told me, through the interest group advice literature (see chapter 6), which underlined that children would develop a gradual understanding of their conception over years.

The confrontations by the children led to seemingly typical dynamics in knowledge-management: the child was told—then the child talked—then the parents took this as a cue to talk about it even more, to the child and to their social circle. This dynamic is apparent in the quotes by the Schneiders above and when the Feldmans added that "maybe it is time" to talk to their son some more, because they felt "slightly strange" with their impression that he was simply retelling the book without making sense of it.

With German mother Maria Lieb, who had an older daughter than most of my interviewees, this step-by-step dynamic became particularly clear. When first interviewed Lieb said about her daughter who was around eight years old at the time:

Maria Lieb: "Now my daughter is starting to tell people, or at least that's the feeling I've got. I think I have to clarify a few things for myself, rather than to keep suppressing that. The other day, at the train, I felt like she talked to some kids she met there really loudly: that she does not know her father and that he donated at a sperm bank. (…). She said that as if it was something special to her, which is actually a good thing. Only, I should be at the point where I could share this. The stupid thing is that I am still uncomfortable with that."

When interviewed two years later, things had changed:

Maren Klotz: "In the last interview you mentioned how you were uncomfortable with your daughter's openness…"
Maria Lieb: "-well, so much has changed! I don't even know why exactly. I worked through the whole issue quite extensively [part of this was going to see a counselor]. And because my daughter was telling so many people, I had to position myself differently. All these funny things happened… The mother of my daughter's best friend, for instance, approached me and said that she found it really interesting what my daughter was telling her and she wanted to let me know, just in case, that they were all completely relaxed with such things: her husband, she said, was donating sperm so that her best friend, who is lesbian, could become pregnant… [laughs]. When she said that I thought 'well, okay, I am living in Großstadt now' [she had lived in another large German city before] and it seems like times have changed much more than I thought."

Lieb's assertion that she had to position herself differently pointedly captures how her daughter's confrontations had actually set in motion a dynamic of further disclosure. These dynamics yielded positive surprises how donor conception was "much less a taboo" than it felt like to the single-mother-by-choice for a while.

Lieb was also the only parent who in her narrative reconstructions combined detailed and reflexive accounts of her awkwardness during such situations with the more commonly adopted joking tone. All apparent framings of the confrontation (depiction as awkward, depiction as comical, depiction as peculiar because of the child's lack of understanding) have to be understood in relation to the aforementioned loss of agency of the parents as exclusive kinship knowledge-managers. While the parents were following the canonic approach to make their children *know all along* (see 6 and 7.3) in practice what was known all along, of course, was ever changing: for young children with neither an understanding of sexuality nor of heredity were knowing things quite differently than their parents along the way. One could say the foundational link between kinship and scientific knowledge as proclaimed through Schneider (1968) was not in place yet for the children.

This exposes how the idea of *knowing all along* is a backward-looking concept of knowledge-management, formulating an intended outcome. The effect of children knowing kinship-by-donation differently from their parents often produced occasions for laughter, as captured in the quotes above. The comical effect was produced through the juxtaposition of these differing ways-of-knowing and shifts in meaning. For example through the blurring of conventionally distinctly adult topics (sperm, ova, clinics) with non-sexualized children's play, for instance centering on "egg and sperm in a kitchen". The parental realization that they "knew differently" than their children commonly prompted further practices of disclosure. This last specific confrontation thus conveyed how kinship knowledge-management also entailed family-internal power-dynamics between parents and children in gradually shaping kinship-knowledge.

9. Conclusions

This book presents an ethnographic exploration of a form of knowing and doing kinship that has only emerged in the last 25 years: through clinically administered sperm or egg donation, within the framework of non-anonymous regulatory set-ups, and openly discussed in families. Taking inspiration from Strathern's (1999) postulate that kinship-knowledge should be viewed as constitutive information, this exploration centers on how kinship-by-donation is constituted within what I came to call kinship knowledge-management. It thus centers on the negotiation of which aspects of kinship-knowledge are validated, which are drawn on in various practices, made accessible or inaccessible, foregrounded or silenced. Kinship is understood as a prime site for the negotiation of what a Western society perceives as the made and the given, and for working out which roles are attributed to biology within practices of human solidarity. The book focuses empirically on four intersecting domains: families, clinics, regulation, and interest group activism. In its theoretical and methodological design, it emphasizes the processual material-semiotic constitution of kinship, taking a multi-sited perspective. In contrast to Britain as academic and empirical center stage of the new kinship studies, empirical engagement with the phenomena here studied has been scarce in Germany. In ensemble, this study hopes to make a comparative contribution to the empirical and theoretical analysis of kin-formation and social change in plural late-modern societies in Europe. The research demonstrates a contemporary re-negotiation of the values of privacy, information-sharing, and connectedness.

Kinship is a *flexible* cultural technology, as parental knowledge management demonstrates (see chapters 4, 7, and 8). Parents actively intervene in its constitution through their knowledge-practices, including use of various "kinship objects" from photographs to children's books. Chapters 4, 7, and 8 also demonstrate *constraints* to the constitution of kinship-by-donation: from lovers' wishes for a shared corporeal continuity, to clinics' advocating DI only as a "last resort" after the utilization of IVF/ICSI, and to outside confrontations of the parents with an assumed genetic relatedness. These confrontations can lead parents to develop reflexive kinship expertise. They explicitly interrogate and observe how kinship is constituted in everyday life and when genetics and heredity are invoked —recognizing the often flexible and ritualized dimensions of this invocation. Parents are not alone in their [k]information work. Clinical actors and practices, interest group activities, and regulatory regimes are also powerful (see chapters 5 and 6). The unique material-semiotic relation of kinship-by-donation to clinical classification practices and standards affects parental knowledge-management. Clinics' administrative practices and associated regulation underline the genetic "link" to the donor as socially relevant, while parental interest group activism offers a canon of knowledge-management that makes disclosure imperative on moral, not genetic grounds. Part of the emergent canon of knowledge-management through interest groups is the output and utilization of children's books, guides, workshop-offers and self-help meetings.

A shift of authority is evident in the way kinship-by-donation is known and managed in Europe, a shift, more minute in Germany than in Britain, towards interest groups, parents, and policy-makers, away from a sometimes high-handed medical profession.

Four of my findings require more detailed discussion:

1. There is a strong co-implication of kinship-by-donation with national and transnational regulation, made visible through comparison between Britain and Germany.
2. Instead of unambiguously discernible *geneticization*, the re-negotiation of the inherent value of information-sharing is moving closer to *transparentization.*
3. David Schneider's original assertion of the foundational link between kinship and biological science requires revision. Kinship-by-donation in Europe is constituted through diverse fields of authoritative knowledge-production, ranging from the "psy-sciences" (invoked by parents and the increasingly influential interest groups), to the fields of governance and administration, to the IT sector, and on to the systems of medical standards and classification.

4. Through knowledge-management, concerned parents actively intervene in the constitution of kinship-by-donation. Aided by their growing reflexive expertise they simultaneously multiply and mitigate what Strathern (1999, 75) calls the immediate (simultaneous) social effects of biological information.

These outcomes hopefully encourage further detailed comparative ethnography. They are meant as an invitation "to be invented around, to forge new relations and to open up new perspectives" (Scheffer and Niewöhner 2010, 11), by pointing to broader discernible patterns in the data and discussing them in relation to existing literatures.

9.1 National and Transnational Regulation and the Constitution of Kinship-by-Donation

This research employs multiple axes of comparison, pertaining to the four intersecting domains under study (families, clinics, regulation, interest groups), among individual cases, and between Germany and Britain. Comparison as a methodological tool makes visible local specificities and thus serves to not approach kinship as "hidden grammar", but to instead focus on how it is constituted in diverse and flexible practices. Germany and Britain are put into focus as distinct regulatory environments—with kinship knowledge-management as *tertium comparationis.* Where gamete donation is clinically administered in Europe, it is bound up with national regimes for not only donor-anonymity or non-anonymity, but also diverging reproductive technology regulation and family law. How these European differences play out locally has barely found empirical attention. To tease out how regulatory regimes are implicated in [k]information was achievable only through cautious ethnographic comparison, seeking to avoid problematic conceptualizations of "container-like national-cultures" that often taint comparative projects (Beck and Amelang 2010, 164), yet answering calls coming out of STS and the new kinship studies to look closely at the local "enactment of regulation" (Wilson-Kovacs et al. 2010, 101) in Europe. Close comparison makes possible the productive exploration of how "technocratic models of kinship" are part of and informed by the local constitution of kinship (Edwards 2006, 137).

Crucially, kinship-by-donation in Germany is not regulated closely. A newly established fragile non-anonymity exists since 2007 (GewebeG 2007), while potential legal connections between child and donor have not been comprehensively severed through the law, as in Britain. In contrast, from 1990 onwards, the UK has established comprehensive though changing regulations of clinical gamete-donation. In 2004–2005 gamete donation became non-anonymous by law (UK Gov 2004). Children born from gamete donation in Britain can access so-called identifying information on the donor from a national registry held at the HFEA when they turn 18.

Foregrounding national difference, my data show that clinical knowledge-management for gamete donation in Germany was far more diverse and open to differing actors' interpretations than in Britain. Through endeavors of evidence-based policymaking, serving as "conveyor belts" between law and local practice in Britain, donor-conception appeared to be taking place in a highly controlled "laboratory setting" in contrast. This led to the consecutive emergence of new problems in knowledge-management, for instance pertaining to access rights of parents to the national registry or, more generally, to data-protection. I argue that the constitution of kinship-by-donation in the two countries is linked to a tight, yet processual approach of "governance at a distance" (Miller and Rose 2008) in Britain compared to a "hands-off" minimal mode of governance in Germany.

German physicians appear to claim a stronger authority in prescribing non-disclosure to patients/clients in the absence of a clear regulatory situation or of a generally stronger public visibility of gamete donation as discernible for Britain. They may assume the authority to intervene more than British doctors in the matching process between donors and receiving patients/clients. This strong involvement of the personal views and attitudes of the clinicians leads to a physical incorporation of their opinions and anticipations of parental knowledge-management into the bodies of the children born through such procedures. In Britain, parents exercise more decision-making authority. In effect the knowledge-management of the parents themselves determines the selection of gametes and thus elements of the physical constitution of the children. Discussions surrounding donor-anonymity, kindled through the regulatory changes, seemed to displace discussions surrounding disclosure *per se* among the British clinicians.

The influence of genetic/genomic considerations on clinical knowledge-management is distinctly different in the two countries (during the period of the study). Genetic tests played an important role for donor selection in British clinics, where donors were routinely subjected to them (e.g. for cystic fibrosis carrier status). In contrast, in one German clinical field site not even a karyotype test was performed, and genetic tests were conducted in neither of the German clinics sampled. The British clinic acted on the encouragement (although not the prescription) of genetic testing in the HFEA guidelines (HFEA 2009a). In contrast, the German working party of sperm bank operators in their recommendations explicitly discourages the genetic testing of donors (Arbeitsgruppe Richtliniennovellierung 2006). Although not directly discernible in my fieldwork materials, the wider public debates on bioethics in Germany, mostly marked through religious and post-Nazism considerations, and finding their expression in the strict German regulations on reproductive medicine and stem cell research, as discernible in the Embryo Protection Law of 1990, allow this abstinence from genetic considerations to be interpreted as one typicality of *German* kinship-by-donation.

The ambivalence of disclosing German parents toward their children's possible future interest in the donation and the donor, I tentatively attribute to the unclear German regulatory situation. However, it was *not* that in the absence of a clear German regulatory situation, German interest group activities filled this perceived gap. At the time of my fieldwork German parents focused on informal private meetings, rather than on attempts at lobbying work. In Britain the DC Network was involved in political advocacy work and policy-making. The British processual mode of governance gave the DC Network members ample entry points into policymaking practices, beyond broad political protests or more classical back-stage lobbying work. For example, prominent members could regularly provide evidence at HFEA meetings and consultations. The DC Network also had a much larger membership than the German internet-based groups, which mainly consisted of bi-parental heterosexual families-by-sperm-donation. German membership was nonetheless growing quickly. In contrast, the DC Network was comprised of heterosexual, homosexual, and single-mother families. In short, in Germany, interest group formation was more related to family form, whereas in Britain group identity was articulated around the method of conception. A likely reason for this difference would be that donor conception has been an intensively debated "regulatory item" in Britain since the 1980s, in contrast to Germany. In Britain gamete donation is thus more likely to be networked around as an available parental or personal identity. Being a donor-conceived person or parent-by-donation has become an "interactive kind" of classification in Ian Hacking's (2000) sense—implying that a classification can have social looping effects.

Foregrounding national differences simultaneously makes visible the limited influence of national regulation on knowledge-management and the co-implication of transnational regulation. All domains under study were highly transnational. The EU Tissue Directive, ISO standards, and the WHO guidelines, for instance, strongly influenced clinical practices, which were embedded in an emergent assemblage of transnational standards and regulation. The parents I engaged with were not passive consumers of the reproductive medicine available in their country of residence, but travelled to conceive or ordered gametes online to be delivered to their home country. Knowledge-transfers between interest groups in Germany and Britain were also common and had an additional transnational dimension through the involvement of key actors such as Olivia Montuschi (manager of the British Donor Conception Network) and Petra Thorn (influential German infertility counselor and group workshop convener) in organizations such as the transnational umbrella interest group ICSI (International Consumer Support for Infertility). And donor-conceived adults and parents established transnational connections in subversive search endeavors. The unofficial German gamete donation register, for instance, was now hosted through a US-American company and website and supported through American donor-conceived activist and blogger Nancy Greenawalt. Transnational communication and networking options thus undermined national regulatory regimes and—along with advancing genetic testing technologies—are likely to make anonymous donation regimes increasingly difficult to maintain beyond the far more prominent rights-based debates.

My findings thus show the minute co-implication of kinship-by-donation with national and transnational regulation, made visible through the comparison between Britain and Germany as distinct regulatory environments. Differing modes of governance affect how actors are bestowed with authority and to which resistant modes of knowledge-management actors resort: when clinicians have more freedom and authority and parents are less legitimized in their disclosure tactics through specific regulatory regimes, uncertainty about how to get knowledge-management "right" may increase. When governmental authority in the shape of *government at a distance* supplements clinical authority, interest groups have clearer entry points for advocacy work within this system, thus gaining a more authoritative position in establishing a canon of knowledge-management. Transnational communication and networking however may serve to reduce these differences.

9.2 Transparentization

When discussing anonymous and non-anonymous donation regimes, Strathern argues:

> "if we do wish to pursue openness then we should know that part of the stimulus comes from certain politics of communication (open information for a free society; truth for the sake of justice), and not from systematic investigation into kinship practices." (Strathern 1999, 80)

This book analyzes, partially along borders of national regulation, how such a stimulus has found entrance into the material-semiotic constitution of kinship-by-donation through clinical standards and "audit cultures" (Strathern 2000) that are particularly pronounced in Britain. Such a stimulus was also part of the constitution of kinship-by-donation in families and interest group activities. Equal information-sharing was viewed as morally imperative in both countries: a conceptualization strongly informed through knowledge-pathways stemming from the "psy-sector".

Also fitting Strathern's hypothesis, the empirically novel phenomena of non-anonymous donation regimes and disclosing parents were, when read through my fieldwork materials, not unambiguously related to an increasing valorization of genetics. Noting the entanglements of kinship with societal and scientific transformations, my research thus suggests that kinship is changed through its resonance with a cultural pattern of *transparentization*: not, or at least not first and foremost, through *geneticization*. Making this argument requires briefly recapitulating claims about diagnoses and the refutation of *geneticization*, and a consideration of transparency as a contemporary moral imperative.

Geneticization is a concept developed in the early 1990s by feminist epidemiologist and health-researcher Abby Lippman (e.g. 1992), as briefly discussed in earlier chapters. Thus, it was coined long *before* the hype leading up to the completion of the mapping of the human genome had given way to a "morning-after feeling" of how exactly to use the produced data and a related strengthening of epigenetics and systems biology. What the concept usually does is to ascribe a growing currency to genetics/genomics within different social arenas. There, genetic explanatory models are argued to unfold a dangerously determinist character and to be colonizing of other, more politically just, emancipatory, or actively chosen social relationships and concepts. In her key article "Led (Astray) by Genetic Maps" Lippman, for instance, cautions against a "genetic colonization—geneticization—we are witnessing in the areas of health and illness" (1992, 1474). She warns of the "ongoing process of geneticization in which differences between individuals are reduced to their DNA codes" (1992, 1470) and genetic interventions are sought instead of addressing medical and social problems brought about through poverty and injustice. This may "lead to the perverse effect of worsening our individual well-being and our collective health directly and indirectly" (Lippman 1992, 1471).

Although reverberating with some of the same themes and sometimes being subject of similar critiques, *geneticization* as an analytical framework of the 1990s was not directly related through literature discussions to the older concept of *medicalization*. This latter concept, originally coined by Irving Kenneth Zola (e.g. 1972), emerged out of sociology and became widely used within the sociology and anthropology of health and illness (for critical discussion, particularly in light of German *Volks-* and *Völkerkunde* see Beck 2007). Broadly summarized, *medicalization* refers to a much longer historical development towards an increasingly medical framing of phenomena formerly understood in, say, religious, moral, or social frameworks in the industrial West. More recent works emerging out of this strand of scholarly work which also focus on changes in medicine brought about through contemporary molecular biology have tended to use terms such as "biomedicalization" (e.g. Clarke et al. 2003; Mamo 2005) or to focus on the "culturalization of medicine" (Beck 2007) instead of geneticization. Such works also have tended to be critical (often from a feminist perspective) of both the passive portrayal of actors assumed to be subjected to geneticization and of the utilization of an insufficiently complex impact model of science and society relations, as also found within some works utilizing the broader medicalization framework (e.g. Gibbon 2002; Knecht and Hess 2008; Lock and Kaufert 1998).

The analytical framework of *geneticization* has also been applied to kinship. As recurrently touched upon in this book, Finkler (e.g. 2000, 2001, Finkler et al., 2003) has been one of its more widely cited proponents.[1] In similar vein to her arguments, Dorothy Nelkin and Susan M. Lindee assert:

> "In the 1990s genetic connections have come to define a new molecular family, one bound together less by history, tradition, or common experience than by shared DNA. The parent-child relationship, particularly, appears in popular culture as dependent less on caring contact than on genetic similarity, as adoptees search for genetic roots and prospective parents endure painful fertility treatments in order to produce a child." (Nelkin and Lindee 1995, 58)

On the surface, many of the phenomena analyzed in this book seem to be resonant with such a trend: for instance non-anonymous donation regimes or sibling and donor searches.

Yet my fieldwork shows that *geneticization* is often rejected as well. Kinship figures as not entirely unhinged from hereditary thinking and the wish for a shared "corporeal continuity" between lovers in my fieldwork materials. However, kinship first and foremost appears as a flexible cultural technology. Families-by-donation do not invariably suffer from not being genetically related, even if they reflexively play along with such confrontations as resemblance-talk. Instances of real or imagined relationships

1 To be precise, Finkler actually uses the term *medicalization*, but seemingly employing it synonymously to the narrower concept of *geneticization* and within its analytical thrust and empirical focus on genetics. For discussion e.g. see Franklin's comments to Finkler (2001, 250–251).

appear to be geneticized in the sense of using genetics "to make connections", such as apparent in the wayward searches and relations endorsed by the donor-conceived. Yet such *wayward relations* do not have to be colonizing, but can be complementary to other relationships. They are characterized by their unprecedentedness and related lack in associated social roles. They can be infused with a strong assertion of agency by the actors who shape these relations aided by expert deployment of IT and of other areas of contemporary science.

In the more general policy discussions surrounding anonymous or non-anonymous donation regimes, Haimes, as early as 1992 (135), reminds us that the *in*accessibility of donor-information can be interpreted as a sign of *geneticization*. What makes this information so special and potentially disruptive that it needs to be withheld through special regulatory regimes? And multiple later ethnographic (recent examples for instance are Carsten 2000; Edwards 2006; Edwards and Salazar 2009) coming out of the new kinship studies about assisted conception, kinship, and biotechnologies, but not focusing exclusively on kinship-by-donation, have underlined how "genetic explanation is neither necessarily nor always a prominent feature of the way in which different publics across Europe make sense of kinship" (Edwards 2006, 132). My findings thus align with such results that refute a simple diagnosis of *geneticization*. Moreover, my findings offer a first exploration of the implication of a yet different cultural pattern which I term *transparentization*. By this term I am pointing to the rise of transparency as moral imperative for various forms of information-sharing and as a framework to manage problems.

Concerning the negotiation of kinship-information in contemporary North America, Kimberley Leighton (2012) has recently pointed to the worrying convergence between conservative and anti-gay family politics with the North American right-to-know activism of the donor-conceived. She does not argue within the *geneticization* framework, but from a perspective of political philosophy and critical bioethics. Unlike the situation in Britain and Germany I portrayed, she points to the tendency of conservative institutions, such as the think-tank Institute for American Values to "exploit their [adoptees and the donor-conceived] lack of knowing (and their desire to know) as a means of promoting their own views of what families are supposed to be" (Leighton 2012, 70). Namely, Leighton argues, not to be transgressive of heteronormative, and more implicitly addressed, also racialized, boundaries to family formation. Thus, even if not assenting to *geneticization* as a descriptive term for the phenomena analyzed in this book, nor as a fruitful wider analytical framework, one nevertheless has to be warned about the specific "resonance machines"[2] (Connoly 2005) the implicit or explicit valorization of genetic kinship-knowledge can enter.

My own empirical findings suggest a different *resonance machine* than the nexus between genetics and changing perceptions of the family (as brought forward within the *geneticization* framework of analysis) or the nexus between right-to-know activism and conservative family values (as Leighton sketches out for the US, where reproductive technologies are mostly unregulated and highly commercialized). Most of the phenomena analyzed in this work rather suggest a resonance with the broader contemporary re-negotiation of the values of privacy, information-sharing, and connectedness. In my empirical materials this nexus became visible in the framings of non-disclosure as "lying" apparent on the level of interest group knowledge-management and among my parental interviewees in both Britain and Germany. *Transparency* here is infused with an explicit moral judgment. This is based on values of equal information-sharing and a belief in the impairment of relationships should such equality be absent, as underlined by counselors, psychologists, and interest group activists.

This nexus also became apparent on the level of institutional knowledge-management. It was particularly pronounced in Britain, where data on the donor but also on clinical practices were constantly collected and then made available in a regime of *government at a distance* and associated *audit cultures*. Transparency here is infused with specific ideas of more efficient and just government and administration in ad-

2 With the suggestive term *resonance machine* Connoly makes use of Deleuze and Guattari to refer to the dynamics of association and amplification at work within public discourse and politics hardly explainable through causal logics: "in politics diverse elements infiltrate into the others, metabolizing into a moving complex—Causation as resonance between elements that become fused together to a considerable degree. Here causality, as relations of dependence between separate factors, morphs into energized complexities of mutual imbrication and interinvolvement, in which heretofore unconnected or loosely associated elements fold, bend, blend, emulsify, and dissolve into each other, forging a qualitative assemblage resistant to classical models of explanation" (Connoly, 2005, 870).

vanced neoliberal shape and with a social-democratic legacy.[3] And it lastly became apparent as result of the above-diagnosed socio-material "incontainability" of kinship-knowledge. Transparency here is infused with the new networking and search capacities of the World Wide Web and advancements in computing power and associated technologies for genetic sequencing and analysis. It is at odds with anonymous donation regimes and the informational gate-keeper status of clinics and regulation. More generally, transparency has become a contemporary political catch-word, carrying with it a utopian promise of democracy and untainted personal relationships (for analysis e.g. see Comaroff and Comaroff 2003; Sperling 2011).

Transparentization, broadly defined, describes the multilevel application of a framework of transparency to manage problems. This pattern is discernible in numerous phenomena: from the activities of the newly surfaced and highly successful German Pirate Party, over initiatives such as WikiLeaks, and NGOs such as Transparency International, to the common baring of personal information that was previously considered private on social networking sites. It is also much used within applied governance research. There it is predominantly interpreted as leading to consumers' empowerment through informed choice, often state-driven, because private companies are assumed self-evidently not to endorse transparency (Fung et al. 2007). The utopian hopes attached to transparency are pointedly captured in the way James Marcquart summarizes *New York Times* columnist William Safire, who has argued that the catch-word transparency captures a

> "momentous, on-going transformation in social affairs from the machinations associated throughout time with the pursuit and the abuse of power to a new and hopeful order in which modernity and the virtues associated with it—reason, objectivity, truth, and democratic and accountable governance—help secure

3 Evidenced-based policymaking as discernible in current HFEA practices has been introduced by the Blair Government, as discussed in chapter 2 above. More broadly spoken, Foucault has actually spent parts of the development of his *Gouvernementality* concept on analysing the neoliberal transformations of the German social democratic party (see Foucault 2000). Stuart Hall is also cited through Strathern (2000, 283) in ironically pointing to the curious nexus between "neoliberalized" social-democracy and audit cultures: "good social-democratic souls…have learned to speak a brand of metallic new entrepreneurialism, a new managerialism".

individual liberty and peace and prosperity among the countries of the world." (Marquardt 2011, 1)

Echoing Ulrich Beck's (1992) diagnosis of the "risk society", German philosopher Byung-Chul Han (2012) has recently published his (critical) appraisal of the "transparency society [Transparenzgesellschaft]" while media activist, consultant, and political scientist Micah Sifry (2011) has affirmatively declared the dawning "age of transparency". Anthropologists and sociologists have tended to keep a critical eye on this elevation of transparency as ambiguous moral imperative, pointing to its previously discussed entanglement with neoliberalism and "the very explicitness of our therapeutically minded culture" (Comaroff and Comaroff 2003, 290–291). They have also pointed to the difficulty of grasping and describing what I call *transparentization* as a cultural pattern and not just a taken-for-granted step towards enlightenment, given the deeply personal and political investment people tend to have in it (e.g. Smart 2011; Strathern 1999).

Edwards (2009a) and Knecht (2009b) note an "imperative to connect" at work within sibling searches and ancestry research, an imperative similar to a tendency that I also consider present in the search endeavors of my interviewees (see 7.4). In Knecht's and Edwards' concept "making connections" becomes a moral imperative and a joy and celebration of the serendipity moment. The authors describe this connection-making as not only a newly elating pastime, but just as much as a form of counter-movement to late-modern experiences of fragmentation. Their concept captures aspects of what I call *transparentization*; our analyses are thus related and, in my view, supportive of each other. What sets our categories apart are three aspects: firstly, *transparentization* more strongly points to the implication of the "psy-sciences" in stressing values of information-sharing. Secondly, *transparentization* points more to the political dimensions of information-sharing. And thirdly, it points more to the attachment of hope and broad utopian visions of a better society.

Knecht (forthcoming), however, also cautions us against an overhasty declaration of the "end of anonymity" in light of the wider cultural patterns resonating in the novel kinship practices analyzed in this book. She instead calls for a research program to address the social productivity of *anonymity* and its more minute adjustments in the contemporary.

Kinship-by-donation in Germany certainly did not appear to be as imbricated with *transparentization* as did kinship-by-donation in Britain and the rest of the English-speaking world, despite displaying a potentially similar development. This development does indeed show how *transparentization* does not bring with it emancipatory politics *per se,* as sometimes hailed. It instead brings certain shifts in power the ethnographer of the contemporary should note closely. *Transparentization* entails a shift of authority about how [k]information is managed in Europe—and a shift of authority, more minute in Germany than in Britain, towards interest groups, parents, and policymakers, away from sometimes high-handed medical professionals.

9.3 Diverse Fields of Authoritative Knowledge-Production

Kinship-by-donation in its constitution through knowledge(-practices) is permeated with diverse strands of scientifically validated knowledge. This *particular diversity* of strands of knowledge, as elaborated below, is the third central finding of my study. Schneider (1968) famously proclaimed a foundational link between Western kinship and the scientific sector of biology. However, he never expanded on how he saw the mediation between the two (for discussion e.g. see Franklin 2001). This book enlarges the list of knowledge strands to include scientifically endorsed notions of information-sharing that stem from the "psy-sciences" (and have a particular impact on families), modes of governance and associated regimes of audit and administration, innovations in the IT sector, and diverse medical classification and standardization practices. All are part of this mediation for the case of gamete donation. For kinship-by-donation, I thus show, the "scientifically discovered facts about biogenetic relationship" that make "kinship into what it is and was all along" (Schneider 1968, 23) were not displaced, but are pervaded with ways-of-knowing bound up with Latourian "centers of calculation" (e.g. 1987) elsewhere, outside of the molecular-biological laboratory. In other words, Schneider underlined that what "nature" i.e. presumed substance of Western kinship, is seen to be, at a certain point in time, is related to science. The other "major cultural order" he saw symbolically at work, in addition to "the order of nature", was "the order of law", related to conduct and jurisdiction (Schneider 1968, 27). My research shows how both the "nature" in kinship-by-donation and the law/conduct are, in part, constituted through strands of diverse, scientifically validated knowledges that do not stem from cutting edge biology.

My empirical findings thus underline the arguments coming out of STS and the new kinship studies which foreground reproductive technologies as transforming "the relationship between substance and code for conduct not only by making the substance the object of conduct, but conduct (e.g. scientific research) the origin of substance" (Franklin 2012, 58). Franklin's statement is one of numerous examples of how the new kinship studies are still extending and re-phrasing Schneider's original assertions from the 1960s to describe the changes they are studying in the contemporary. Franklin underlines in her above cited analysis of the legacy of IVF how substance is regulated and how conduct nowadays produces biological substance in the laboratory. She foregrounds how this specific legacy of IVF has fostered understandings of the human as "biologically relative" (2012, 58).

My empirical findings extend such arguments from STS and the new kinship studies in light of the specific case of kinship-by-donation. It is the donor who links the constitution of kinship-by-donation to *particularly diverse* fields of authoritative knowledge-production. Importantly, the low-tech nature of sperm donation in comparison to other reproductive technologies minimizes its relation to cutting edge biological research. The IVF sector, in contrast, has a close connection to stem cell science, at least in Britain (e.g. Franklin 2006; Hauskeller 2004). And although the link to stem cell research is not strongly developed in Germany due to strict bioethical regulations, IVF still warrants far more complex laboratory equipment and training of personnel in both countries. In contrast, the Sperm Bank Friedhausen, for example, operated only with laboratory and physician's assistants trained through the German vocational education system. Only the clinic owner, Dr. Dettmaringen, had studied medicine at a university. Moreover, IVF, in comparison to using a gamete donor, concentrates heavily on "making babies" despite, or because of, a couple's gametes falling short of various scientific quality indicators. IVF/ICSI is far more involved at the level of high-tech "working" upon procreational substance, rather than in judging and classifying it. In contrast, when a donor is used, particularly a sperm donor (but to a more limited extent, the egg donor also) is measured against various scientific standards in place for judging procreative substances, such as the WHO guidelines, and classification systems of human physiognomic variation, which are involved in the matching process. The use of a donor thus becomes the entry point of various scientific standards, classifications, and considerations of parents and doctors. Those standards, classifications, and parental and medical "kinship values" all become physically incorporated in the resulting children.

Because German and British parents attach social significance to the use of a donor, they join interest groups and buy guides on how to raise the donor-conceived child. They thereby establish a foundational link to the psy-sector and to the growing lay-expertise currently producing authoritative knowledge on "how to get it right" when raising a donor-conceived child. The social significance attached to the use of a donor also lets regulation and the medical institutions pay attention to kinship-by-donation in specific ways. Knowledge about the donor becomes a subject of governance and administration. Knowledge about the donor, ranging from DNA data to index cards simply recording an address, also becomes implicated in various information-infrastructures. The existence of this information in authoritatively governed information-infrastructures, as well as the new subversive and IT-endorsed means to access or bypass them, exacerbates power struggles on who has a right to what knowledge. Such power-struggles over kinship information do not occur for IVF, but sometimes for adoption. The latter is however not infused with all the scientific classifications and standardizations at work for gamete donation.

9.4 Agency and Reflexive Expertise

Individuals personally affected in the constitution of kinship-by-donation actively intervene *through knowledge-management*. Related to this active intervention I also note an emergent *reflexive expertise* on kinship, as elaborated below. Parents and the donor-conceived thereby simultaneously multiply and mitigate what Strathern (1999, 75) calls the immediate (simultaneous) "social" effects of "biological" information.

Strathern's (1999) concept of constitutive information (as explored in chapter 2) informs this finding of active intervention. Her discussion of kinship-knowledge as constitutive information is based on her combined analysis of the status of scientific knowledge in Western societies and of identity formation for Westerners, as bound up with knowledge of genetic relatedness. She analyzes how Schneider (1968, 23) asserts science's foundational link to kinship, thereby disclosing an inherently Western concept of knowledge. This is a concept of knowledge that is externally verifiable and simultaneously internalized into relational configurations of personhood. Strathern sees the constitutive effects of kinship-knowledge on *identity* as leaving no choice for those personally affected:

> "In the right to know comes a (regulative) enablement: being able to choose the right course of action. In the case of kinship, as Euro-Americans construe it, there are (constitutive) areas in which there are no choices." (Strathern 1999, 80)

But individuals evidently can assert choice, and hence agency, in how they actively pursue kin relationships (Strathern 2005, 26). As discussed in chapter 2, Carsten called for an empirical study of how persons actively manage kinship-knowledge, not in order to reject Strathern's overall argument, but rather "to put to work the antithesis Strathern draws out between the implications of acquiring information and refusing it" (Carsten 2007, 405). For her own empirical work, Carsten asks whether there are "degrees" of kinship-knowledge "or different trajectories of processing it", and then focuses on the role temporality plays in managing kin relationships (2007, 406).

My analysis, inspired by Strathern's concept and Carsten's call for empirical study, addresses the detailed management of kinship-knowledge, mediated in various ways, through regulations, physiologies, infrastructures, and practices. My findings highlight the situational constitution of kinship-by-donation within processes of validation, storage and representation, and distribution, drawing on the anthropology of knowledge (e.g. Barth 2002) and STS (e.g. Latour 1999; Star 2002). This speaks to yet another research *desideratum* formulated in the new kinship studies (e.g.

Edwards 2009b), to look more closely below at what underpins the broad concepts of nature and culture, examining kinship "in the making".[4]

Focusing on knowledge-management reveals how knowing about kinship may be mediated through various materialities and informally compiled "kinship-archives": through photographs, collected memorabilia, pedigrees, and also the observation of children's changing bodies, which were seen to display different resemblances to different persons at different times. Kinship talk appears as a "connector" between not only persons, but also places, bodies, and different temporalities. Part of this active construction of connections involves seeking out and commenting on physical resemblances and shared mannerisms between family members. *Not* knowing the donor as an embodied person may in this context be addressed as uncanny and can lead to moments where parents are unsure how to "read" their children, for instance, as if "someone else" appeared to be looking at them "through the child", or some physical feature or behavior of the child appeared "alien". Out of the scarce clinical information the parents have, the donor then "re-materializes" in the parents' imagination (Mamo 2005) into an amicable person, thereby mitigating against such effects of the uncanny.

Further notable knowledge-management strategies and tactics of parents and donor-conceived children include:

a) the active intervention into how kinship-by-donation should and could be known among children, family and friends through choosing and advocating specific kin terminology. For example when the heterosexual parents took great care that the sperm donor would not be addressed with a parental or patchwork-family idiom, such as "biological father", but as "donor".
b) The active intervention into how kinship would be known "all along" by the children, through the usage of children's books on gamete donation emerging from the interest group and counseling sector. The narratives the books conveyed were not as extensively interrogated by the parents as was the case for other areas of knowledge-management. In the books, kinship is symbolically portrayed as brought into being through non-sexual parental love, powerful enough to enroll doctors, a volunteering donor, and biological substances. Heredity as a concept or "connector" between people does not figure in such accounts.

4 For a more general discussion and literature review pertaining to a relational anthropology "below" the nature /culture divide see Beck (2008).

c) The active subversion of official regimes of knowledge-management, apparent in the sibling- and donor-searches described. Those sometimes implied the highly professional utilization of complex infrastructures and DNA-testing technologies that are hardly noticed by the media or social science research.
d) The tactical management of situations in which families were reminded of the donation, such as apparent in situations of "playing along" with resemblance-talk, where parents lightheartedly join in chatting about physical similarities without disclosing the donation.

As suggested by Carsten's research (e.g. 2000, 2007), *temporality* figures crucially in how individuals try to assert agency through managing kinship-knowledge. For example where adults experienced their own donor-conception as a deprivation of knowledge in the past, setting up or researching about genetically endorsed kin-relationships in the contemporary is infused with efforts to reclaim agency over this very past. Viewed predominantly from the parents' perspective (and not from the perspective of the affected children, such as in Carsten's discussions) my research moreover shows the following: in order to intervene directly into how kinship can and should be known, parents draw on both the social novelty of openly acknowledged and non-anonymous kinship-by-donation (as apparent in a lack of established terminology) and on the power that time and proximity grants them to inform children in certain ways.

Both active interventions into the constitution of kinship-by-donation and the reactions to confrontations produced a reflexive expertise on kinship among parents. The development of strategies for knowledge-management and of tactics for dealing with confrontations led parents to explicitly debate, sensitively observe, and carefully reflect upon otherwise taken-for-granted aspects of kinship. These include the ubiquity of resemblance-talk in everyday life, and whether and how this is related to heredity, which kin terms imply which kind of relationships, or how femininity and masculinity relate to reproduction. In a process that is quite analogous to the one used by the researcher of kinship, parents inquire into the constitution of kinship, but on the basis of their own experiences with kinship-by-donation.

That the utilization, sometimes even only the awareness, of methods for assisted conception leads to actor's more reflexive approaches to family formation has been discussed in several recent works out of the new kinship studies (e.g. Bestard 2009; Howell 2001; Knecht and Hess 2008; Knecht et al. 2011). These works also stress a simultaneous gain in reflexivity and lay-expertise. My findings align with such outcomes, which together describe diverse practices of reflexive "meaning making" around assisted conception and the inherent challenge of the classic heterosexual reproductive model (combining romantic heterosexual relationship, sexual intercourse, and joint reproduction).

This book teases out what the *specific reflexive expertise* of families-by-donation is: namely a certain constructivism by practical experience when it comes to the role of heredity in everyday life, as is apparent in the recognition of resemblance-talk as "stubborn" everyday practice of interaction and not straightforward cognitive activity. Importantly, the growing reflexive expertise of those personally affected finds its extension and professionalization in the increasing influence of interest groups on policymaking and clinical practice. Unlike the activities of the interest groups analyzed by Epstein (e.g. 1996) or Callon and Rabeharisoa (e.g. 2008), the parents in my study do not so much intervene with the knowledge-production in the domain of clinical practice, but rather introduce a new strand of knowledge into clinical practice and policymaking: a combination of professional and experiential "psy" expertise.

Clinics, regulations, and interest groups contribute, but personally affected parents play a decisive role in making and managing the knowledge they receive and draw from these sources. When they use their knowledge-management to actively intervene in the constitution of kinship-by-donation, they reveal a simultaneous effect of recognition and attempted normalization. The donor may, for example, be recognized with a specific kin-name, but at the same time within such naming practices, is also allocated a relational space that the parents view as non-disruptive to their family. The donation may be disclosed early, in the hope that this early disclosure, and the associated usage of the children's books stressing love rather than genetic kinship, leads to biological information *not* unfolding any disruptive potential. *All* such practices of [k]information simultaneously multiply and mitigate the immediate social effects of biological kinship knowledge.

To summarize, this research demonstrates a contemporary renegotiation of the values of privacy, information-sharing, and connectedness.

Additionally, this research points to an evident shift in authority towards policymakers and interest groups in the management of kinship-knowledge in Europe. These trends are apparent in the above-discussed four central results of my study, focusing on changing intersections between families, clinics, regulation, and interest group activism. Firstly, they are apparent in the strong co-implication of kinship-by-donation with national and transnational regulation. Second, they are apparent in kinship-by-donation's resonance with the emerging cultural pattern and moral imperative of *transparentization*. Third, they appear in kinship-by-donation's link to *particularly diverse* fields of authoritative knowledge-production, ranging from the "psy-sciences" (invoked by parents and interest groups), to the fields of governance and administration, to the IT sector, and on to the systems of medical standards and classification. Fourth, the way individuals personally affected in the constitution of kinship-by-donation intervene actively *through knowledge-management* highlights this shift in values and authority. Kinship-by-donation was thus used as a tool to probe into the (re-)negotiation of relationships in late-modern Europe. This book shows how kinship-by-donation is constituted within hybrid practices and contested politics of communication —within practices of [k]information.

Abbreviations

ANT	Actor Network Theory
BICA	British Infertility Counselling Association
BKid	Beratungsnetzwerk Kinderwunsch Deutschland
CMV	Cytomegalovirus
DCN	Donor Conception Network
DI	Donor Insemination
DNA	Deoxyribonucleic Acid
DSR	Donor Sibling Registry
EDI	Electronic Data Interchange
EGENIS	ESRC Centre for Genomics in Society
HFE Act	Human Fertilisation and Embryology Act
HFEA	Human Fertilisation and Embryology Authority
HIV	Human Immunodeficiency Virus
HTL Viruses	Human T-Lymphotropic Viruses
HU Berlin	Humboldt University Berlin
ICSI	Intracytoplasmic Sperm Injection
IfEE	Institut für Europäische Ethnologie [Department for European Ethnology]
ISO	International Organization for Standardization
IVF	In Vitro Fertilization
LFH	Largecity Fertility Hospital (Pseudonym)
LSVD	Lesben- und Schwulenverband Deutschland [Lesbian and Gay Federation in Germany]
NDPB	Non-Departmental Public Body
NHS	National Health Service
NRTs	New Reproductive Technologies
OTR	Opening the Register

QM	Quality Management
SFB	Sonderforschungsbereich [Collaborative Research Cluster]
SNPs	Single Nucleotide Polymorphisms
STRs	Single Tandem Repeats
STS	Science and Technology Studies
UKDL	United Kingdom Donorlink
WHO	World Health Organisation

List of Figures

Bibliography

Almeling, Rene (2011). *Sex Cells: The Medical Market for Eggs and Sperm*. Berkeley: University of California Press.

Amann, Klaus, and Stefan Hirschauer (eds.) (1997). *Die Befremdung der eigenen Kultur. Zur ethnographischen Herausforderung soziologischer Empirie*. Frankfurt a. M.: Suhrkamp.

Arbeitsgruppe Richtliniennovellierung (2006). *Richtlinien des Arbeitskreises für donogene Insemination*. Retrieved from http://www.donogene-insemination.de/downloads/Richtl_Druckfassung.pdf (last accessed: 5.7.2010).

Aspinall, Peter J. (2009). The Future of Ethnicity Classifications. *Journal of Ethnic and Migration Studies*, 35 (9), 1417–1435.

Aull Davis, Charlotte (1999). *Reflexive Ethnography. A Guide to Researching Selves and Others*. London and New York: Routledge.

Barad, Karen (1998). Getting Real: Technoscientific Practices and the Materialization of Reality. *Differences: A Journal of Feminist Cultural Studies*, 10, 87–126.

Barad, Karen (1999). Agential Realism. Feminist Interventions in Understanding Scientific Practices. In M. Biagioli (ed.) *The Science Studies Reader*, 67–83. New York: Routledge.

Barth, Fredrik (1995). Other Knowledge and Other Ways of Knowing. *Journal of Anthropological Research*, 51 (1), 65–68.

Barth, Fredrik (2002). An Anthropology of Knowledge. *Current Anthropology*, 43 (1), 1–18.

Bateman Novaes, Simone (1998). The Medical Management of Donor Insemination. In Ken Daniels and Erica Haimes (eds.) *Donor Insemination: International Social Science Perspectives*, 105–131. Cambridge; New York: Cambridge University Press.

Baxter, Nicola, and DCN (2002a). *Our Story: A Book for Young Children About Their Conception through Donor Sperm to Lesbian Parents*. Nottingham: Donor Conception Network.

Baxter, Nicola, and DCN (2002b). *Our Story: For Children Conceived through DI into Single Parent Families*. Nottingham: Donor Conception Network.

Baxter, Nicola, and DCN (2002c). *Our Story: For Children Conceived through Double or Embryo Donation*. Nottingham: Donor Conception Network.

Baxter, Nicola, and DCN (2002d). *Our Story: For Children Conceived through Egg Donation*. Nottingham: Donor Conception Network.

Beck, Stefan (2007). Medicalizing Culture(S) or Culturalizing Medicine(S). In Regula Valerie Burri and Joe Dumit (eds.) *Medicine as Culture. Instrumental Practices, Technoscientific Knowledge, and New Modes of Life*, 17–33. London: Routledge.

Beck, Stefan (1996). *Umgang mit Technik: Kulturelle Praxen und kulturwissenschaftliche Forschungskonzepte*. Berlin: Akademie Verlag.

Beck, Stefan (2008). Natur | Kultur. Überlegungen Zu einer relationalen Anthropologie. *Zeitschrift für Volkskunde*, 104 (2), 161–199.

Beck, Stefan (2012). Biomedical Mobilities: Transnational Lab-Benches and Other Space-Effects. In Michi Knecht, Maren Klotz and Stefan Beck (eds.) *Reproductive Technologies as Global Form. Ethnographies of Knowledge, Practices, and Transnational Encounters*, 357–375. Frankfurt: Campus.

Beck, Stefan, and Katrin Amelang (2010). Comparison in the Wild and More Disciplined Usages of an Epistemic Practice. In Thomas Scheffer and Jörg Niewöhner (eds.) *Thick Comparison. Reviving the Ethnographic Aspiration*, 155–180. Leiden and Boston: Brill.

Beck, Stefan, Nevim Cil, Sabine Hess, Maren Klotz, and Michi Knecht (eds.) (2007a). *Verwandtschaft machen. Reproduktionsmedizin und Adoption in Deutschland und der Türkei* (Vol. 42). Berlin: LIT.

Beck, Stefan, Sabine Hess, and Michi Knecht (2007b). Verwandtschaft neu ordnen. Herausforderungen durch Reproduktionstechnologien und Transnationalisierung. In Stefan Beck, Nevim Cil, Sabine Hess, Maren Klotz and Michi Knecht (eds.) *Verwandtschaft machen. Reproduktionsmedizin und Adoption in Deutschland und der Türkei*. Münster und Berlin: LIT.

Beck, Ulrich (1992). *Risikogesellschaft: Auf dem Weg in eine andere Moderne*. London: Sage Publications.

Becker, Gay, Anneliese Butler, and Robert D. Nachtigall (2005). Resemblance Talk: A Challenge for Parents Whose Children Were Conceived with Donor Gametes in the US. *Social Science and Medicine*, 61 (6), 1300–1309.

Bergmann, Sven (2012). Resemblance That Matters: On Transnational Anonymized Egg Donation in Two European IVF Clinics. In Michi Knecht, Maren Klotz and Stefan Beck (eds.) *Reproductive Technologies as Global Form. Ethnographies of Knowledge, Practices, and Transnational Encounters*, 331–356. Frankfurt: Campus.

Bergmann, Sven (2014 forthcoming). *Ausweichrouten der Reproduktion*. Wiesbaden: VS Verlag.

Bestard, Joan (2009). Knowing and Relating: Kinship, Assisted Reproductive Technologies and the New Genetics. In Jeanette Edwards and Carles Salazar (eds.) *European Kinship in the Age of Biotechnology*, 19–28. Oxford: Berghahn.

BICA (2007). *Guidelines for Good Practice in Infertility Counselling. British Infertility Counselling Association.* Retrieved from http:// www.bica.net/ sites/ default/ files/ file_attach/Guidelines_for_good_practice.pdf (last accessed: 10.1.2012).

BKiD (2008). Leitlinie für die psychosoziale Beratung bei Gametenspende. *BKiD Beratungsnetzwerk Kinderwunsch Deutschland*, 1–11. Retrieved from www.bkid.de/ gs_leitlinien.pdf (last accessed: 11.1.2012)

Blake, Lucy, Polly Casey, J. Readings, Vasanti Jadva, and Susan Golombok (2010). Daddy Ran out of Tadpoles: How Parents Tell Their Children That They Are Donor Conceived, and What Their 7-Year-Olds Understand. *Human Reproduction*, 25 (10), 2527–2534.

Blyth, Eric (2008). Donor Insemination and the Dilemma of the 'Unknown Father'. In Gisela Bockenheimer-Lucius, Petra Thorn and Christiane Wendehorst (eds.) *Göttinger Schriften zum Medizinrecht*, 3, 157–175. Göttingen: Universitäts-Verlag Göttingen.

Bourdieu, Pierre (1976). *Entwurf einer Theorie der Praxis.* Frankfurt a. M.: Suhrkamp.

Bourdieu, Pierre (1996). On the Family as a Realized Category. *Theory, Culture and Society*, 13 (3), 19–23.

Bowker, Geoffrey C., and Susan Leigh Star (1999). *Sorting Things Out: Classification and Its Consequences.* Cambridge, MA: MIT Press.

Boyer, Dominic (2005). Visiting Knowledge in Anthropology. *Ethnos*, 70 (2), 141–148.

British Fertility Society (2004). *British Fertility Society Response to Donor Anonymity Paper in Human Reproduction.* British Fertility Society Press Release 10.11.2004. Retrieved from http:// www.fertility.org.uk/ news/ pressrelease/ 04_11-donor_-anonymity.html (last accessed: 12.7.2008).

Bundesärztekammer (2006). (Muster-)Richtlinie zur Durchführung der assistierten Reproduktion. Novelle 2006. *Deutsches Ärzteblatt*, 103, A1392-A1403.

Bunton, Robin, and Alan R. Petersen (2001). *The New Genetics and the Public's Health.* London: Routledge.

Butler, Judith (1990). *Gender Trouble: Feminism and the Subversion of Identity.* New York: Routledge.

BVerfGE. (1989). German Constitutional Court 31.01.1989. *Kenntnis der eigenen Abstammung.* (BVerfGE 79, 256).

Callon, Michel (1999). Some Elements of a Sociology of Translation. Domestication of the Scallops and the Fishermen of St. Brieuc Bay. In Mario Biogioli (ed.) *The Science Studies Reader*, 67–83. New York and London: Routledge.

Callon, Michel, and Vololona Rabeharisoa (2008). The Growing Engagement of Emergent Concerned Groups in Political and Economic Life: Lessons from the French Association of Neuromuscular Disease Patients. *Science, Technology, Human Values*, 33 (2), 230–261.

Carsten, Janet (2000). 'Knowing Where You've Come From': Ruptures and Continuities of Time and Kinship in Narratives of Adoption Reunions. *The Journal of the Royal Anthropological Institute*, 6 (4), 687–703.

Carsten, Janet (2003). *After Kinship*. Cambridge: Cambridge University Press.

Carsten, Janet (2007). Constitutive Knowledge: Tracing Trajectories of Information in New Contexts of Relatedness. *Anthropological Quarterly*, 80 (2), 403–426.

Clarke, Adele E., Janet K. Shim, Laura Mamo, Jennifer Ruth Fosket, and Jennifer R. Fishman (2003). Biomedicalization: Technoscientific Transformations of Health, Illness, and U.S. Biomedicine. *American Sociological Review*, 68 (2), 161–194.

Clifford, James (1986). On Ethnographic Allegory. In James Clifford and George E. Marcus (eds.) *Writing Culture: The Poetics and Politics of Ethnography*, 98–121. Berkeley: University of California Press.

Clifford, James, and George E. Marcus (eds.) (1986). *Writing Culture: The Poetics and Politics of Ethnography*. Berkeley: University of California Press.

Collier, Stephen J. (2006). Global Assemblages. *Theory Culture Society*, 23 (2–3), 399–401.

Comaroff, Jean, and John Comaroff (2003). Transparent Fictions or the Conspiracies of a Liberal Imagination. In Harry G. West and Todd Sanders (eds.) *Transparency and Conspiracy. Ethnographies of Suspicion in the New World Order*, 287–300. Durham: Duke University Press.

Connoly, William E. (2005). The Evangelical-Capitalist Resonance Machine. *Political Theory*, 33 (6), 869–886.

Cook, Rachel (1999). Donating Parenthood: Surrogacy, Gamete Donation. In Andrew Bainham, Shelley Day Sclater, Martin Richards and Cambridge Socio-Legal Group. (eds.) *What Is a Parent? A Socio-Legal Analysis*, 25–46. Oxford: Hart.

Cooper, Trevor G., and et al (2009). World Health Organisation Reference Values for Human Semen Characteristics. *Human Reproduction Update*, 1–15.

Crick, Malcom R. (1982). Anthropology of Knowledge. *Annual Review of Anthropology*, 11 (1), 287–313.

Cussins (Thompson), Charis (1998). Producing Reproduction: Techniques of Normalization and Naturalization in Infertility Clinics. In Sarah Franklin and Helena Ragoné (eds.) *Reproducing Reproduction. Kinship, Power, and Technological Innovation*, 66–101. Philadelphia: University of Pennsylvania Press.

Daniels, Ken (2004). *Building a Family with the Assistance of Donor Insemination*. Palmerston North: Dunmore Press.

Daniels, Ken, and Erica Haimes (eds.) (1998). *Donor Insemination: International Social Science Perspectives*. Cambridge; New York: Cambridge University Press.

Daniels, Ken, and Petra Thorn (2001). Sharing Information with Donor Insemination Offspring: A Child Conception Versus a Family-Building Approach. *Human Reproduction* 16, 9 (9), 1792–1796.

David, Miriam E. (2002). Introduction: Themed Section on Evidence-Based Policy as a Concept for Modernising Governance and Social Science Research. *Social Policy and Society*, 1 (3), 213–214.

Davidoff, Leonore, Megan Doolittle, Janet Fink, and Katherine Holden (1999). *The Family Story: Blood Contract and Intimacy*, 1830–1960. London and New York: Longman.

DCN (2012). So How Did It All Begin? Sheila Cooke Describes How the Dc Network Began. *Donor Conception Network Website.* Retrieved from http:// www.donor-conception-network.org/ dcn_history.htm (last accessed: 19.7.2012).

Delaney, Carol (1986). The Meaning of Paternity in the Virgin Birth Debate Man. *Man*, 21 (3).

Dewey, John, and Arthur F. Bentley (1945). A Terminology for Knowings and Knowns. *The Journal of Philosophy*, 42 (9), 225–247.

DI Kind (2007). *DI Kind.* [DI child – website of a donor conceived German woman in her thirties]. Retrieved from www.di-kind.de (last accessed: 30.03.2008).

Diedrich, Klaus, Ricardo Felderbaum, Georg Griesinger, Hermann Hepp, Hartmut Kreß, and Ulrike Riedel (2008). Reproduktionsmedizin im internationalen Vergleich. Wissenschaftlicher Sachstand, medizinische Versorgung und gesetzlicher Regelungsbedarf. *Gutachten im Auftrag der Friedrich-Ebert-Stiftung*. Berlin: Stabsabteilung der Friedrich-Ebert-Stiftung.

Dietzsch, Ina, Wolfgang Kaschuba, and Leonore Scholze-Irrlitz (eds.) (2009). *Horizonte Ethnografischen Wissens. Eine Bestandsaufnahme.* Wien: Böhlau.

Donovan, Catherine (2006). Genetics, Fathers, and Families: Exploring the Implications of Changing the Law in Favour of Identifying Sperm Donors. *Social and Legal Studies*, 15 (4), 449–510.

Dreaper, Jane (13.08.2006). Meeting the Sperm Donor Family. *BBC News Online.* Retrieved from http:// news.bbc.co.uk/ 2/ hi/ health/ 4785187.stm (last accessed 7.9.2010).

Duster, Troy (2003). Buried Alive: The Concept of Race in Science. In Alan H. Goodman, Deborah Heath and M. Susan Lindee (eds.) *Genetic Nature/Culture: Anthropology and Science Beyond the Two-Culture Divide*, 258–278. Berkeley: University of California Press.

Edwards, Jeanette (1999). Explicit Connections: Ethnographic Inquiry in North West England. In Jeanette Edwards, Sarah Franklin, Eric Hirsch, Frances Price and Marilyn Strathern (eds.) *Technologies of Procreation: Kinship in the Age of Assisted Conception*, 61–87. London: Routledge.

Edwards, Jeanette (2000). *Born and Bred: Idioms of Kinship and New Reproductive Technologies in England.* Oxford: Oxford University Press.

Edwards, Jeanette (2006). Reflecting on the 'Euro' in 'Euro-American Kinship': Lithuania and the United Kingdom. *Acta Historica Universitatis Klaipendensis*, XIII, 129–139.

Edwards, Jeanette (2009a). The Ancestor in the Machine. *CRESC Working Paper Series*, 71, 2–21. Retrieved from http:// www.cresc.ac.uk/ sites/ default/ files/ wp %2071.pdf (last accessed: 15.8.2011).

Edwards, Jeanette (2009b). The Matter in Kinship. In Jeanette Edwards and Carles Salazar (eds.) *European Kinship in the Age of Biotechnology*, 1–19. Oxford: Berghahn.

Edwards, Jeanette, Sarah Franklin, Eric Hirsch, Frances Price, and Marilyn Strathern (eds.) (1999). *Technologies of Procreation: Kinship in the Age of Assisted Conception.* London: Routledge.

Edwards, Jeanette, and Carles Salazar (eds.) (2009). *European Kinship in the Age of Biotechnology.* Oxford: Berghahn.

Elliott, Shean J. (2011). Congenital Cytomegalovirus Infection: An Overview. *Infectious Disorders-Drug Targets*, 11 (5), 432–436.

Emerson, Robert M., Rachel I. Fretz, and Linda L. Shaw (1995). Processing Fieldnotes: Coding and Memoing. In Robert M. Emerson, Rachel I. Fretz and Linda L. Shaw (eds.) *Writing Ethnographic Fieldnotes*, 142–168. Chicago: University of Chicago Press.

Epstein, Steven (1995). The Construction of Lay Expertise: Aids Activism and the Forging of Credibility in the Reform of Clinical Trials. *Science, Technology and Human Values*, 20 (4), 408–437.

Epstein, Steven (1996). *Impure Science. Aids, Activism, and the Politics of Knowledge.* Berkeley: University of California Press.

ESchG. (1990). German Government 13.12.1990. *Embryonenschutzgesetz.*

Färber, Alexa (2009). Das unternehmerische ethnografische Selbst. Aspekte der Intensivierung von Arbeit im ethnologisch-ethnografischen Feldforschungsparadigma. In Ina Dietzsch, Wolfgang Kaschuba and Leonore Scholze-Irrlitz (eds.) *Horizonte Ethnografischen Wissens.* Eine Bestandsaufnahme, 178–203. Böhlau.

Faubion, James D., and George E. Marcus (2009). *Fieldwork Is Not What It Used to Be: Learning Anthropology's Method in a Time of Transition.* Ithaca: Cornell University Press.

Featherstone, Katie (2006). *Risky Relations: Family, Kinship and the New Genetics.* Oxford: Berg.

Finkler, Kaja, Cecile Skrzynia, and James P. Evans (2003). The New Genetics and its Consequences for Family, Kinship, Medicine and Medical Genetics. *Social Science and Medicine*, 57 (3), 403–412.

Finkler, Kaya (2000). *Experiencing the New Genetics. Family and Kinship on the Medical Frontier.* Philadelphia: University of Pennsylvania Press.

Finkler, Kaya (2001). The Kin in the Gene. The Medicalization of Family and Kinship in American Society. *Current Anthropology*, 42 (2), 235–263.

Finkler, Kaya (2005). Family, Kinship, Memory and Temporality in the Age of the New Genetics. *Social Science and Medicine*, 61 (5), 1059–1071.

Firth, Raymond (1954). Social Organisation and Social Change. *The Journal of the Royal Anthropological Institute*, 84 (1/2), 1–20.

Fishburne Collier, Jane, and Silvia Junko Yanagisako (eds.) (1987). *Gender and Kinship. Essays toward a Unified Analysis.* Stanford, California: Stanford University Press.

Foucault, Michel (2000). Die "Gouvernementalität" (Vorlesung 1. Februar 1978). In Ulrich Bröckling, Susanne Krasmann and Thomas Lemke (eds.) *Gouvernemental-*

ität der Gegenwart. Studien zur Ökonomisierung des Sozialen, 41–67. Frankfurt a. M.: Suhrkamp.

Fox Keller, Evelyn (1995). The Body of a New Machine: Situating the Organism between Telegraphs and Computers. In Evelyn Fox Keller (ed.) *Refiguring Life. Metaphors of Twentieth-Century Biology*, 79–118. New York: Columbia University Press.

Fox, Renee C., and Judith P. Swazey (1992). *Spare Parts: Organ Replacement in American Society*. New York: Oxford University Press.

Franklin, Sarah (1995). Science as Culture, Cultures of Science. *Annual Review of Anthropology*, 24, 163–184.

Franklin, Sarah (1997a). Conception among the Anthropologists. *Embodied Progress: A Cultural Account of Assisted Conception*, 17–73. London: Routledge.

Franklin, Sarah (1997b). *Embodied Progress: A Cultural Account of Assisted Conception*. London: Routledge.

Franklin, Sarah (2001). Biologization Revisited: Kinship Theory in the Context of the New Biologies. In Sarah Franklin and Susan McKinnon (eds.) *Relative Values: Reconfiguring Kinship Studies*, 302–328. Durham, NC: Duke University Press.

Franklin, Sarah (2006). Embryonic Economies: The Double Reproductive Value of Stem Cells. *BioSocieties*, 1 (1), 71–90.

Franklin, Sarah (2012). Five Million Miracle Babies Later: The Biocultural Legacies of IVF. In Michi Knecht, Maren Klotz and Stefan Beck (eds.) *Reproductive Technologies as Global Form. Ethnographies of Knowledge, Practices, and Transnational Encounters*, 27–60. Frankfurt: Campus.

Franklin, Sarah, and Susan McKinnon (eds.) (2001). *Relative Values: Reconfiguring Kinship Studies*. Durham, NC: Duke University Press.

Frean, Alexandra (21.04.2004). Register Can Trace Donor Relatives. *The Times*.

Freeman, Tabitha, Vasanti Jadva, Wendy Kramer, and Susan Golombok (2009). Gamete Donation: Parents' Experiences of Searching for Their Child's Donor Siblings and Donor. *Human Reproduction*, 24 (3), 505–516.

Fung, Archon, Mary Graham, and David Weil (2007). *Full Disclosure: The Perils and Promise of Transparency*. Cambridge: Cambridge University Press.

Gamble, Natalie, and Louisa Ghevaert (2009). The Human Fertilisation and Embryology Act 2008: Revolution or Evolution? *Family Law*, 8, 730–733.

Gay y Blasco, Paloma, and Huon Wardle (2007a). Comparison. The Ethnographic Outlook. In *How to Read Ethnography*, 13–35. Abingdon [England]; New York: Routledge.

Gay y Blasco, Paloma, and Huon Wardle (2007b). *How to Read Ethnography*. Abingdon [England]; New York: Routledge.

Geertz, Clifford (1988). *Works and Lives: The Anthropologist as Author*. Palo Alto: Stanford University Press.

GewebeG. (2007). German Government 20.7.07. *Transplantationsgesetz (Revision): Gesetz über die Spende, Entnahme und Übertragung von Organen und Geweben* (BGBl. I S. 1574).

GEZEIT (1994). Gender is not Something which one puts on – an Interview with Judith Butler. *GEZEIT Zeitschrift der Fakultätsvertretung Geisteswissenschaften Universität Wien*, 3.

Gibbon, Sahra (2002). Re-Examining Geneticization: Family Trees in Breast Cancer Genetics. *Science as Culture*, 11 (4), 429–457.

Gingrich, André, and Richard Gabriel Fox (2002). *Anthropology, by Comparison*. London: Routledge.

Golombok, Susan, Anne Brewaeys, M.T. Giavazzi, D. Guerra, Fiona Mac Callum, and John Rust (2002). The European Study of Assisted Reproduction Families: The Transition into Adolescence. *Human Reproduction*, 17, 830–840.

Golombok, Susan, Emma Lycett, Fiona MacCallum, Clare Murray, John Rust, Hossam Abdella, and Raoul Margara (2004). Parenting Infants Conceived by Gamete Donation. *Journal of Family Psychology*, 18, 443–452.

Goodenough, Ward H. (1986). Navigation in the Western Carolines: A Traditional Science. In Laura Nader (ed.) *Naked Science. Anthropological Inquiry into Boundaries, Power, and Knowledge*, 29–42. New York and London: Routledge.

Goodman, Alan H., Deborah Heath, and M. Susan Lindee (2003). *Genetic Nature/Culture: Anthropology and Science Beyond the Two-Culture Divide*. Berkeley: University of California Press.

Goody, Jack (ed.). (1971). *Kinship: Selected Readings*. Harmondsworth: Penguin Books.

Göttsch, Silke, and Albrecht Lehmann (eds.) (2007). *Methoden der Volkskunde. Positionen, Quellen, Arbeitsweisen der Europäischen Ethnologie*. Berlin: Reimer.

Grabow, Karsten, and Uwe Jun (2008). *Mehr Expertise in der deutschen Politik? Zur Übertragbarkeit des "Evidence-Based Policy Approach"*. Gütersloh: Bertelsmann Stiftung.

Graumann, Sigrid. (2007). Risiken und Belastungen für die betroffenen Frauen. Paper presented at the Workshop: "Umwege zum eigenen Kind: Verfügbarkeit donogener Reproduktionstechniken", Zentrum für Medizinrecht Göttingen, Göttingen (22.7.2007).

Green, Sarah, Penny Harvey, and Hannah Knox (2005). Scales of Place and Networks: An Ethnography of the Imperative to Connect through Information and Communications Technologies. *Current Anthropology*, 46 (5), 805–826.

Griffiths, John (2003). The Social Working of Legal Rules. *Journal of Legal Pluralism*, 48, 1–84.

Haarhoff, Heike (6.10.2007). Vater: Unbekannt. *taz*.

Hacking, Ian (2000). *The Social Construction of What?* Cambridge, Mass.: Harvard University Press.

Haimes, Erica (1990). Recreating the Family. Policy Considerations Relating to the 'New' Reproductive Technologies. In Maureen McNeil, Ian Varcoe and Steven Yearley (eds.) *The New Reproductive Technologies*, 154–172. London: Macmillan.

Haimes, Erica (1998). The Making of 'the DI Child': Changing Representations of People Conceived through Donor Insemination. In Ken Daniels and Erica

Haimes (eds.) *Donor Insemination: International Social Science Perspectives*, 53–76. Cambridge ; New York: Cambridge University Press.

Haimes, Erica (2003). Embodied Spaces, Social Places and Bourdieu: Locating and Dislocating the Child in Family Relationships. *Body and Society*, 9 (1), 11–33.

Haimes, Erica (2006). Social and Ethical Issues in the Use of Familial Searching in Forensic Investigations: Insights from Family and Kinship Studies. *Journal of Law, Medicine and Ethics*, 34 (2).

Haimes, Erica, Kenneth Taylor, and Ilke Turkmendag (2012). Eggs, Ethics and Exploitation? Investigating Women's Experiences of an Egg Sharing Scheme. *Sociology of Health and Illness*, 34 (8).

Hall, Stuart (1996). New Ethnicities. In David Morley (ed.) *Stuart Hall*, 440–450. London: Routledge.

Hamra, Sulamith (2007). Eltern-TÜV? – Standardisierung und Normalisierung von Elternschaft am Beispiel von Adoptionsbewerbern und Adoptiveltern. E-Publishing Humboldt-Universität zu Berlin, Magisterarbeit. Retrieved from http:// nbn-resolving.de/ urn:nbn:de:kobv: 11–10081278 (last accessed: 15.4.2009).

Han, Byung-Chul (2012). *Transparenzgesellschaft*. Berlin: Matthes and Seitz Berlin.

Haraway, Donna (1997). *Modest_Witness@Second:Millenium*. New York: Routledge.

Hargreaves, Katrina (2006). Constructing Families and Kinship through Donor Insemination. *Sociology of Health and Illness*, 28 (3), 261–283.

Harris, Christopher Charles (1990). *Kinship. Concepts in Social Science*. Buckingham: Open University Press.

Hastrup, Kirsten (2004). Getting It Right: Knowledge and Evidence in Anthropology. *Anthropological Theory*, 4 (4), 455–472.

Hauser-Schäublin, Brigitta, Vera Kalitkus, Imme Peterson, and Iris Schröder (eds.) (2000). *Der Geteilte Leib. Die kulturelle Dimension von Organtransplantation und Reproduktionsmedizin in Deutschland*. Frankfurt a. M. : Campus.

Hauskeller, Christine (2004). How Traditions of Ethical Reasoning and Institutional Processes Shape Stem Cell Research in Britain. *Journal of Medicine and Philosophy*, 29 (5), 509–532.

Hauskeller, Christine (2006). Human Genomics as Identity Politics. Cornell University Center for Ethics and Public life. Retrieved from http:// www.genomicsnetwork.ac.uk/ media/ Microsoft %20Word %20-%20Identity %20Politics%20revised%20acknowl%20(2).pdf (last accessed: 18.03.2012).

Hauskeller, Christine (2009). The Genetic Re-Making of Human Identity and Why It Should Not Be Trusted. *Photo-ID: Photographers and Scientists Explore Identity*, 37–49. Norwich: Wellcome Trust/Norfolk Contemporary Art Society.

Heimerdinger, Timo (2011). Pacifiers and Fairies: Family Culture as Risk Management—a German Example. *Journal of Folklore Research*, 48 (2), 197–211.

Helfferich, Cornelia (2005). *Die Qualität qualitativer Daten*. Wiesbaden: VS Verlag für Sozialwissenschaften.

Hertz, Rosanna, and Jane Mattes (2011). Donor-Shared Siblings or Genetic Strangers: New Families, Clans, and the Internet. *Journal of Family Issues*, 32 (9), 1129–1155.

HFEA (2002). *Response to the Department of Health's Consultation on Donor Information.* Human Fertilisation and Embryology Authority. Retrieved from http:// www.hfea.gov.uk/ AboutHFEA/ Consultations/ Donor%20Info%20response.pdf (last accessed: 01.08.2006).

HFEA (2009a). *Code of Practice (8th Edition).* Human Fertilisation and Embryology Authority in accordance with section 26(4) of the Human Fertilisation and Embryology Act 1990. (Revisions April 2010, April 2011).

HFEA (2009b). *Opening the Register Policy – a Principled Approach.* HFEA Authority Paper. Retrieved from www.hfea.gov.uk/ docs/ AM_Item_9_Jan09.pdf (last accessed: 22.11.2011).

HFEA (2009c). *Summary of Access Rights.* Human Fertilisation and Embryology Authority. Retrieved from http:// www.hfea.gov.uk/ docs/ Summary_of_Access_-Rights.pdf (last accessed: 9.6.2012).

HFEA (2011a). *Business Plan 2012/2013.* Retrieved from www.hfea.gov.uk/ docs/ 2012–03–30_-_Business_Plan_-_DH_approved_publication_v1_pdf_-_-2012–2013.PDF (last accessed: 9.07.2012).

HFEA (2011b). *Facts and Figures: New Donor Registrations.* Retrieved from http:// www.hfea.gov.uk/3411.html (last accessed: 18.5.2012).

HFEA (2011c). *HFEA Agrees New Policies to Improve Sperm and Egg Donation Services.* Press Release 19.10.2011. Retrieved from http:// www.hfea.gov.uk/ 6700.html (last accessed: 25.10.2011).

Hirschauer, Stefan (2001). Ethnographisches Schreiben und die Schweigsamkeit des Sozialen. Zu einer Methodologie der Beschreibung. *Zeitschrift für Soziologie*, 30 (6), 429–451.

Hoeyer, Klaus (2010). An Anthropological Analysis of European Union (EU) Health Governance as Biopolitics: The Case of the EU Tissues and Cells Directive. *Social Science and Medicine*, 70, 1867–1873.

Homer, Nils, Szabolcs Szelinger, Margot Redman, David Duggan, Waibhav Tembe, Jill Muehling, et al. (2008). Resolving Individuals Contributing Trace Amounts of DNA to Highly Complex Mixtures Using High-Density SNP Genotyping Microarrays. *PLoS* Genetics, 4 (8), e1000167.

Howell, Signe (2001). Self-Conscious Kinship. Some Contested Values in Norwegian Transnational Adoption. In Sarah Franklin and Susan McKinnon (eds.) *Relative Values: Reconfiguring Kinship Studies*, 203–223. Durham, NC: Duke University Press.

Howell, Signe (2006). *The Kinning of Foreigners: Transnational Adoption in a Global Perspective.* Oxford and New York: Berghahn Books.

Human Rights Act. (1998). UK Government. *Human Rights Act.*

Ilkilic, Ilhan (2002). *Die aktuelle Biomedizin aus der Sicht des Islam.* Ein Gutachten erstellt im Auftrag der AG Bioethik und Wissenschaftskommunikation des Max-Delbrück-Centrums für molekulare Medizin, Berlin-Buch.

Imber-Black, E. (ed.). (1993). *Secrets in Family and Family Therapy.* New York: W.W. Norton.

Ingold, Tim (2000). *The Perception of the Environment: Essays on Livelihood, Dwelling and Skill.* London; New York: Routledge.

Ingold, Tim (2007). *Lines: A Brief History.* New York: Routledge.

Ingold, Tim (2008). Anthropology Is Not Ethnography. *Proceedings of the British Academy,* 154, 69–92.

Jasanoff, Sheila (2005). *Designs on Nature: Science and Democracy in Europe and the United States.* Princeton, N.J.: Princeton University Press.

Jeggle, Utz (ed.). (1984). *Feldforschung.* Tübingen.

Johnson, Martin (1999). A Biomedical Perspective on Parenthood. In Andrew Bainham, Shelley Day Sclater, Martin Richards and Cambridge Socio-Legal Group. (eds.) *What Is a Parent? A Socio-Legal Analysis.* Oxford: Hart.

Jones, Howard W., Ian Cooke, Roger Kempers, Peter Brinsden, and Doug Saunders (2010). International Federation of Fertility Societies Surveillance 2010. *Fertility and Sterility,* 95 (2), 43–62.

Katz Rothman, Barbara (2005). *Weaving a Family: Untangling Race and Adoption:* Beacon Press.

Katzorke, Thomas (2008). Entstehung und Entwicklung der Spendersamenbehandlung in Deutschland. In Gisela Bockenheimer-Lucius, Petra Thorn and Christiane Wendehorst (eds.) *Göttinger Schriften zum Medizinrecht,* 3, 89–103. Göttingen: Universitätsverlag.

Kay, Lilly (2000). *Who Wrote the Book of Life? A History of the Genetic Code.* Palo Alto: Stanford University Press.

Keesing, Roger M. (1975). *Kin Groups and Social Structure.* New York: Holt.

KindRVerbG. (2002). German Government 09.04.2002. *Kinderrechteverbesserungsgesetz* (BGBl I, 1239).

Kittles, Rick, and Charmaine Royal (2003). The Genetics of African Americans: Implications for Disease Gene Mapping and Identity. In Alan H. Goodman, Deborah Heath and M. Susan Lindee (eds.) *Genetic Nature/Culture: Anthropology and Science Beyond the Two-Culture Divide,* 219–234. Berkeley: University of California Press.

Klock, Susan (1997). The Controversy Surrounding Privacy or Disclosure among Donor Gamete Recipients. *Journal of Assisted Reproduction and Genetics,* 14 (7), 378–380.

Klotz, Maren (2006). *Hello Daddy! The Construction of Gamete Donors and Their Kin-Relations in UK Regulatory Discourse on Donor Anonymity.* Unpublished MSc Thesis, University of Exeter, Exeter.

Klotz, Maren (2007). Doing Kinship in British Parliament: Selfish Parents – Disruptive Children? In Stefan Beck, Nevim Cil, Sabine Hess, Maren Klotz and

Michi Knecht (eds.) *Verwandtschaft machen. Reproduktionsmedizin und Adoption in Deutschland und der Türkei*, 80–91. Berlin: LIT.

Klotz, Maren (2009). Verwandtschaft wissen. Regulatives und familiäres "Wissens-Management" im Bereich assistierter Reproduktion. In Michael Simon, Thomas Hengartner, Timo Heimerdinger and Anne-Christin Lux (eds.) *Bilder, Bücher, Bytes – zur Medialität des Alltags.*, 128–137. Münster: Waxmann.

Klotz, Maren (2011). Wissensmanagement bei Keimzellspende. *Journal für Reproduktionsmedizin und Endokrinologie*, 8 (1), 1.

Klotz, Maren (2012). Making Connections: Reflecting on Trains, Kinship, and Information Technology. In Michi Knecht, Maren Klotz and Stefan Beck (eds.) *Reproductive Technologies as Global Form. Ethnographies of Knowledge, Practices, and Transnational Encounters*, 111–138. Frankfurt: Campus.

Klotz, Maren, and Michi Knecht (2009). Wissenswege Lokal – Global: Zur Ethnographie von Wissenspraxen und Regulationsformen im Umgang mit Reproduktionstechnologien. In Sonja Windmüller, Beate Binder and Thomas Hengartner (eds.) *Kultur – Forschung: Zum Profil einer volkskundlichen Kulturwissenschaft*, 211–237. Münster: LIT.

Klotz, Maren, and Michi Knecht (2012). What Is Europeanization in the Field of Assisted Reproductive Technologies? In Michi Knecht, Maren Klotz and Stefan Beck (eds.) *Reproductive Technologies as Global Form. Ethnographies of Knowledge, Practices, and Transnational Encounters*, 283–305. Frankfurt: Campus.

Knecht, Michi (2003). Die Politik der Verwandtschaft neu denken. Perspektiven der Kultur- und Sozialanthropologie. In Zentrum für transdisziplinäre Geschlechterstudien der Humboldt Universität zu Berlin (ed.) *Warum noch Familie?*, 52–70.

Knecht, Michi (2009a). Contemporary uses of Ethnography. Zur Politik, Spezifik und gegenwartskulturellen Relevanz ethnographischer Texte. In Michael Simon, Thomas Hengartner, Timo Heimerdinger and Anne-Christin Lux (eds.) *Bilder, Bücher, Bytes – zur Medialität des Alltags.*, 148–155. Münster: Waxmann.

Knecht, Michi (2009b). Der Imperativ, sich zu verbinden: Neue kulturanthropologische Forschungen zu Verwandtschaft in europäischen Gegenwartsgesellschaften. *Österreichische Zeitschrift für Volkskunde*, 112 (2), 27–51.

Knecht, Michi (2010). Ethnographische und Historische Zugänge zu Samenbanken und Samenspendern. In Michi Knecht, Anna Frederike Heinitz, Scout Burghardt and Sebastian Mohr (eds.) *Samenbanken – Samenspender. Ethnographische und Historische Perspektiven auf Männlichkeiten in der Reproduktionsmedizin*, 6–29. Münster: LIT.

Knecht, Michi (forthcoming). Die soziale Produktivität von Anonymität – Ein Forschungsprogramm (Antrittsvorlesung 24.4.2012). *Deutsche Zeitschrift für Volkskunde.*

Knecht, Michi, Anna Frederike Heinitz, Scout Burghardt, and Sebastian Mohr (eds.) (2010). *Samenbanken – Samenspender. Ethnographische und Historische Perspektiven auf Männlichkeiten in der Reproduktionsmedizin.* Berlin: Panama.

Knecht, Michi, and Sabine Hess (2008). Reflexive Medikalisierung im Feld moderner Reproduktionsmedizin. Zum aktiven Einsatz von Wissensressourcen in gendertheoretischer Perspektive. In Nikola Langreiter and Elisabeth Timm (eds.) *Wissen und Geschlecht*, 169–194. Wien: Veröffentlichungen des Instituts für Europäische Ethnologie.

Knecht, Michi, Maren Klotz, and Stefan Beck (eds.) (2012). *Reproductive Technologies as Global Form. Ethnographies of Knowledge, Practices, and Transnational Encounters*. Frankfurt: Campus.

Knecht, Michi, Maren Klotz, Nurhak Polat, and Stefan Beck (2011). Erweiterte Fallstudien zu Verwandtschaft und Reproduktionstechnologien: Potentiale einer Ethnographie von Normalisierungsprozessen. *Zeitschrift für Volkskunde*, 107 (1), 21–48.

Knoll, Eva-Maria (2012). Reproducing Hungarians: Reflections on Fuzzy Boundaries in Reproductive Border Crossing. In Michi Knecht, Maren Klotz and Stefan Beck (eds.) *Reproductive Technologies as Global Form. Ethnographies of Knowledge, Practices, and Transnational Encounters*, 255–283. Frankfurt: Campus.

Konrad, Monica (1998). Ova Donation and Symbols of Substance: Some Variations on the Theme of Sex, Gender and the Partible Body. *Journal of the Royal Anthropological Institute*, 4 (4), 643–667.

Konrad, Monica (2005a). *Nameless Relations: Anonymity, Melanesia and Reproductive Gift Exchange between British Ova Donors and Recipients*. New York and Oxford: Berghahn.

Konrad, Monica (2005b). *Narrating the New Predictive Genetics: Ethics, Ethnography, and Science*. Cambridge, UK; New York: Cambridge University Press.

Lambert, Victoria (21.12.2009). Challenging Donor Anonymity: Tracing My Father Could Save My Life. *Daily Telegraph*. Retrieved from http://www.telegraph.co.uk/health/ 6840705/ sperm-donor-IVF-mantle-cell-lymphoma.html (last accessed 20.04.2012).

Latour, Bruno (1987). *Science in Action: How to Follow Scientists and Engineers through Society*. Milton Keynes: Open University Press.

Latour, Bruno (1993). *We Have Never Been Modern*. Cambridge, Massachusetts: Harvard University Press.

Latour, Bruno (1999). *Pandora's Hope*. Cambridge, Massachusetts: Harvard University Press.

Latour, Bruno (2004). How to Talk About the Body? The Normative Dimension of Science Studies. *Body and Society*, 10 (2–3), 205–229.

Latour, Bruno (2005). *Reassembling the Social*. Oxford; New York: Oxford University Press.

Lave, Jean, and Etienne Wegner (1991). *Situated Learning*. Cambridge: Cambridge University Press.

Leighton, Kimberly (2012). Addressing the Harms of Not Knowing One's Heredity: Lessons from Genealogical Bewilderment. *Adoption and Culture*, 3, 63–107.

Levinson, Jack (2010). *Making Life Work. Freedom and Disability in a Community Group Home.* Minneapolis: University of Minnesota Press.

Liberty (2002). *Donor Insemination Case – Children Can Claim Right to Personal Identity* (Press Release 26.07.2002). Retrieved from http://www.liberty-human-rights.org.uk/press/press-releases-2002/index.shtml (last accessed: 1.8.2005).

Liesnard, Corinne, P. Revelard, and Yvonne Englert (1998). Is Matching between Women and Donors Feasible to Avoid Cytomegalovirus Infection in Artificial Insemination with Donor Semen? *Human Reproduction*, 13 (suppl 2), 25–31.

Liew, Anthony (2007). Understanding Data, Information, Knowledge, and Their Interrelationships. *Journal of Knowledge Management Practice*, 8 (2).

Lipp, Carola (2005). Kinship Networks, Local Government, and Elections in a Town in Southwest Germany, 1800–1850. *Journal of Family History*, 30 (4), 347–365.

Lippman, Abby (1992). Led (Astray) by Genetic Maps: The Cartography of the Human Genome and Health Care. *Social Science and Medicine*, 35, 1469–1476.

Lock, Margret M., and Patricia Alice Kaufert (1998). *Pragmatic Women and Body Politics.* Cambridge: Cambridge University Press.

LSVD (ed.). (2007). *Regenbogenfamilien – alltäglich und doch anders.* Köln: Selbstverlag des Familien- und Sozialvereins des Lesben- und Schwulenverbandes in Deutschland e.V.

Lycett, Emma, Ken Daniels, Ruth Curson, B. Chir, and Susan Golombok (2004). Offspring Created as a Result of Donor Insemination: A Study of Family Relationships, Child Adjustment, and Disclosure. *Fertil Steril*, 82, 172–179.

Malinowski, Bronislaw (1948). Baloma. The Spirits of the Dead in the Trobriand Islands. In Bronislaw Malinowski (ed.) *Magic, Science and Religion*, 149–274. New York: Anchor Books.

Malinowski, Bronislaw (1957). *The Sexual Life of Savages in North Western Melanesia.* London: Routledge.

Mamo, Laura (2005). Biomedicalizing Kinship. Sperm Banks and the Creation of Affinity-Ties. *Science as Culture*, 14 (3), 237–264.

Marquardt, James J. (2011). *Transparency and American Primacy in World Politics.* Farnham: Ashgate.

Marre, Diana, and Joan Bestard (2009). The Family Body: Persons, Bodies and Resemblance. In Jeanette Edwards and Carles Salazar (eds.) *European Kinship in the Age of Biotechnology*, 64–78. Oxford: Berghahn.

Mattes, Jane (1994). *Single Mothers by Choice: A Guidebook for Single Women Who Are Considering or Have Chosen Motherhood.* New York: Times Books.

Mauss, Marcel (1990). *The Gift: Forms and Functions of Exchange in Archaic Societies.* New York: Norton.

McCarthy, Doyle E. (1996). *Knowledge as Culture. The New Sociology of Knowledge.* London and New York: Routledge.

McKinnon, Susan (2001). The Economies in Kinship and the Paternity of Culture: Origin Stories in Kinship Theory. In Sarah Franklin and Susan McKinnon (eds.)

Relative Values: Reconfiguring Kinship Studies, 277–302. Durham, NC: Duke University Press.

Miller, Peter, and Nikolas Rose (2008). *Governing the Present: Administering Economic, Social and Personal Life*. Cambridge: Polity.

Mol, Annemarie (2002). *The Body Multiple: Ontology in Medical Practice*. Durham: Duke University Press.

Mol, Annemarie, and John Law (2004). Embodied Action, Enacted Bodies: The Example of Hypoglycemia. *Body and Society*, 10 (2–3), 43–62.

Montuschi, Olivia (2006a). *Telling and Talking: Telling and Talking About Donor Conception with 0–7 Year Olds. A Guide for Parents*. Nottingham: Donor Conception Network.

Montuschi, Olivia (2006b). *Telling and Talking: Telling and Talking About Donor Conception with 8–11 Year Olds. A Guide for Parents*. Nottingham: Donor Conception Network.

Morrison, Blake (11.03. 2006). A Generous Donation. *The Guardian*. Retrieved from http://www.guardian.co.uk/lifeandstyle/2006/mar/11/familyandrelationships.family2 (last accessed 10.08.2006).

Moss, Lenny (2003). *What Genes Can't Do*. Cambridge, Massachusetts: MIT Press.

Motluk, Alison (2005). Anonymous Sperm Donor Traced on Internet. *The New Scientist*, 2524, 6.

Murray, Clare, Fiona MacCallum, and Susan Golombok (2006). Egg Donation Parents and Their Children: Follow-up at Age 12 Years. *Fertility and Sterility*, 85 (3), 610–618.

Nahman, Michal (2012). Making Interferences: The Cultural Politics of Transnational Ova "Donation". In Michi Knecht, Maren Klotz and Stefan Beck (eds.) *Reproductive Technologies as Global Form. Ethnographies of Knowledge, Practices, and Transnational Encounters*, 305–331. Frankfurt: Campus.

Nahmann, Michal (2006). Materializing Israeliness: Difference and Mixture in Transnational Ova Donation. *Science as Culture*, 15 (3), 199–213.

Nash, Catherine (2005). Geographies of Relatedness. *Transactions of the Institute of British Geographers*, 30, 449–462.

NatureNews (2008). DNA Databases Shut after Identities Compromised. *Nature*, 455, 13.

Nelkin, Dorothy, and M. Susan Lindee (1995). The Molecular Family. In *The DNA Mystique*, 58–78. New York: Freeman.

Niewöhner, Jörg, and Thomas Scheffer (2010). Thickening Comparison: On the Multiple Facets of Comparability. In Thomas Scheffer and Jörg Niewöhner (eds.) *Thick Comparison. Reviving the Ethnographic Aspiration*, 1–17. Leiden and Boston: Brill.

Novas, Carlos, and Nikolas Rose (2000). Genetic Risk and the Birth of the Somatic Individual. *Economy and Society*, 29 (4), 485–513.

O'Donovan, Katherine (1990). "What Shall We Tell the Children?": Reflections on Children's Perspectives and the Sexual Revolution. In D. Morgan and R. Lee (eds.) *Birthrights: Law and Ethics at the Beginnings of Life*, 96–114. London: Routledge.

Offord, Jane, Angela Mays, Sheila Cooke, and Julie Heath (Illustrations) (1991). *My Story: For Children Conceived by Donor Insemination*. Infertility Research Trust. Jessop Hospital for Women. Sheffield: J.W. Northend Ltd.

Ortner, Sherry B. (1984). Theory in Anthropology since the Sixties. *Comparative Studies in Society and History*, 26 (1), 126–166.

Peletz, Michael G. (1995). Kinship Studies in Late Twentieth-Century Anthropology. *Annual Review of Anthropology*, 24, 343–372.

Petersen, Imme (2000). *Konzepte und Bedeutung von "Verwandtschaft": Eine ethnologische Analyse der Parlamentsdebatten zum bundesdeutschen Embryonenschutzgesetz*. Herbolzheim: Centaurus.

Pickering, Andrew (1995). *The Mangle of Practice – Time, Agency and Science*. Chicago: Chicago University Press.

Polanyi, Michael (1973). *Personal Knowledge: Towards a Post-Critical Philosophy*. London: Routledge and Kegan Paul.

Polat, Nurhak (2012). Concerned Groups in the Field of Reproductive Technologies: A Turkish Case Study. In Michi Knecht, Maren Klotz and Stefan Beck (eds.) *Reproductive Technologies as Global Form. Ethnographies of Knowledge, Practices, and Transnational Encounters*, 197–228. Frankfurt: Campus.

PräimpG. (2011). German Government 8.12.11. *Gesetz zur Regelung der Präimplantationsdiagnostik* (BGBl. I S. 2228).

Pratt, Mary (1986). Fieldwork in Common Places. In James Clifford and George E. Marcus (eds.) *Writing Culture: The Poetics and Politics of Ethnography*, 27–50. Berkeley: University of California Press.

Price, Frances (1995). Conceiving Relations – Egg and Sperm Donation in Assisted Procreation. In Andrew Bainham, David Pearl and Ros Pickford (eds.) *Frontiers of Family Law*, 176–186. Chichester: Wiley and Son.

Pryer, Nick (22.2.2010). Despair of the DNA Sisters: In Terrible Mistake That Casts New Doubt on DNA Profiling, It Turns out They Weren't Related at All. *Daily Mail*. Retrieved from http://www.dailymail.co.uk/femail/article-1252590/Despair-DNA-sisters-In-terrible-mistake-casts-new-doubt-DNA-profiling-turns-werent-related-all.html (last accessed 10.11.2011).

Pulman, Bertrand (2004/5). Malinowski and Ignorance of Physical Paternity. *Review Française de Sociologie*, 45, 121–142.

Rabeharisoa, Vololona, and Michel Callon (2002). The Involvement of Patients' Associations in Research. *International Social Science Journal*, 171, 57–67.

Rabinow, Paul (1996). Artificiality and Enlightenment. From Sociobiology to Biosociality. In Mario Biagioli (ed.) *Essays on the Anthropology of Reason*, 99–103. Princeton: Princeton University Press.

Rabinow, Paul, and Niklas Rose (2006). Biopower Today. *BioSocieties* (1), 195–217.

Ragoné, Helena (2004). Surrogate Motherhood and American Kinship. In Robert Parkin and Linda Stone (eds.) *Kinship and Family: An Anthropological Reader*, 342–361. Malden, Mass., Oxford: Blackwell.

Rapp, Rayna (1999). *Testing Women, Testing the Fetus: The Social Impact of Amniocentesis in America.* New York: Routledge.

Reinecke, Christiane, Jörg Feuchter, Regina Finsterhölzl, Andrea Fischer-Tahir, Friedhelm Hoffmann, Simone Holzwarth, et al. (2010). Wissen und soziale Ordnung. Eine Kritik der Wissensgesellschaft. Mit einem Kommentar von Stefan Beck. *Working Papers des Sonderforschungsbereiches 640*, 1. Retrieved from http://edoc.huberlin.de/series/sfb-640-papers/2010–1/(last accessed: 12.10.2011).

Resolve (2011). *Risks to the Recipient.* Resolve: The National Infertility Association USA. Retrieved from http:// www.resolve.org/ family-building-options/donor-options/using-donor-egg.html (last accessed: 2.8.2012).

Richardt, Nicole (2003). A Comparative Analysis of the Embryological Research Debate in Great Britain and Germany. *Social Politics: International Studies in Gender, State and Society* 10 (1), 86–128.

Roberts, Elizabeth (2011). Abandonment and Accumulation: Embryonic Futures in the United States and Ecuador. *Medical Anthropology Quarterly*, 25 (2), 232–253.

Rose and Anor vs HFEA. (2002). England and Wales High Court. *Rose and Anor Vs Secretary of State for Health Human Fertilisation and Embryology Authority* (1593 (Admin)).

Rubin, Herbert J., and Irene S. Rubin (1995). Qualitative Interviewing. The Art of Hearing Data. London: Sage.

Rumball, Anna, and Vivienne Adair (1999). Telling the Story: Parents' Scripts for Donor Offspring. *Human Reproduction*, 14 (5), 1392–1399.

Rütz, Eva Maria K. (2008). *Heterologe Insemination – Die rechtliche Stellung des Samenspenders.* Berlin: Springer.

Sabean, David Warren, and Simon Teuscher (2007). *Kinship in Europe. Approaches to Long-Term Development.* Oxford: Berghahn.

Scheffer, Thomas, and Jörg Niewöhner (eds.) (2010). *Thick Comparison. Reviving the Ethnographic Aspiration.* Leiden and Boston: Brill.

Schneider, David M. (1968). *American Kinship: A Cultural Account.* Englewood Cliffs: Prentice-Hall.

Schneider, David M. (1984). *A Critique of the Study of Kinship.* Ann Arbor: University of Michigan Press.

Schultze, Ulrike, and Charles Stabell (2004). Knowing What You Don't Know? Discourses and Contradictions in Knowledge Management Research. *Journal of Management Studies*, 41 (4), 549–573.

Searle, John (1969). *Speech Acts.* Cambridge: Cambridge University Press.

Segalen, Martine (2001). The Shift in Kinship Studies in France: The Case of Grandparenting. In Sarah Franklin and Susan McKinnon (eds.) *Relative Values: Reconfiguring Kinship Studies*, 302–328. Durham, NC: Duke University Press.

Sheldon, Sally (2005). Fragmenting Fatherhood: The Regulation of Reproductive Technologies. *The Modern Law Review*, 68 (4), 523–553.

Sifry, Micah L. (2011). *Wikileaks and the Age of Transparency*. New Haven: Yale University Press.

Silverman, David (1993). *Interpreting Qualitative Data*. London: Sage.

Smart, Carol. (2009). Family Secrets: Law and Understandings of Openness in Everyday Relationships. Paper presented at the Workshop: We Are Family? The Genetics and Identity Politics of Parenthood and Family (Fourth workshop of the EGN Work stream on 'Genomics and Identity Politics,' 19th – 20th February 2009), Edinburgh (19.02.2009).

Smart, Carol (2011). Families, Secrets and Memories. *Sociology*, 45 (4), 539–553.

Sperling, Stefan (2011). The Politics of Transparency and Surveillance in Post-Reunification Germany. *Surveillance and Society*, 8 (4), 396–412.

Star, Susan Leigh (1991). Power, Technologies and the Phenomenology of Conventions: On Being Allergic to Onions. In John Law (ed.) *A Sociology of Monsters: Essays on Power, Technology and Domination*, 26–56. London and New York: Routledge.

Star, Susan Leigh (2002). Infrastructure and Ethnographic Practice. Working on the Fringes. *Scandinavian Journal of Information Systems*, 14 (2), 107–122.

Star, Susan Leigh, Geoffrey C. Bowker, and L. J. Neumann (2003). Transparency Beyond the Individual Level of Scale: Convergence between Information Artifacts and Communities of Practice. In Anne Peterson Bishop, Nancy A. Van House and Barbara. P. Buttenfield (eds.) *Digital Library Use: Social Practice in Design and Evaluation*, 241–270. MIT Univ. Press.

Stehr, Nico (1994). *Knowledge Societies*. London: Sage.

Steinke, Ines (2000). Gütekriterien qualitativer Forschung. In Uwe Flick (ed.) *Qualitative Forschung. Ein Handbuch*, 319–331. Reinbek: Rowohlt Taschenbuch.

Strathern, Marilyn (1992a). *After Nature: English Kinship in the Late Twentieth Century*. Cambridge and New York: Cambridge University Press.

Strathern, Marilyn (1992b). *Reproducing the Future: Essays on Anthropology, Kinship and the New Reproductive Technologies*. Manchester: Manchester University Press.

Strathern, Marilyn (1999). Refusing Information. In *Property, Substance, and Effect: Anthropological Essays on Persons and Things*, 64–88. London: Athlone Press.

Strathern, Marilyn (2005). *Kinship, Law and the Unexpected: Relatives Are Always a Surprise*. Cambridge, UK; New York, NY: Cambridge University Press.

Strathern, Marilyn (ed.). (2000). *Audit Cultures: Anthropological Studies in Accountability, Ethics, and the Academy*. London New York: Routledge.

Strauss, Anselm L. (1987). *Qualitative Analysis for Social Scientists*. Cambridge: Cambridge University Press.

Sturdy, Steven. (2009). Genetic Suspects: DNA and Forensic Identification. Paper presented at the Genomics and Identity Politics Workshop Exeter (24.09.2009).

TallBear, Kimberly (2003). DNA, Blood, and Racializing the Tribe. *Wicazo Sa Review*, 18 (1), 81–107.

Thompson, Charis (2001). Strategic Naturalizing: Kinship in an Infertility Clinic. In Sarah Franklin and Susan McKinnon (eds.) *Relative Values: Reconfiguring Kinship Studies*, 175–202. Durham, NC: Duke University Press.

Thompson, Charis (2005). *Making Parents: The Ontological Choreography of Reproductive Technologies.* Cambridge, MA: MIT Press.

Thompson, Charis (2009). Skin Tone and the Persistence of Biological Race in Egg Donation for Assisted Reproduction. In Evelyn Nakano Glenn (ed.) *Shades of Difference: Why Skin Color Matters*, 131–147. Stanford: Stanford University Press.

Thorn, Petra (2008a). Eine Familie… Ist Eine Familie… Ist Eine Familie? In Dorothee Kleinschmidt, Petra Thorn and Tewes Wischmann (eds.) *Kinderwunsch und professionelle Beratung. Das Handbuch des Beratungsnetzwerkes Kinderwunsch Deutschland* (BKiD), 99–106. Stuttgart: Kohlhammer.

Thorn, Petra (2008b). *Familiengründung mit Spendersamen. Ein Ratgeber zu psychosozialen und rechtlichen Fragen.* Stuttgart: Kohlhammer.

Thorn, Petra, and Ken Daniels (2000). Psychosoziale Fragestellungen, Die bei der Familienbildung mit donogener Insemination entstehen. *Reproduktionsmedizin*, 16 (3), 202–207.

Thorn, Petra, and Ken Daniels (2006). Vorbereitung auf die Familienbildung mit donogener Insemination – die Bedeutung edukativer Gruppenseminare. *Reproduktionsmedizin und Endokrinologie*, 3 (1), 49–53.

Thorn, Petra, and Lisa Herrmann-Green (2009). *Die Geschichte unserer Familie. Ein Buch für lesbische Familien mit Wunschkindern durch Samenspende.* Mörfelden: FamArt.

Thorn, Petra, Thomas Katzorke, and Ken Daniels (2008). Semen Donors in Germany: A Study Exploring Motivations and Attitudes. *Human Reproduction*, 23 (11), 2415–2420.

Thorn, Petra, and Tiziana Rinaldi (2006). *Die Geschichte unserer Familie. Ein Buch für Familien, die sich mit Hilfe der Spendersamenbehandlung gebildet haben.* Mörfelden: FamArt.

Timm, Elisabeth (2010). "Ich fühle mich absolut verwandt." Entgrenzung, Personalisierung und Gouvernementalität von Verwandtschaft am Beispiel der populären Genealogie. In Erdmute Alber, Bettina Beer, Julia Pauli and Michael Schnegg (eds.) *Verwandtschaft heute: Positionen, Ergebnisse und Perspektiven*, 47–71. Berlin: Reimer.

Timm, Elisabeth (2011). Genealogie ohne Generationen. Verwandtschaft in der populären Forschung. In Ruth-E. Mohrmann (ed.) *Generationenbeziehungen in Familie und Gesellschaft*, 147–179. Münster: Waxman.

Timm, Elisabeth (2012). Von wem man ist. Ontologien von Familie und Verwandtschaft in Wissenschaft und Alltag. *Recherche: Zeitung für Wissenschaft* (1). Retrieved from www.recherche-online.net/ elisabeth-timm.html (last accessed: 3.12.2013)

Titmuss, Richard M. (1997). *The Gift Relationship: From Human Blood to Social Policy.* London: LSE Books.

Tober, Diane (2001). Semen as Gift, Semen as Goods: Reproductive Workers and the Market in Altruism. *Body and Society*, 7 (2–3), 137.

Turkmendag, Ilke (2012). The Donor-Conceived Child's 'Right to Personal Identity': The Public Debate on Donor Anonymity in the United Kingdom. *Journal of Law and Society*, 39 (1), 58–75.

Tyler, Katharine (2007). Race, Genetics and Inheritance. Reflections Upon the Birth of "Black" Twins to a "White" IVF Mother. In Peter Wade (ed.) *Race, Ethnicity and Nation: Perspectives from Kinship and Genetics*, 33–53. Oxford: Berghahn.

UK Government (1999). *Modernising Government White Paper*. London: Cabinet Office. Retrieved from http://www.archive.official-documents.co.uk/document/cm43/4310/4310.htm (last accessed: 3.10.2010).

UK Government (2004). Human Fertilisation and Embryology Authority. *Disclosure of Donor Information* (Sl 1511).

UKDL (2012). Annual Report 2009/2010. *UK Donorlink. Voluntary Information Exchange and Contact Register Following Donor Conception Pre-1991*. Retrieved from www.ukdonorlink.org.uk (last accessed: 03.04.2012).

Walker, Iain, and Pia Broderick (1999). The Psychology of Assisted Reproduction – or Psychology Assisting Its Reproduction. *Australian Psychologist*, 34 (1), 38–44.

Wallbank, Julie (2004). The Role of Rights and Utility in Instituting a Child's Right to Know Her Genetic History. *Social and Legal Studies*, 13 (2), 245–264.

Warnock, Mary, and Committee of Inquiry into Human Fertilisation and Embryology (1985). *A Question of Life: The Warnock Report on Human Fertilisation and Embryology*. Oxford; Cambridge, Mass: Blackwell.

Welz, Gisela (1998). Moving Targets. Feldforschung unter Mobilitätsdruck. *Zeitschrift für Volkskunde*, 94, 177–194.

Wendehorst, Christiane (2008). Die rechtliche Regelung donogener ART in Deutschland und Österreich. In Gisela Bockenheimer-Lucius, Petra Thorn and Christiane Wendehorst (eds.) *Göttinger Schriften zum Medizinrecht*, 3, 103–133. Göttingen: Universitätsverlag.

Weston, Kath (1991). *Families We Choose: Lesbians, Gays, Kinship*. New York: Columbia University Press.

WHO (2010). *WHO Laboratory Manual for the Examination of Human Semen and Sperm-Cervical Muscus Interaction* (5th Edition): World Health Organisation.

Wilson-Kovacs, Dana M., Susanne Weber, and Christine Hauskeller (2010). Stem Cell Clinical Trials for Cardiac Repair: Regulation as Practical Accomplishment. *Sociology of Health and Illness*, 32 (1), 89–105.

Woolf, Marie (30.6.2006). Sperm; Your Country Needs You. *Independent on Sunday*.

Wuttke, Gisela, and Terre des Hommes (1995–1996). *Ein Kind um jeden Preis? Eine Studie zum Adoptionskinderhandel*. Terre des Hommes Germany. Retrieved from www.adoption.de/pdf/studie_tdh.pdf (last accessed: 21.10.2010).

Zola, Irving Kenneth (1972). Medicine as an Institution of Social Control. *Sociological Review*, 20, 487–504.

Index